Medical Devices: Use and Safety

Associate Editor: Mairi McCubbin
Project Manager: David Fleming, Christine Johnston
Designer: Stewart Larking
Illustrations Manager: Bruce Hogarth

Medical Devices:
Use and Safety

Bertil Jacobson MD PhD
Emeritus Professor of Medical Engineering, Karolinska Institute,
Karolinska University Hospital, Stockholm, Sweden

Alan Murray PhD
Professor of Cardiovascular Physics, Medical Physics Department,
Newcastle University, Freeman Hospital, Newcastle upon Tyne, UK

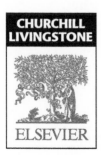

Edinburgh   London   New York   Oxford   Philadelphia   St Louis   Sydney   Toronto   2007

CHURCHILL LIVINGSTONE

An imprint of Elsevier Limited

First published 2007

ISBN-10: 0 443 10259 7
ISBN-13: 978 0 443 10259 2

British Library Cataloguing in Publication Data
A catalogue record for this book is available from the British Library

Library of Congress Cataloging in Publication Data
A catalog record for this book is available from the Library of Congress

Transferred to Digital Print 2011

Contents

Preface

Medical Devices: Use and Safety deals with the practical use of medical equipment and the safety risks involved. The book is intended for everyone working in the healthcare sector who is responsible for the safety of patients where medical devices are involved.

Without medical devices, the success of modern medicine would be poorer and many lives now saved would have been lost. This book, in part, praises their success. But medical devices can also cause accidents, which can be avoided by an understanding of the underlying principles. With greater knowledge, people are more prepared for the unexpected and more ready to act quickly when patient care is not going to plan. *Medical Devices: Use and Safety* encourages safe use by increasing awareness of how medical equipment functions and what can go wrong. Readers who are experts in particular devices will find that the descriptions provide only the details necessary for that purpose; the book is not intended to replace instruction booklets or safety manuals.

At the heart of this book are the case histories, which are both enthralling and appalling. All are based on factual reports recorded in various publications, and all refer anonymously to real people, apart from one case history in Chapter 13 created from a number of separate incidents. The authors have carefully avoided changing any of the details in these reports and have adhered to what was actually reported for the sake of credibility, as certain cases include some unlikely events. The majority of cases have been retrieved from annual publications and medical journals, and some from publications such as *Health Devices, Biological Safety and Standards*, and the reports from the Medicines and Healthcare products Regulatory Agency. Where the accidents occurred is irrelevant; the human propensity to make mistakes is unfortunately universal.

Since the text is intended for readers with varying levels of background knowledge, certain sections are presented in "Fundamentals" and "Techniques" boxes. Readers can, therefore, choose their own level of required knowledge to some extent, but all are advised to read the case histories, which promote the primary purpose of the book: to achieve quality and safety in modern medicine.

As a scientific advisor in medical engineering to the Swedish Board for Health and Welfare for 20 years, the first author was appalled by the observation that the same types of accidents were occurring over and over again. This was the incentive to write the book in the hope that it will contribute to reducing the number of accidents. Although originally written for a Swedish audience, the text has general applicability, since medicine is practised in much the same way in most developed countries. This English edition has been revised and expanded from the second Swedish edition, and recent case histories have been included.

All figures and illustrations are intended to show only general principles; detail has purposely been omitted in favour of comprehensibility.

The authors would appreciate any comments or suggestions for improvements.

Stockholm, Sweden and   Bertil Jacobson
Newcastle upon Tyne, UK   Alan Murray
2006

Acknowledgements

The authors are deeply indebted to many colleagues for helpful advice and positive criticism. Without their input we could not have covered this vast subject as fully, and hopefully as accurately, as we now do. So many have assisted in some way with the content of this book that it is not possible to identify everyone, but we want to express our sincere gratitude to all who might have helped in any way. Also countless students for over a decade have been an endless source of inspiration.

Special thanks are owed to Pia Alm Basu, MD, who translated the text. Her experience within cardiology and clinical physiology made it possible for her to do much more than a mere translation; she suggested many textual improvements and additions.

1

Safety in health care

Physicians of antiquity were well aware that, during physical examination and treatment, they must not cause any deterioration of the patient's condition. They considered this to be more important than anything else – their primary medical ethical rule was *Primum non nocere* ("First, do no harm"). The patient must not, under any circumstances, be harmed, or caused any unnecessary suffering.

Life-saving and life-enhancing procedures beyond the imagination of our parents would not have been possible without the development of so many new medical devices. Those advances, by their very nature, bring risks, but the benefits far outweigh the risks. Many would not be alive today had they not accepted such risks.

The annual number of fatal accidents related to the use of medical devices within countries with well-developed safety procedures can be counted on one hand per million inhabitants. If calculated on the basis of hours of activity, the risk of perishing due to a medical-device accident is of the same order of magnitude as that of suffering a fatal accident in the workplace, or at home. Thus the risk is generally small. This, however, does not absolve health care professionals, as the responsible parties, from doing everything within their power to prevent accidents. This is especially so as the number of nonfatal accidents leading to injuries is much higher. In retrospect, most accidents involving medical devices appear to have been entirely avoidable.

Many of the devices used within the health care system are technically advanced. This means that patients benefit more. But staff are often forced to use these devices without having a thorough understanding of how they work. Health care professionals need to accept that they will learn about this technology solely from the perspective of the user.

Most accidents occur within technology-intensive areas, such as surgery, anaesthesia and intensive care, but one third occur within other areas, Figure 1:1. About half of the reported accidents and incidents are probably caused by the human factor, Figure 1:2. However, this proportion is probably even larger, as many cases are not reported in spite of legal requirements. When reporting was done anonymously, it was found in a British study that 80% were due to user errors.

To be able to use technical devices with confidence and avoid the feeling of uncertainty, which could also make the patient feel anxious, staff must be aware of their responsibilities. Each country issues directives and general guidelines dealing with safety of medical devices. By way of example, in the UK all device accidents and incidents must be reported to the Medicines and Healthcare products Regulatory Agency (MHRA). As well as formal reports staff working in hospitals or other medical centres are encouraged to report any incident anonymously to the National Patient Safety Agency (NPSA) to allow a fuller and independent assessment. The most important legal aspects of this responsibility will be discussed in greater detail in Chapter 13; here we will instead concentrate on how high-quality health care can be given in a practical manner.

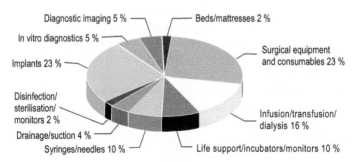

Figure 1:1 Relative percentages of the most commonly reported hospital-related incidences by device group (excludes incidents involving wheeled mobility equipment)

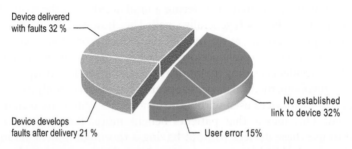

Figure 1:2 Of the number of reported accidents, about half are caused by factors not related to the device; that is, they were likely caused by human error

Quality assurance

The key to providing safe health care for every patient is **quality assurance**. By definition, this involves using methods and equipment to "maintain an adequate work quality level". This would only be both a vague and empty objective if we did not have a number of regulations that actually specify how this is to be achieved. This book is intended to assist health care personnel in accomplishing what these regulations are designed to achieve.

It is essential to be able to anticipate and thus avoid risks. This is the reason why risk analysis is such an important part of the quality assurance process. Just as a driver of a car must anticipate that a child might suddenly run across the street at a place where visibility is reduced, personnel must, when using technical devices, always anticipate what could possibly go wrong.

Here we will discuss the problems in connection with all applicable areas: **acquiring** suitable equipment, **manufacturers' defects**, **initial inspections** upon delivery, **maintenance, training, handling and operation** of the equipment, the need for vigilant **patient monitoring**, and finally, what needs to be done, and what must not be done, when an **accident** has occurred.

SAFE MEDICAL DEVICES

Medical-Technical Products (MTPs) are divided into three groups as specified in the European Medical Devices Directive (MDD, Chapter 13). The majority belong to the group just called "Medical Devices". These are generally used in direct contact with the patient – examples are passive, implantable products, such as hip prostheses and cardiac valves, infusion pumps, defibrillators, surgical diathermy and X-ray equipment, as well as the large group of low-risk products that are being used in health care. The division into groups is mainly of benefit to the manufacturer. For most health care personnel, these groups are of lesser interest, as long as the devices are being used for their intended purpose.

The manufacturer must specify for what specific use the product is intended. If the product is used for a different purpose, the manufacturer ceases to have liability.

All health care personnel naturally have the right to demand that all products in hospitals and other health care facilities are suitable. The most important issue is whether the device complies with the so-called "essential requirements" for a specified type of use according to the Medical Devices Directive. This, among other things, means that the manufacturer has assumed the responsibility for the accuracy of stated performance data and has described the potential adverse effects and risks. If the manufacturer has complied with the **harmonized standards**

(Chapter 13) during the manufacturing of the medical device, the essential requirements are considered fulfilled.

Labelling

It is important to know whether a device is safe for a certain type of application. Since 1998 all new commercially available medical devices in the European Union must have a **CE label** (French: Conformité Européenne). Although specifically intended for the European Union, other countries throughout the world find the symbol valuable. The CE symbol indicates that the device complies with the significant requirements applicable to the specified use. The manufacturer also warrants that the device will comply with these requirements during its entire life, not just during the warranty period. The CE label must conform to the specific design shown in Figure 1:3.

The manufacturer must also specify how the product is to be maintained. If a product is not used or maintained as per the instructions, the liability may be transferred to the user. If two CE-labelled devices that are not supposed to be used together are connected to each other, the assurance provided by the CE-labelling becomes invalid. Here, too, the liability is transferred to the person who carried out or ordered the connection of the two devices.

Customized medical-technical products and new products under clinical trials may not be CE-labelled. This also applies to "internally manufactured devices": that is, devices manufactured at the hospital for in-hospital use only. Then other rules, which are discussed below, apply.

In addition to the general CE symbol, devices are often labelled with various specific symbols. The **date of manufacture** for products of limited stability is shown by a symbol of a factory building with the date of manufacture displayed underneath, as illustrated in Figure 1:3. Likewise, "use by" is designated by a symbol of an hourglass with the date underneath.

Yet another example is the symbol for **single use,** which consists of a crossed-out "2", indicating that it must not be used twice. For example, if a tubing set is labelled with this symbol, it must not be re-used. If this happens, the user assumes the liability and, should an accident occur, the manufacturer could not be held responsible.

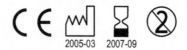

Figure 1:3 Medical device labelling

A great many other symbols exist, depending on the areas of product use. The most important of these will be discussed in the following sections.

Device requirements

It is the obligation of the care provider to ensure that only suitable devices are acquired. Within the public health sector, for example, the care provider could consist of one or more designated authorities at the national level as well as public or private hospitals, plus the clinician in charge of the patient. In the UK there is the NHS (National Health Service), along with the individual trust management board, and the clinician in charge of the patient. Within the private sector it consists of the owner of the health care facility. In general, devices should be acquired in consultation with all personnel who will be using the device. Clinical engineers should of course always be consulted, as they will bear the primary responsibility for the service and preventive maintenance of the devices.

Before a device is ordered, the requirements should be analysed. This analysis should result in a **requirement specification** consisting of a list of desired performance features. It is crucial that the **intended use** is specified. If this is not clearly specified, it may later be impossible to claim that the device is not fulfilling the desired requirements.

In addition to medical and technical requirements, those regarding availability, ergonomics, environmental factors, ease of maintenance and safety issues should also be specified. The requirement specification is extremely important to ensure that neither the purchaser nor the user will be held liable in the case of an accident or damage when the device was used as specified.

Although the care provider is obliged to provide suitable devices, this does not exempt the appropriate **director** (such as the medical director of a hospital or trust, the nursing director, or the director of allied health care professions) from the responsibility of ensuring that unsuitable devices are not being used. A line of communication has to be established, whereby the facility/department/ward director is informed whether newly acquired devices actually comply with all requirements regarding suitability in their area. Such communication often takes place via **nurses**, who are in direct contact with the hospital equipment management service. It is important that the opinions of the nurses, who are going to be using the devices, are taken into account.

Devices of varying age

Newly acquired devices must be inspected upon delivery to have an acceptance test carried out before being turned over to the various departments and laboratories. Wrongly constructed or assembled devices pose accident hazards in two instances: **old non-CE marked devices** still available in the hospital, and **internally manufactured devices** constructed or modified for special purposes by nonqualified persons.

Newly acquired devices

In some very unusual cases, newly acquired devices are inadvertently sent directly to the hospital departments or laboratories, as illustrated by the following example:

CASE 1:1 Loose control knob

Patients suffering from pains in the neck and arms are sometimes treated with traction to relieve the pressure on nerves, which are compressed by the cervical spine. For this purpose, a traction device is used. This device consists of a harness that is fastened around the chin and head, an electrically powered traction device and a control knob that regulates the desired traction force.

On one such occasion, where a traction device was to be used, the force was set to that produced by a 2 kg mass. The force delivered, however, was that of a 30 kg mass. The reason was that the control knob, by which the traction force was supposed to be set, was sitting loose on the shaft. This caused the knob to slide along the shaft, which in turn resulted in the incorrect traction force.

The traction device, which had been delivered directly to the health care centre in question at least three years earlier, had never been inspected, neither at the time of delivery, nor through any periodic maintenance. According to current standards, these knobs must be designed in such a way that they lock into place in a certain position on the shaft.

Thanks to the vigilance of the medical staff at this health care centre an accident was avoided. However, the risk was great. This is sadly illustrated by the fact that a designer of such a device died the last time he tested his own construction.

Some patients require customized devices – this is often the case for handicapped people. Such devices are not to be CE-labelled and are not to be used for other patients.

Old devices

Older devices are not CE-labelled. It is important to check that no old, unsuitable or obsolete devices remain:

CASE 1:2 Short-circuit

Neonates, especially those with low birth weight, have difficulty maintaining their body temperature. This is one of the reasons that newborns are often placed in incubators. The incubator consists of a box, either closed or open on top. The incubator is equipped with heating elements to maintain a reasonably constant temperature. The temperature is regulated by an electronic circuit that increases or reduces the current to the heating element whenever the temperature falls below or rises above a certain preset value.

When electronic control technology was new, several accidents occurred because of malfunctioning circuits, and infants were severely burned. For this reason it was required that incubators must be equipped with over-heating safety relays, which disconnect the heating element, and have an acoustic alarm system that sounds if the temperature becomes too high.

In spite of this regulation, another incubator incident occurred. The temperature rose to 47°C because of a short-circuit in the regulating circuit that prevented the alarm from being triggered, which in turn was due to the fact that it was possible to disconnect the alarm. To construct a medical device in such a way that it is possible to disconnect an alarm is in itself a questionable practice. The most serious defect, however, was that the incubator had not been equipped with an overheating safety limit, resulting in the incubator overheating.

Neither the hospital director, nor the senior physician, who at this time were formally responsible, had set up the purchasing procedures so as to include an inspection by a clinical engineer to ensure that the device complied with the specified performance requirements.

Luckily, the paediatric nurse was vigilant and rescued the baby from being seriously injured.

Although the majority of nurses responsible for the medical care are not formally accountable for medical-technical devices, they are often able to reduce the risks of accidents by maintaining informal contacts with the clinical engineering departments. In some hospitals, special "technology responsible nurses" have been appointed, and thus are responsible for medical-technical safety.

Older devices previously deemed suitable are unsuitable for use if they cause electrical interference (EMC, Chapter 3) to such an extent that they interfere with the proper functioning of newly acquired devices.

Internally manufactured devices

Internally manufactured products can be divided into three categories:

- **One-of-a-kind devices** only manufactured in single numbers, such as devices intended for research purposes.

- CE-labelled devices, **the construction of which has been modified.** This category includes software that is modified following delivery from the manufacturer.

- Several CE-labelled devices that are **connected** in a fashion not approved by the manufacturer.

Internally made devices can offer desirable and valuable product development, and they are contrived by creative people who on their own initiative endeavour to improve the quality of health care. But this enthusiasm can sometimes be greater than the degree of sound judgement:

CASE 1:3 Cheap transformer

A technician with no education in the field of biomedical engineering wanted to reduce the cost of powering a rectoscope of an older design, which used dry cells. Consequently, he put together a battery eliminator of inferior technical design.

The first time the battery eliminator was to be used during rectoscopy, the assisting nurse grasped the rectoscope with one hand, and grasped a wall-mounted lamp with the other. The shaft was made of metal, and had been correctly earthed (grounded, Chapter 3). Both hands cramped and she was unable to move away as current from 230 volts passed through her body via her arms. The nurse suffered a major heart attack as well as burns on her hands and arms, but recovered after a long convalescence.

The faith of an individual in his or her own technical skills sometimes seems unlimited:

CASE 1:4 Endotracheal tube explodes in the larynx

General anaesthesia is often administered by supplying gaseous anaesthetics to the lungs via an endotracheal tube that is inserted via the larynx. To avoid gas leakage, the tube is equipped with an inflatable cuff, designed to create a seal between the tube and the larynx inner wall. It is of course very important to avoid exposing the cuff to excessive pressure levels, as this might cause tissue damage.

In connection with a surgical procedure, where a laser was used in close proximity to the endotracheal tube, a commercially available plastic endotracheal tube had been modified and equipped with a metal tube to avoid the possibility of the plastic melting and catching fire. A leak, however, was present between the metal tube and the thin plastic tubing which normally connects the cuff with the small syringe used to inflate the cuff. For this reason, it was decided to compensate for the air leak by continuously administering air.

A "pressure controller" had been designed and connected to the wall-mounted medical grade air outlet, which is usually pressurized to a level of about 4 bar. To regulate the pressure, among other things, a three-way stopcock had been attached, with the intention of setting an adequate opening for separating the airflow and releasing the excess air. Furthermore, a pressure gauge had been attached for pressure measurement. In addition, various unnecessary components "accompanied" the construction.

When the construction was to be used, the air stopcock was opened, but the pressure gauge gave no reading. The cuff, however, "exploded", and "certain injuries to the patient's larynx were noted".

One possible explanation as to why the pressure gauge gave no readings could be that the connecting tube was bent, thus obstructing the airflow.

A three-way stopcock is much too imprecise a method for pressure regulation. In addition, a major error in this construction was the lack of a safety valve, which could have prevented the excessive pressure build-up.

There are special regulations that apply to **internally made devices**: (1) In the EU, they must meet the essential requirements of the Medical Devices Directive. (2) The details must be recorded. (3) The devices must be designed and constructed by a properly qualified person. (4) A risk analysis must be conducted before any such product is put into use. (5) A qualified person other than the one who constructed it must inspect it objectively and with great expertise. The inspection must not only include the construction as such, but also the training of the medical staff, the scheduling for when the product is to be put into use, and how the maintenance is to be carried out. Hence strict requirements are in place for internally made devices.

For the care-providing personnel, it is important to check that:

- technical documentation is available, demonstrating that a risk analysis has been carried out and that the product fulfils the significant requirements

- the construction has been approved by a clinical engineer

- there are established routines for patient information prior to use

- there are established routines for the reporting of incidents and accidents, should these occur.

Because of these requirements, the development of new devices is cumbersome and restrictive – but this is the price that must be paid for increased safety.

Internally made devices do not have to be very complicated to pose a hazard:

CASE 1:5 Mixed-up tubes

A patient had been admitted for intensive care due to a rupture of the oesophagus with penetration to the pleura. A gastric tube had been inserted with slight suction applied, to keep the stomach emptied. The patient was resting on an antidecubitus mattress – a mattress with adjacent sections being alternately filled and emptied of air for the prevention of bedsores.

At midnight, an assistant nurse noticed that the suction tube to the gastric tube was disconnected, and inadvertently attached the suction tube used for pumping air to the mattress. The staff that came on the next shift soon noticed that the patient's abdomen was inflated, quickly localized the cause, and were able to correct the tube connections. The patient recovered immediately.

Initially, the gastric tube and mattress connections had been designed in such a way as to make it impossible to get them mixed up, but the mattress attachment had broken, and someone had replaced it with a simple plastic connector of a type intended for other purposes. Thus, the cause of this incident was that some helpful person had attempted to mend a tube connection without having a qualified clinical engineer inspect the repair work.

 Remember that the appropriate department in the hospital responsible for medical devices, usually the equipment management department, must be consulted regarding safety and reliability, before devices are acquired. Home-made or modified devices must never be used until they have been approved in writing by qualified experts in the facility.

Initial inspection

Even when new devices are free of any defect regarding their design, it is still necessary to check that there are no manufacturing errors. It is therefore mandatory that all devices be inspected by qualified clinical engineering personnel upon delivery.

CASE 1:6 Faulty electrical connection

Surgical diathermy devices are used for cutting tissues by electric arc and for achieving haemostasis. An assistant nurse was asked to connect such a machine in preparation for a surgical procedure. When attempting to do this, she received a powerful electrical shock but survived.

The ensuing investigation revealed that an electric connection inside the device had been carried out incorrectly, resulting in the housing becoming live. No initial inspection of this device had been done.

Faulty electrical connections happen, and many times the lives of both patients and personnel have been threatened upon connecting the new devices to the power supply. Even when initial inspections have been carried out, faults may still exist:

CASE 1:7 Missing washer in anaesthetic machine

A six-week-old infant was about to undergo surgery and became cyanotic during induction of the anaesthetic, which was being administered via an anaesthetic machine. The gas mixer was set at 60% nitrous oxide and 40% oxygen. When the setting was quickly changed to 100% oxygen, the baby's skin colour returned to normal. In spite of normal breathing sounds, it was suspected that the cyanosis had been caused by some airway obstruction. The gas mixer was again set at 60% nitrous oxide, whereupon the infant again became cyanotic. The nitrous oxide was shut off, and the surgery was performed without nitrous oxide, using a different anaesthetic.

Upon inspection of the machine, it was found that when the control knob was set at 100% oxygen, 100% oxygen was indeed delivered. However, when set at 50% oxygen and 50% nitrous oxide, no oxygen delivery could be detected. The machine was taken out of service. Upon disassembly, it was discovered that an O-ring, a type of rubber washer, was missing from the oxygen flow meter, resulting in the oxygen leaking out instead of being delivered to the patient.

In spite of the gas mixer having passed through the clinical engineering department at the time of delivery, the defect had not been discovered before the device was put into use. Following this incident, the manufacturer devised a testing procedure for detecting possible faults at the time of the initial delivery inspection.

This example demonstrates that particular vigilance is needed every time a device is being used for the first time. Chapter 3 contains advice on how to avoid electrical accidents. When using anaesthetic machines, it is a good rule always to disconnect the machine as soon as a malfunction is suspected. Do not wait too long.

Tip Remember that new devices must be acceptance-tested and inspected by the equipment management department and by an appropriately qualified person (such as a clinical engineer, but it could just as well be an appropriately qualified clinical technologist) at the time of delivery. Even after such inspection, it is prudent to be extra watchful during the initial period that the device is being used.

Maintenance

Accidents often happen because of wear and tear, and insufficient maintenance. Hence, it is important to ensure that preventive maintenance is carried out regularly, and is done by clinical engineers. Even if the formal responsibility is thus assumed by this person, it does not exempt the facility/department director from having to make sure that only such devices that have actually been inspected are used. A good system is to have the clinical engineering department label each device with the inspection date (see Chapter 13 for further discussion).

A large proportion of accidents that are caused by insufficient maintenance lead to injuries because of devices falling on the patient, or the patient falling on the floor. Such accidents are not uncommon during X-ray examinations. As the following example illustrates, frequent maintenance may indeed be necessary:

CASE 1:8 Chain breaks five times

X-ray machines are becoming increasingly more sophisticated, partly to reduce the work that has to be carried out by the X-ray personnel when changing the patient's position. Nowadays, this is often done using power-driven beds. With this type of design, it is possible to use fluoroscopy with the patient in the supine position, and then raise the table so that the investigation can continue with the patient in the standing position. At the same time, the table is elevated, so that the patient is hoisted up to the level of the X-ray tube.

At one such occasion, the chain elevating the table broke. The patient fell on the floor, from a height of half a metre. The chain had previously broken no less than four times when the poorly designed bed had become stuck.

Poor device maintenance can prove to be fatal in cases where the very life of the patient depends on proper function:

CASE 1:9 Ventilator battery not charged

During abdominal surgery, total muscle relaxation is needed to facilitate the procedure. Muscle relaxants that paralyse all striated musculature are administered. As the patients are thus rendered incapable of spontaneous respiration, they are normally attached to a ventilator.

A newly delivered ventilator was being used, but ceased to function after 15 minutes. The ventilator was not connected to the main power supply, but was being powered by a battery unit.

It was suspected that the ventilator had stopped because of debris particles in the pressurized air that had to be used to run the ventilator. Later, however, it was discovered that the battery unit had not been charged before the first use. The charging of the battery unit at the factory had been sufficient for the ventilator to pass the initial inspection. However, the staff did not read the instructions for use, where it was stated that the ventilator needed to be charged for a total of 10 hours prior to use.

Defibrillators (Chapter 10) are located in various places in hospitals as a safety measure, so that they are readily available in case of an emergency to stop sudden ventricular fibrillations. They are often unused for long periods of time, during which the batteries become discharged, and for this reason defibrillators pose some of the greatest incident hazards, unless these batteries are regularly recharged.

The fact that a device has been recently serviced is no excuse to be less vigilant – on the contrary:

CASE 1:10 Woman in labour paralysed

For supplying pain relief during childbirth, epidural anaesthesia is sometimes administered using an infusion pump; anaesthetics are infused into the spinal canal, around the nerves supplying the uterus and other structures. This anaesthetic has to be administered by an anaesthetist, who will personally set the pump infusion rate, or delegate this task to a midwife.

In one such case, the infusion pump had been sent to the clinical engineering department for periodic maintenance and was returned with the infusion rate set at 99.9 ml per hour. After the epidural catheter had been inserted, the physician activated the pump, thinking that it must be fully functional, since it had just come back from maintenance.

The woman was quickly anaesthetized all the way up to the upper part of her chest, and thus completely paralysed in the lower part of her body. She was unable to move her legs or participate actively during the labour.

Inspection revealed that the patient had been given the anaesthetic infusion at 20 times the normal rate, due to the fact that the correct infusion rate was never set. The staff had been used to having the pumps always set at "the normal rate", and thus believed this to be the case here as well.

The woman did not suffer any permanent damage because of this incident.

Tip Devices must receive regularly scheduled maintenance. But be prepared that a malfunction can recur in spite of repairs and maintenance. Be extra watchful whenever a device is used for the first time following maintenance.

SAFE HANDLING AND OPERATION

About 50% of all reported accidents and incidents within health care are probably due to the human factor in direct relation to the care of patients, Figure 1:2. Although the individual physician or nurse is personally responsible, many times the cause is insufficient administrative management.

Training

Whoever is responsible for medical care, **the facility/department director** has the obligation to ensure that the personnel possess the adequate level of competency required to operate all devices. The distribution of responsibility in general is discussed further in Chapter 13.

The following examples illustrate some, not entirely uncommon, handling and operational errors. These cases – **involving mechanical injury, wrong gas dosage** and **thermal injury** – all illustrate the possible consequences of such errors.

Mechanical injuries

Every year, many patients are injured by accidents where device components fall on the patient, or where the patient falls off an examination table or out of a bed or a wheelchair.

CASE 1:11   Patient hoisted up too high – fell on the floor

A patient was going to be lifted from his wheelchair to his bed using a patient lift. Before the patient had been positioned over the bed, it was found that he had been hoisted up too high. The assistant nurse let go of the patient's legs, and left him dangling in the lift-harness alone, whereupon the patient started swinging. Suddenly, one of the four straps by which the harness was attached to the lift came loose, and the patient fell on the floor. The patient suffered a fractured rib, contusion of the lung and died after one week.

The cause of the accident was that two additional hoops had been hung on the lift, contrary to the instructions given by the manufacturer during the training session. Thus wrong handling caused the accident.

Further examples of various types of mechanical injuries are given in Chapter 2.

Wrong gas dosage

While administering gases, the risks are small thanks to established routines and the fact that the personnel involved are well aware of the consequences of wrong dosage. The following two accidents serve as good reminders.

CASE 1:12   Surgery without anaesthesia

A 17-year-old patient, who was to undergo surgery for appendicitis, was to be administered general anaesthesia, using a combination of intravenous sedatives, nitrous oxide and muscle relaxants. Following intubation, her heart rate immediately rose from 95 to 155 beats per minute.

It was suspected that this was due to the anaesthetic being too shallow, and after 15 minutes additional intravenous sedatives were given. As the heart rate still remained high, at the end of the surgical procedure, halothane, a volatile anaesthetic, was administered. Only when the surgery was almost complete, did the anaesthetist discover that she had inadvertently not administered any nitrous oxide to the patient during the earlier stages of the anaesthetic.

After the operation it was discovered that the patient had felt the pain during the major part of the procedure, ever since the incision was made. She had tried to move but had been unable because of the muscle relaxant.

The reason for this accident was that the anaesthetist had mixed up the rotameter control knobs for the nitrous oxide and the oxygen. She was used to a different kind of anaesthetic machine at another hospital, where the gas flow control knobs were placed in their usual location, with the oxygen knob located on the far left, and that for nitrous oxide on the far right. But this hospital had ordered a different type of machine, where the control knobs were placed differently.

The anaesthetist had operated the machine out of habit, without realizing that she was operating an unusual type of anaesthetic machine.

CASE 1:13 Instrument misread

Underdeveloped infants often need to receive extra oxygen in the incubator. But 100% oxygen must never be administered since it is toxic for the infant and can lead to injuries, including blindness.

A number of newborn infants were inadvertently given pure oxygen, in spite of the intention being to administer only air, that is, 21% oxygen. The cause was a poorly designed incubator, which was equipped with a mixing gauge that was very hard to read when the dial was at the maximum 100% oxygen level. In spite of this poor design, the clinicians directly involved with patient care were responsible for these errors.

Further examples of the various types of risks involving gas equipment are given in Chapter 4.

Thermal injuries

Various types of devices used for heating pose hazards. Particular medical aspects of thermal injuries are described in Chapter 4. From a technical standpoint, special caution should always be exercised when using **incubators, heating pads** and **heating lamps**.

CASE 1:14 Improperly attached heating lamp

To prevent hypothermia in a newborn infant, a heating lamp was used, attached to a floor stand which was next to the child, because an incubator was unavailable. But the heating lamp slid down towards the infant and thereby came closer than the stated safe distance of 80 cm. Because of this the baby died from prolonged overheating.

A contributing factor was that the attachment of the heating lamp to the floor stand was unreliable. But wrong handling must be regarded as the most significant cause, as it should have been easy to check that the heating lamp was properly attached to the stand.

Further examples of thermal injuries are given in Chapter 4.

Read the instructions for use

All devices used in health care must be accompanied by **instructions for use**, and these must be readily available to the personnel. In cases where it is especially important that the instructions be read, the product is labelled with the following symbol:

However, the instructions for use must always be read; failure to do so can have catastrophic consequences:

CASE 1:15 Burned cornea

The pressure within the eyeball should be within a certain normal range. It is considered that high pressure if left untreated could lead to blindness from glaucoma. The pressure is therefore measured in elderly patients using a tonometer (Chapter 6). A force is applied against the cornea and the distance that the cornea is pushed inwards by a known force is measured. The less the cornea is pushed inwards, the higher the pressure in the eyeball. In old tonometers the pressure was applied with a metal disc.

In order to prevent contamination, the disc had to be sterilized for each patient. This was achieved by heating the disc to 250°C, and during this heating process a red lamp was lit, with a text stating that sterilization was in process. When the sterilization process was completed, a green lamp with the text "READY" lit up. But the disc was still hot when the green light came on and had to cool down before it could be used again.

A doctor who was familiar with a different type of tonometer placed the hot tonometer disc on the eye of a patient, and thereby burned the cornea.

This accident would never have happened if the doctor had read the instructions for use prior to the procedure. The same type of accident occurred a year later in another hospital.

Remember that medical devices require training. Never start to operate a device before you have read the instructions for use.

Alarms and indicators

Alarms are supposed to alert us when hazardous situations arise. But because of the ever-increasing number of devices and difficulties in correctly setting the alarm limits, alarms are not only helpful, but have also become a source of disturbance. When several alarms go off simultaneously, it is hard to know which one to attend to first, and this increases work stress. Finally people get tired, and routinely disconnect alarms that go off too frequently and for no significant reason. Sometimes, it can also be hard to distinguish between alarm signals and other sounds in hospitals and ambulances.

For these reasons, standards have been proposed, whereby new devices are supposed to be equipped with alarm systems emitting signals that are clearly different from other sounds. Various tones are mixed, so as to form a characteristic chord that is easy to recognize. To facilitate the interpretation, it has been suggested that the alarm signals should have different sound characteristics, depending on the level of urgency:

- **High priority:** The pulse rate of alarm signal burst is high.

- **Medium priority:** The pulse rate of alarm signal burst is low.

- **Low priority:** The alarm signal has one or two pulses only.

The different acoustic characteristics of the alarm signals are intuitively grasped so that the level of urgency is understood.

The messages indicated by indicator lights should also be of uniform meaning:

- **Red:** Danger or error requiring immediate action.

- **Yellow:** Attention or caution.

- **Green:** The device is safe and can be used.

- **Other colour:** Message related to issues other than safety or danger.

Unexpected malfunctions

It is harder to avoid errors when devices are not functioning properly. Some accidents happen in this way. Some devices are even still inadequately constructed.

CASE 1:16 Control knob turned too many times

During surgical procedures on the extremities, it is common practice to shut off the flow of blood to the operation area. This can be accomplished easily by placing an inflatable tourniquet around the arm or leg, and applying a pressure higher than the arterial pressure, thereby creating a bloodless operating field.

During surgery on a finger, a pressure regulator was used in conjunction with a tourniquet to achieve a bloodless operating field. After the operation, it was discovered that the pressure delivered from the regulator was 850 mmHg, which corresponded to the set pressure-gauge pressure, 230 mmHg, plus an additional turn on the pressure regulator setting knob. The setting knob had been turned once too many times.

The patient suffered a nerve injury due to the high pressure used during the operation. If the pressure of the inflatable tourniquet had been checked during inflation, the accident could have been avoided.

 Be suspicious. Always observe and assess the readings whenever changes are made to any device settings.

Investigations of accidents and incidents show that the risks increase during stress, for example, interruption by a telephone call or by questions from colleagues and patients' relatives. The risks also increase when the patient is connected to several devices simultaneously – in the confusion of tubes and cables it can be hard to discern just what may be wrong. Situations involving personal conflict among staff are especially hazardous.

 Try to be particularly alert in stressful situations and if you have had a conflict with a colleague or been upset by some adverse behaviour on the part of a patient.

Watch over the patient

Although ceiling-mounted devices should always be securely attached, operating tables secured and powered devices never allowed to run amok, unfortunately this is not always the case. Since unexpected accidents can happen, staff must be prepared to intervene quickly. Fortunately, most of these episodes do not turn into anything more serious than a near incident, thanks to vigilant personnel who react quickly. However, the outcome is not always this fortunate.

CASE 1:17 Patient's toe crushed

During an X-ray examination of a patient, the X-ray tube/cassette holder was being power manoeuvred. Despite having released the power control button, the downward movement continued due to a technical construction error in combination with a defect in the material. As a consequence, one of the patient's toes was crushed.

This case too is just one of many. All devices with power-manoeuvred parts connected to patients carry the potential hazard of causing injuries by crushing.

Staff members often run a smaller risk than the patients, as they are familiar with the devices in their departments and can anticipate and avoid accidents.

The responsibility for making sure that patients themselves do not cause any calamities naturally has to remain with the staff. Patients should, if possible, never be left unattended when technical devices are being employed within the patient's reach. It is particularly important to instruct patients, so that they do not try to operate devices themselves without being aware of the potential hazards. Such accidents are fortunately rare. Two cases ended well:

CASE 1:18 Patient shuts off infusion alarm

A blood clot is often treated by administering heparin, which reduces the ability of the blood to coagulate and prevents the clot from growing. Heparin must not be overdosed, however, as it can cause bleeding, for example, in the brain.

A patient, receiving a heparin infusion for the treatment of a blood clot, was sent to the X-ray department for an examination. While the patient was waiting to be examined, the infusion pump alarm went off, and the patient pressed the button used for shutting off the alarm. Shortly thereafter, the alarm went off again, and the patient again shut it off, without notifying any staff member. After the X-ray examination, the patient was kept in the waiting room, in spite of the fact that the infusion pump alarm kept going off.

The patient returned to his ward after several hours. During the clinical rounds, it was discovered that the infusion bag containing the heparin was completely empty. The patient had received 25,000 IU of heparin instead of the intended 3000 IU. The infusion pump had been set at the intended number of drops per minute.

Luckily, the patient did not exhibit any symptoms or signs of bleeding, but was at great risk until an antidote could be given to counter the large dose of heparin.

CASE 1:19   Senile patient hoists his bed to the ceiling

A room with four elderly patients had been equipped with a permanently mounted ceiling lift that could be repositioned to serve all beds. In the instructions for use, it was stated that the lift should be moved to its "parking position" after use, but nobody understood what this really meant.

When this incident occurred, the remote control, which was attached to the lift motor by a cable, had inadvertently been left hanging over a patient. The patient probably thought this was the bell, and pressed a button, whereby the lift fork was lowered. When no one came, the patient pressed another button that raised the lift fork. This now became stuck in the left side of the bed and lifted the bed towards the ceiling, hanging with the left side up. The patient fell towards the right side of the bed while the bed remained about one metre above the floor. The patient suffered bruises to the forehead and one leg, but no further injuries, thanks to the fact that the bed railing caught him.

 When technical devices are being used, watch over the patient. If the patient has to be left unattended, it is necessary to tell the patients what they may and may not do. Elderly or confused patients need to be watched more closely. A device can never replace a human being. It can only serve as an aid.

Believe the patient

It can often be hard to discern what a patient is really trying to say. Perhaps it is all too easy to interpret what a patient is saying as uncalled-for complaints. But in everything patients express, there is some kind of message, even if it is not always conveyed with easily understood words. An observant doctor or nurse is able to interpret the words and comprehend what really troubles the patient.

Whenever technical devices are being used, staff must always regard what the patient is saying as being accurate. The following case, which occurred in 1968, is one of the most tragic examples of the information given by a patient having been ignored.

CASE 1:20   Patient fried on the operating table

Before the patient was to undergo a knee operation, it was not clear whether surgical diathermy (Chapter 11) was going to be needed, but to be on the safe side, the diathermy unit was connected. This was apparently done correctly, with proper application of the dispersive electrode. During the operation, surgical diathermy was never used – or so it was thought.

The patient had received spinal anaesthesia, and was anaesthetized from the waist down. During the surgical procedure, that lasted about one hour, the patient initially complained that he felt "warm and sweaty". He then changed the wording to saying that "he was being fried as in a frying pan". Everyone present tried to persuade the patient that everything was in order, and that the operation would soon be over.

After the operation, palm size, third degree burns were discovered over the buttocks, and in addition there were burns of lesser degree on the forearms. Nine months after the accident, the burns had still not healed.

A reconstruction of the accident showed that the diathermy active electrode most likely had slid down and come into contact with a metal part of the operating table. In addition, the surgeon had very probably used the footswitch as a footrest during the procedure, without realizing that he thereby had been activating the electrosurgical unit. The electrosurgical current had thus been conducted from the return electrode, around one thigh and up towards the body, where it had been distributed with the major part going through the buttocks and a minor part being conducted through the arms.

This accident happened using a diathermy unit that, at the time, was considered modern. It did not issue any buzzer signal during use. This and similar accidents in other countries led to surgical diathermy generators being equipped with such a buzzer signal to facilitate detection of any inadvertent activation.

Even if it is fairly unlikely that this type of accident would happen again, this case teaches us an important lesson – that the patient may actually be telling the truth, even when he is saying something as absurd as that he is being "fried" on the operating table.

 Listen to what the patient is saying, and assume it to be true.

The most important measures for minimizing the risk of accidents are summarized in Figure 1:4.

REPORTING

When an accident or incident does happen, it is important that the situation is handled responsibly. The incident or accident could, for example, be caused by an inappropriate device being chosen, and then such devices may need to be taken out of service. If the accident is due to an operational error, it is of course equally important to learn from this experience. For all accidents and near incidents, several things must be remembered.

All cables and other detachable device components must be left untouched, so that it will be possible afterwards to know just what

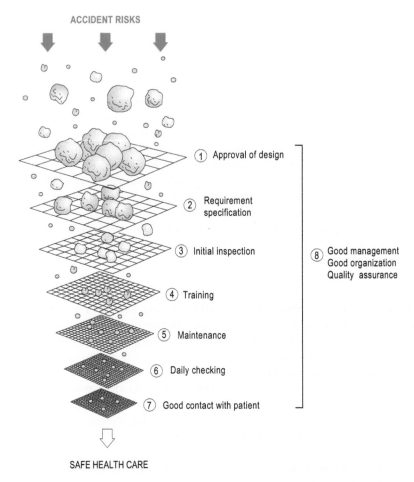

ACCIDENT RISKS

① Approval of design

② Requirement specification

③ Initial inspection

④ Training

⑤ Maintenance

⑥ Daily checking

⑦ Good contact with patient

⑧ Good management
Good organization
Quality assurance

SAFE HEALTH CARE

Figure 1:4 The eight most important measures for shifting away the risk of accidents

combination of devices was being used. Only then will it be possible for technical experts to investigate the cause. Ask a clinical engineer, or an appropriately qualified clinical technician for assistance. There may be reasons to take photographs, or in other ways document the accident before touching the equipment. The manufacturer must be notified, preferably by a clinical engineer.

CASE 1:21 Loose contact kills three patients

Patients with acute myocardial infarction are at great risk of dying from ventricular fibrillation after the onset. Many patients have been saved thanks to ambulance personnel being able to defibrillate the patient during transportation to the hospital.

During one such transport, the defibrillator was not working, and the patient died. It was assumed that the malfunction was due to defective batteries, and the batteries were replaced. No report regarding the accident was ever sent to the clinical engineering department. A few months later, the defibrillator again refused to work, and another patient died. Due to incomplete documentation of the accident, the technical error was still not discovered. Six months later the scenario was again repeated, and a third patient died on the way to the hospital.

Technical investigation revealed that the batteries were intact, but that the battery contact was simply loose.

Tip When an accident happens, remember that all technical equipment must be secured. Leave all accessories where they are, and do not change any settings, if at all possible. All equipment must be quarantined.

In the upset and confused situation that ensues after an accident, it can be hard to describe what really happened. In addition, there is a great risk that details of great importance may be forgotten. For these reasons, as detailed an account as possible of what has happened must be written without delay.

Tip Immediately write down your version of what happened and what you did.

When a patient has died or been injured, or has been subjected to such risk, the facility director and hospital safety officer must immediately be notified, and they will in turn decide how the matter is to be handled further. The information regarding the incident must be reported onwards. For this purpose, every health care facility or hospital must appoint a person in charge of all clinical incident reporting on the part of the hospital. This responsibility is sometimes borne by the head of the clinical engineering department.

A special "clinical incident form" has to be filled out. An adverse incident report should immediately be sent to the national authorities that oversee medical safety. Furthermore, the health and safety executive would want to be told in certain situations.

In addition, according to the **vigilance system**, the manufacturer or distributor must be informed. They should be invited to the investigation, although they must not touch or interfere with the equipment. If the problem with the equipment is due to incompetent hospital personnel, then an independent investigator from outside the hospital could be consulted.

The purpose of the reporting is not to find scapegoats; the purpose is to prevent incidents from being repeated.

SUMMARY

In a UK study made at an intensive care unit in 1991, anonymous reporting of incidents was introduced. Serious situations that could have had disastrous consequences, but which never occurred thanks to appropriate actions taken, were reported anonymously. The reports were analysed by a small number of investigators and then destroyed, to prevent any tracking of the report.

Other countries carried out similar studies, which have resulted in formal and anonymous incident reporting, as well as guidelines on the prevention of accidents involving the use of technical methods in health care. These can be summarized as follows:

* Regularly check the device functions.

* Be especially watchful when responsibilities are handed over between personnel when changing shifts and in stressful situations.

* Use written checklists.

* Never ignore an alarm signal.

* Suspect more than one cause of an error.

* If you are unsure, ask. Accidents are prevented by experienced staff members helping and checking the less experienced.

2

Mechanics and safety

Gravity is both a blessing and a nuisance. It keeps the earth comfortably close to the sun, resulting in a suitable temperature that prevents us from freezing to death. But gravity is a problem not only for high jumpers. For health care personnel it causes patients to fall if not supported, and it pulls heavy equipment down if not adequately fastened, potentially striking both patients and staff with disastrous results.

When considering incidents that might injure patients, we usually think of complex devices such at heart–lung machines and infusion pumps running amok. We rarely think of simple mechanical causes. But mechanical injuries are surprisingly common in health care. This warrants a short description of a few risks before going on to more technically complex issues. We will discuss the hidden dangers of **bed rails, flawed mechanics, removable parts** and **packaging**.

BED RAILS

When bed rails are mounted on hospital beds, it might be assumed that patients are safe. But rails can also turn into deadly traps. In the USA it has been reported (Bed Rail Entrapment Statistics 2001) that between 1985 and 1999, patients were entangled or strangled in beds with side rails on 371 occasions. Of these, 228 people died, 87 had nonfatal injuries and 56 were saved thanks to the intervention of the staff.

Improved bed designs have reduced the risks somewhat, but many old beds are still in use. Two principally different situations can be distinguished. First the patient can become entrapped between the mattress and the side rail or headboard/footboard, Figure 2:1. The outcome can be disastrous:

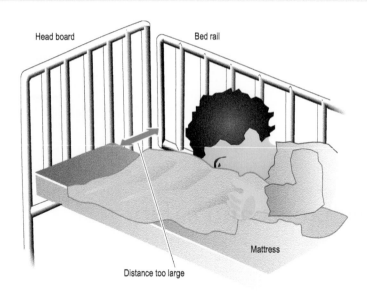

Figure 2:1 Entrapment between mattress and bed rail

CASE 2:1 Nursing home violent death

An elderly woman in a nursing home was found dead shortly after midnight. Her head was wedged between the mattress and side rail and her nose had become smashed and discoloured. The woman's legs were positioned under the rails. Urine, blood and excrement were found on the floor of the room, indicating that she had probably suffered a painful death struggle before she succumbed from asphyxiation.

The other situation is when parts of the patient's body are caught by the rails, Figure 2:2. Rail entanglement can occur in several ways, for example, between the individual bars of the side rail if the gap between two adjacent rails is larger than the patient's head, or between the two sections of a split side rail. If the patient's head gets between the bars when turned in a certain position it might be impossible to avoid entrapment when turned again. Children, as well as old people, might not have the muscular strength to avoid suffocation before help arrives.

Patients at risk include those with altered mental states, frail or elderly patients, or those with general restlessness, as well as infants or children. It is essential to assess the patient's physical and mental status and closely monitor high-risk patients. Apart from avoiding the use of badly designed beds, it is particularly important to avoid mattresses that are improperly sized, resulting in a gap-trap between the mattress and the side rail.

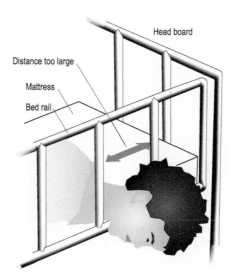

Figure 2:2 Entrapment between two bars in a bed rail

FLAWED MECHANICS

Mechanical injuries constitute about half of all patient-related accidents in radiology departments, and they occur within virtually all other specialties as well. The accidents result either from **unexpected movements** or from **malfunctions**.

One common type of accident is when some part of the patient's body is crushed. A particularly insidious type is when the patient puts his hands or feet in unexpected positions, where an injury could result. This can easily happen, for example, when a patient regains consciousness and grasps for something to hold on to, Figure 2:3. Children are curious and want to explore everything by sticking their fingers and hands in holes and crevices.

Some modern devices are very heavy and could not be operated were they not **power driven**. It is the operator's responsibility to check that the patient does not have any part of their body, such as hands or feet, between the moving structure and any rigid surface, such as the floor or device part, Figure 2:3.

CASE 2:2 Patient's toe crushed

During a radiology examination of a patient, the X-ray tube with its cassette holder was being power operated. Despite the power control button having been released, the downward movement continued due to a technical construction error in combination with a defect in the material. As a consequence, one of the patient's toes was crushed.

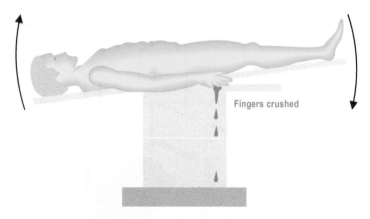

Fingers crushed

Figure 2:3 When patients have recovered from shock, and the table is tilted to its normal level position, the patients might put their hands in potentially dangerous positions

This case too, is just one of many. All devices with power driven parts connected to patients carry the potential hazard of causing injuries by crushing.

 When actuating any power driven part from a position where you cannot see the far side of the patient, who is placed on or near a potentially dangerous mechanical device, take the time to check the far side before operating the device.

CASE 2:3 Patient kills herself

A patient in the UK activated the control of an electrically operated bed. She was found with her head on the foot control, which had resulted in the movement of the bed. She crushed herself to death.

As a result, hospitals were asked to consider whether foot controls could be operated accidentally, and whether they could be covered or locked out.

Sometimes failures occur with **mounting equipment** which supports examination lights, therapy units, radiation shields and contrast media injectors. The risk can be reduced by avoiding rough handling, such as slamming units into their stop points. But when accidents do occur, quick reactions by the personnel can help prevent injuries.

CASE 2:4 Admirable presence of mind

During an X-ray examination the 21-inch monitor broke loose from a ceiling-mounted swing arm. A staff member was able to catch the 23 kg monitor in his arms. No personal injury resulted from the incident, which apparently was caused by a jamming of the swing arm.

CASE 2:5 Fatal falling equipment

A patient was going to be investigated with a nuclear imaging system. When the heavy equipment was moved towards the patient it became dislodged by a footstool and turned over. The patient was crushed to death.

Special attention is essential whenever removable parts are to be repositioned and then retained by **safety latches**. When patients are lifted with such devices, it is particularly important that no latches are left in an open position. Textiles or washcloths may prevent proper latching.

CASE 2:6 Elderly patient falls to the ground

Lifting immobile patients is physically very hard work for health care personnel. Various patient lifts have been designed; some have serious flaws.

A newly delivered patient lift for a car had only been used about 20 times when the snap latch between the strap and the seat did not close. The patient fell to the ground and suffered a fractured femur.

CASE 2:7 Loose film cassette

During an X-ray examination of the stomach, the film cassette in a spot-film device came loose. The cassette fell to the floor, brushing against the patient's head. If the heavy cassette had hit the patient, he could have been seriously injured.

The cause of this incident was that the X-ray assistant had not inserted the film cassette properly into the camera housing. The assistant had not pushed the cassette all the way so as to activate the safety latch. When the cassette is inserted correctly, an audible click indicates that the safety latch has been activated. Thus, wrong handling caused the incident.

CASE 2:8 Newborn baby falls on the floor

As a newborn baby was put on the scale, the scale tray came loose; the baby fell to the floor and suffered a serious concussion.

This accident occurred because the scale had been constructed with unreliable snap latches for the attachment of the scale tray. Just a light tug could easily open the snap latch.

Tip Whenever a removable part of a device locks into its seat by a safety latch, you should hear a "click". If you do not, remove the part, check if any foreign object prevents the latch from engaging and try again. You must hear the typical "click".

Loose screws, bolts and **nuts** are a recurring problem. Even if the manufacturers' maintenance requirements are followed, devices may become loose. In these situations, only the medical personnel might be able to anticipate an accident. Loose bolts are a major problem, particularly for patient lifts.

Tip If you notice that any bolts or nuts seem loose, never use the equipment before it has been checked by qualified personnel in charge of preventive maintenance.

REMOVABLE PARTS AND PACKAGING

In other situations it is essential to remove certain parts before using a device. Liquids are sometimes given to elderly patients and children using an **oral syringe** or a standard hypodermic syringe without a needle. Such syringes are often delivered with a protective plastic cap. The oral syringes may be supplied pre-filled with the medication, or a syringe may be filled on-site and the cap then replaced (some syringes may even be filled with the cap in place). On several occasions life-threatening incidents have occurred because the cap was not removed before administering the medication – the cap was ejected off the end of the syringe into the patient's airways:

CASE 2:9 Six-month-old girl in respiratory distress

The girl was given a decongestant syrup with a syringe when she suddenly developed respiratory distress. During the cardiopulmonary resuscitation the girl was intubated. A small plastic syringe cap was discovered and removed.

It was concluded that the syringe user had probably not removed the cap, which was propelled into the girl's airways.

Batteries are often delivered with a clear shrink-wrap packaging to prevent them from accidental short-circuiting. On several occasions nurses have replaced such 9-volt batteries in temporary pacemakers and ambulatory telemetric transmitters without removing the shrink-wrap. The situation is insidious since the battery compartment in some of these devices differs from those in standard consumer devices, where a battery clips into the battery leads. In some medical devices the battery connections are pressed against the conductive plates in the battery compartment by spring tension. This unfortunately allows a wrapped battery to be inserted, and hence no power is provided to the device.

3

Electricity and safety

Despite an ever-increasing use of electric appliances the annual number of fatal electrical accidents has steadily gone down from about 5 to 1 per million persons in countries with well-established safety regulations. In other industrial countries the number is more than 3 per million. The number of nonfatal accidents is of course greater; approximately 30 times as many, and they often lead to long sick-leave. Of the total number of accidents, about 60% occur among those working professionally with electricity and 40% among laymen. But despite the fact that the professionals often work with high-voltage installations, the number of fatal accidents among them is only a third of that among laymen. Professional knowledge saves lives.

A large number of the medical accidents and near accidents that are reported annually are associated with faults in electric appliances or in their use.

Health care is special in three ways. First of all, patients are often placed in vulnerable situations where they are unable to protect themselves; they may, for example, be unconscious or connected to medical-technical devices. Second, staff use devices that can never be considered electrically safe, such as defibrillators, where the desired effect of the treatment is based on conducting a large current through the body. Third, patients are subjected to treatments where catheters and electrodes are inserted into or near the heart, which greatly increases the risk, as the heart muscle is an especially sensitive part of the body. Thus special routines and regulations for electrical medical devices have been developed.

Ordinary electrical accidents are called **macroshocks**. Those that occur when appliances are used near the heart, inside the body, are called **micro-**

shocks. In order to understand how to avoid these risks, it is essential to know what is meant by **current, voltage** and **conductivity**. The concepts of **earth (ground)** and **leakage currents** are central to an understanding of safety issues within health care. The possible **biological effects** on the body exerted by electromagnetic fields are causes for concern and will be discussed. An important problem is the effect on sensitive electric devices due to inadequate **electromagnetic compatibility (EMC)**. Finally, some of the **symbols** used for medical-technical devices are described.

Here we will primarily deal with the risks at power-line frequency, the alternating current at 50 or 60 Hz (hertz = cycles per second) distributed over the power supply system. This frequency was chosen because of economic considerations in order to reduce the cost of transferring electricity between power plants and consumers. Unfortunately, this frequency also happens to be the most dangerous.

MACROSHOCK AND MICROSHOCK

Electric current that passes through the body can create two different effects: **heating** and **stimulation** of nerves and muscles. Apart from one particular risk during electrosurgery, the thermal effect is not a great medical problem; such high currents that can cause burns occur mostly within the power industry.

The stimulating effect does, however, constitute a larger problem. The current affects both nerves and muscles, causing **contractions** in muscle, but also causes **ventricular fibrillation** in the heart. In fatal cases, both effects usually happen simultaneously. When people receive an **electric shock** this can cause muscles to contract so that they become unable to free themselves from the source of the current, and ventricular fibrillation is triggered.

The effect on the tissues, and thus the risk, is primarily dependent on the current density. If the current is concentrated in a small tissue volume, for example, around the tip of a cardiac catheter, the risk is much greater than if the same current is distributed over the entire chest cage. It is important to distinguish between two types of electric shock.

Macroshock

During macroshock, the current passes between two different skin areas, Figure 3:1. Unless contact occurs on the chest directly over the heart, which is rare, the most dangerous situation is when current passes between the two hands. In this situation, a relatively large portion of the current passes through the heart. It is also dangerous when the current passes between the left hand and the feet. Both situations result in a large current density in the heart muscle.

The magnitude of the effect depends on the current strength, Figure 3:2, and the current distribution. At current strengths below about 1 mA

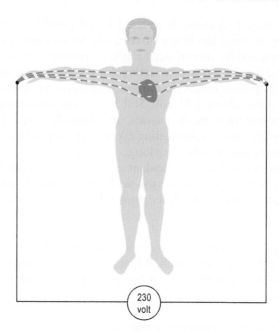

Figure 3:1 In macroshock, electric current from arm to arm is most dangerous

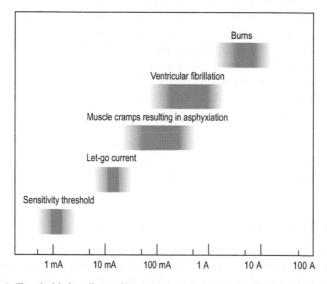

Figure 3:2 Thresholds for effects of 50 or 60 Hz electric current. All values are approximate; the higher limits are rough estimates, since experiments on humans are ethically impossible

(milliampere) the current is not even noticed, at least not as something unpleasant. At a few milliamperes a tingling sensation can be felt – the **sensitivity threshold** has been reached. With increasing current strength, muscles start contracting to the point at which it is impossible to let go.

The maximum current strength where it is still possible to break loose from this grip is called the **let-go current**. The let-go current for women is about 10 mA and for men about 15 mA. Increasing the current further to about 20–30 mA causes contractions of the breathing muscles and death by asphyxiation unless the current is reduced. **Ventricular fibrillation** occurs above about 100 mA. Still higher currents cause **burns** in addition to contractions in all muscles, including the heart. The injuries are often very extensive as the heating takes place deep within the tissues, and the recovery time can be very long.

If a person in an electrical accident is found to be stuck because of contractions, never touch the person with unprotected hands or touch the live device or cord. Instead, try these following alternatives, sequentially:

 Interrupt the electric current: for example, pull out the plug or switch off the power switch. If that cannot be achieved, consider if you can interrupt the current by switching off a power-line circuit breaker.

If this is not possible, consider the following:

 Try to intervene using an insulating material, for example, a dry blanket, coat or an unconnected electrical cord (which of course has insulation). Hold at extreme ends, and put or throw it over the person that is stuck and try to jerk him/her loose using your body weight. Your own life may depend on not accidentally touching the electrically live object with any unprotected part of your body. You also must absolutely avoid touching the person with your bare hands.

Resuscitation after an electrical accident is performed as in other cases of cardiac arrest, using artificial respiration and heart massage until a medically competent person can take over.

CASE 3:1 Elderly couple killed while cutting down a tree

The husband had cut down a tree. He did not notice that the tree had pulled down a 10,000 V (volt) cable in the fall. While chopping off the branches, the wife came into contact with the fallen cable and was killed instantly. The husband tried to help his wife and grabbed hold of her but was also killed.

During ventricular fibrillation, consciousness is lost only after about 10 s (seconds). During that time, the person can move:

CASE 3:2 Electrician was not asleep

An electrician was working at an installation in a new building. His colleagues thought he was taking a lunchtime nap, sitting on the floor and leaning against the wall. He was, however, dead.

The investigation showed that he had been working on a cable, which he apparently thought was not live but unfortunately turned out to be. He had received an electric shock, climbed down from the ladder he was using for this work, taken several steps, sat down and leaned against the wall before he lost consciousness.

Tip Observe a person who has had an electric shock – if someone has an electric shock and does not become immobilized by contractions, you should still observe the person to watch for reactions. Be prepared to give mouth-to-mouth resuscitation and heart massage.

Microshock

Whenever electrodes or catheters are inserted into or near the heart, the risk of microshock exists. The current is then conducted between a contact surface on the body and an area concentrating current flow in or near the heart, Figure 3:3. Thus, this risk also exists when, for example, electrodes are inserted into the oesophagus at heart level, for example, during temperature measurement. A current of 50 µA (microamperes) concentrated to a small area in the heart muscle can trigger **ventricular fibrillation**. The safety limit, the maximum current in normal conditions allowed in patients undergoing procedures in close proximity to the heart, is set at 10 µA.

CURRENT, VOLTAGE AND CONDUCTANCE

The current strength, and hence the current density, is the essential factor. High voltage is not in itself dangerous; for example, 100,000 V is not dangerous in combination with a current strength of just a few microamperes. The voltage from a small watch battery, on the other hand, may be fatal if the voltage is connected to a pacemaker lead and the current is a few hundred microamperes. One does not even need a battery for an accident to happen:

CASE 3:3 Patient dies when nurse touches pacemaker leads

To test for a suitable pacemaker type before the actual implantation, a lead had been inserted with one end connected to the heart and the other exiting through the skin on the patient's chest.

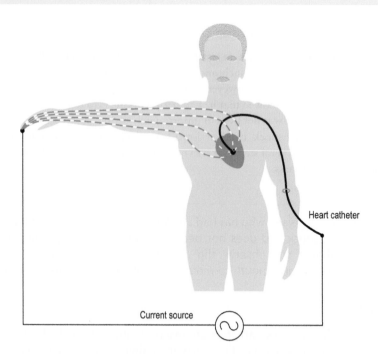

Figure 3:3 A microshock is caused by a high current density in the heart

A nurse who was new to the department had never seen a patient with a pacemaker lead. She asked what it was and touched the electrode. She happened to be charged with static electricity, and this resulted in a current that travelled from her hand via the electrode to the patient's heart muscle. The patient developed ventricular fibrillation and died.

Current strength, which from a safety standpoint is the essential factor, can, as shown in Box 3:1, be derived as:

current = voltage × conductance

If the voltage is doubled, the current becomes twice as high. If the conductance is doubled, the current also becomes twice as high. The least favourable situation is when both voltage and conductance are high. When considering the mains, we cannot do much about the voltage, it is 230 V in most countries; instead we must minimize the conductance.

Conductance

Electric devices are constructed with insulating layers with very low conductance, such as the plastic around the copper wires in an electric cord. This normally gives protection against electric shocks.

Fundamentals · Box 3:1

Introduction to Ohm's law

The current in an electric wire can be compared to water running down a tube. Current strength, which is measured in **amperes**, corresponds to the quantity of water running down per unit of time – the more that runs through the tube per second, the larger the current.

The voltage, measured in **volts**, corresponds to the difference in height between the tube entry and exit openings – the higher the drop, the higher the voltage. Resistance, measured in **ohms**, corresponds to the hindrance to the passage of the water caused by the tube; the flow depends on the tube dimensions – the smaller the diameter of the tube, the smaller the flow and the greater the resistance.

According to Ohm's law, there is a relation between the voltage V measured in volts, the current strength I measured in amperes, and the resistance R measured in ohms:

$$V = R \times I$$

From a clinical engineering perspective, rather than the resistance, it is more practical to speak of the conductance, G, which is measured in **siemens** (S) = 1/ohm and equal to the resistance inverted, $G = 1/R$. If the resistance is 100 ohms, then the conductance is 0.01 S. If R is replaced by G in Ohm's law, we get the relation

$$I = V \times G$$

If the voltage is 230 V and the conductance 0.01 S then current strength is 2.3 A.

The body has a similar protection against electric currents, provided that the skin is dry – the conductance is then low. When the skin is wet, its conductance increases as water has high conductance. Hence it is more dangerous to accidentally touch electrically live objects with wet hands than dry hands.

It is the high conductance of water that allows electric current to pass through the body – we consist of almost 70% water. Because of the properties of water it is dangerous to use electric appliances in rooms where the floor could be wet or damp during normal use. In such areas all electric outlets must be earthed, except for those with special isolation, such as for electric shavers. Do not try to bypass these regulations by using unearthed extension cords.

CASE 3:4 Thirteen-year-old girl killed in bathtub

A girl was playing with her doll in the bathtub. She wanted to dry the doll's hair with a hair dryer, and brought into the bathroom an extension cord of the old type without an earth conductor.

While playing in the water with the hair dryer she got an electric shock, became unconscious and drowned.

Bringing any electric cord into the bathroom is against safety regulations. As the cord in this case was not earthed, the current flowed through the water and the girl – rather than the more direct path via an earth conductor – had it been present. Because there was no short-circuit to earth the fuse did not blow.

For a current to flow, the circuit to and from the power source must form a complete circuit, Figure 3:4. Often our clothes or the properties of the room afford protection against electric circuits unintentionally forming when we inadvertently touch live objects. Shoes with rubber soles and floors with plastic coverings are poor conductors. In such situations nothing happens if we touch live objects. Often we don't even realize it happened.

CASE 3:5 Electric installation lethal for three months

A nurse's assistant was going to put away a bedpan on a heated rack in the washing room. When she touched the heated rack she received an electric shock, fell down and suffered a crush wound to the upper arm.

The investigation showed that an electrician had interchanged the earth and the live wires, resulting in the casing of the heated rack becoming live. The faulty connections had been carried out three months prior to the accident.

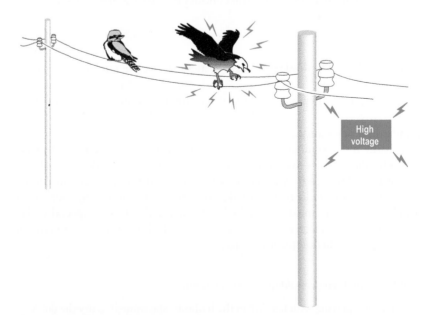

High voltage

Figure 3:4 The bird in contact with two wires forms a closed circuit, and receives a shock. The bird in contact with one wire does not

The reason that the faulty connections had not been discovered earlier was that the staff had previously always been wearing clogs with rubber soles. When the accident happened, the nurse's assistant was wearing shoes with leather soles.

CASE 3:6 One out of three dies

A plumber, a supervisor and a co-worker were going to install a water heater. As they were pushing the water heater across the floor, an electric cord became stuck under it. The heavy water heater damaged the cord insulation, and the heater then became live.

All three had their hands on the water heater. The plumber, who had thin shoes with worn-out leather soles, received an electric shock and died. His colleague, with thick leather soles, had electric shocks but was not hurt by them. The supervisor, who had shoes with thick rubber soles, did not feel a shock at all.

Many accidents happen when we accidentally touch an object at mains voltage and simultaneously are in contact with a earthed object. Our body then serves as a return path for the current to the power source. If someone with damp leather soles stands on a conductive surface, such as a wet floor, the current may, as per Figure 3:5, take the path: power plant – live device – hands – arms – body – floor – earth – power plant.

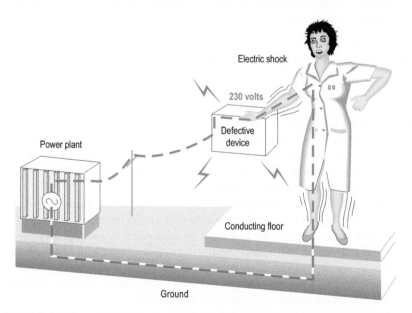

Figure 3:5 A damp floor closes the current to the power plant, which may cause an electric shock

But if we are not electrically connected to earth, for example, if we are wearing shoes with rubber soles, the current cannot pass as easily through the body. As described in Case 3:6, we may not even notice anything if the circuit is open. As stressed above, it is especially dangerous to touch a live object with one hand and be in contact with a earthed object with the other hand.

 Use ONE hand only. As an extra precaution when handling cords and plugs or touching a switch to operate a device, don't touch the device casing or any other conducting object (sink, operating table, rinse tub etc.) with your other hand. Keep it out of the way to avoid the electric circuit from any potential defect flowing between your arms, resulting in a high current density in the heart.

A few facts worth keeping in mind when working with electric devices:

- Metals have high conductance. Metallic objects with high voltage are dangerous to touch.

- Water conducts electricity. Electric devices in damp spaces must be handled with great caution.

- Using damaged cords and damaged electric connectors in damp areas is particularly dangerous.

- In most cases of electric shock, the person will survive. However, having an understanding of the concept of conductance will greatly increase their chances.

EARTH AND PROTECTION CLASSES

The earth (ground) concept is used in two ways. When a voltage value is to be indicated, it is measured in volts relative to the functional earth potential, which is zero. Functional earth is a concept used by constructors of devices; the concept is of lesser interest in practical health care. What is more important is that electrical hazards can be avoided by using a separate earth wire, by connecting outer electrically conducting device parts, **exposed parts**, to earth.

One example of an exposed part is the hotplate of an electric cooker. The metal plate, which conducts electricity, could become live if it did not have a separate earth wire. It must be connected to earth at all times, so that the electricity will short-circuit in case of a fault, and blow a fuse or open a circuit breaker. A plastic or ceramic knob on the cooker is not an exposed part, since it cannot conduct electricity. Should a fault happen, the knob could never become dangerous.

The most important means for avoiding electric shocks is therefore always having devices with exposed parts adequately connected to earth.

Such devices are fitted with **Class I** connectors, that is they have a third lead for connection to earth. When plugged into a wall outlet with an earth lead the exposed part of the device becomes earthed.

Some household devices are fitted with **Class 0** connectors. Such connectors have only two conductors: a live wire for conducting the current to the appliance, and a neutral wire for conducting the return current away from it. A Class 0 connector cannot be plugged into an earthed wall outlet.

It would be dangerous to use Class 0 equipment in damp areas, such as close to a stainless-steel sink in a kitchen. The metal is connected to earth via the plumbing. Touching a live object with one hand and the sink with the other would enable the current to pass through the object

---

 Fundamentals • Box 3:2

Capacitance

The current from a battery always flows in one direction, so-called **direct current**. The **alternating current** of the power distribution grid changes direction 50 or 60 times per second, i.e., the **power-line frequency** is 50 or 60 Hz (hertz). The reason for this is that transferring alternating current is easier and cheaper than transferring direct current.

A **capacitor** can conduct an alternating current. A capacitor consists of two conducting plates separated by an insulator, Figure 3:6. The size of the capacitor, and hence its capacity to conduct alternating current is expressed as its **capacitance**, which is measured in farads (F). The capacitance increases when the area of the plates increases or the distance between them decreases.

A capacitor's capability to conduct alternating current depends upon the frequency of the current. Capacitance can also exist between any two conducting objects separated by an insulator. At low frequencies, the conducting capacity is poor, but it increases with increasing frequency. For example, at 1 MHz (megahertz = 1,000,000 cycles per second) the conductance is so high that warts can be burned away using a current that completes the circuit to the device from the patient without any wire, which is described in Chapter 11. The current travels through the capacitance formed by the body, the air, and the device.

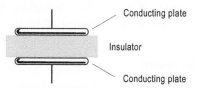

Figure 3:6 A capacitor has an insulator sandwiched between two conduction plates

– hand/arm – chest and heart – the other arm/hand – sink – earth – power station – back to the object.

CASE 3:7 Barefoot woman electrocuted

Contrary to existing safety regulations, a wall outlet without an earth connection had been installed in a kitchen in an apartment. A lamp with a metal shade holder was connected to the outlet. One day, the lamp would not light, and to investigate the problem a woman, who was barefoot at the time, climbed up onto the sink, touched the shade holder, received an electric shock and died.

Due to a faulty installation of the lamp cord, the shade holder had become live because of worn insulation.

If the lamp had been earthed, the current would have travelled via the earth wire when the insulation wore off. This would have resulted in such a high current that the circuit breaker would have tripped, and the current would have been interrupted. At the same time, it would have been discovered that the lamp was defective. The additional third earth wire has great advantages.

Electrical appliances with **double insulation** have power cords with two conductors, and they are safe to use in all indoor environments, as for cords with three conductors which always have three-prong plugs. **Class II** appliances can be plugged into an earthed outlet. They are labelled with the following symbol:

Some devices utilize a low voltage in order to reduce the risk. If the voltage does not exceed 60 V direct current or 25 V alternating current, the device does not need to be furnished with any protection against direct touch. Low voltage is common in many devices for general use, such as alarm clocks, toys, laptop computers and mobile telephones, as well as for battery chargers. Most often the current is supplied from a power adapter, containing a transformer, Box 3:3, integrated with the plug that is directly plugged into the wall outlet. Such power adapters intended for general use may not be used in clinical areas unless CE-marked as part of a medical device. For clinical use special designs are required, but should be avoided, as illustrated by the following case:

CASE 3:8 Nurse grabs live parts

A nutrition pump was being powered by a power adapter, which was plugged directly into the wall socket. When the device was to be shut off, the nurse wanted to pull the adapter out of the wall outlet. However, the adapter cover

Fundamentals • Box 3:3

Transformers

Alternating currents can easily be changed to different voltages by a **transformer**. In the cables from the power plants, the voltage is very high, for example 40,000 V, while at the normal power outlet it has been transformed down to 230 or 120 V. In most medical devices it is stepped down further from 230 or 120 V to 5 V, for example.

A transformer consists of an iron core with two coils of insulated copper wires, Figure 3:7. Current is fed to the transformer via the primary coil and exits via the secondary coil. The relative number of windings in the two coils, the so-called **transformer ratio** determines by what factor the voltage is transformed. If 230 V is to be transformed to 5 V, then the number of windings must be 230:5 = 46 times more in the primary coil than the secondary coil. The transformer ratio has to be 46:1.

Isolation transformers utilize special insulation between the primary and secondary coils to reduce leakage current.

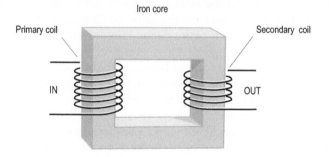

Figure 3:7 A transformer for conversion of alternating currents. If a transformer has fewer turns on the secondary coil, the output voltage will be smaller than the input voltage

came off and the nurse instead accidentally grabbed the loose transformer, which had fallen out of the holder in the cover. The transformer was connected by wires to the metal prongs that were still connected to the wall outlet.

The nurse received an electric shock but luckily survived. The transformer had fallen to the floor on an earlier occasion, and the cover had cracked, but since this had gone unnoticed, the adapter had just been plugged back into the wall as usual.

Devices with unearthed plugs may not be used in areas requiring earthed connections. Making extension cords with connections of a different class at the two ends is not allowed.

EARTH FAULT CIRCUIT BREAKERS AND ISOLATION TRANSFORMERS

Electric circuit breakers provide protection primarily against fire, but do not provide efficient protection against personal injuries caused by defective electric devices or cords. To avoid electrical accidents, **earth (ground) fault circuit interrupters** (**GFCIs**) can be permanently installed in the central electricity supply to the building. Circuit interrupters are also available to be temporarily inserted between the wall outlet and the plug of the device being used. Such GFCIs have become very popular for general use. They work by ensuring that no current escapes on the way to and from the device. In a properly working electricity supply, the same amount of current must of course travel in both directions. If there is a difference, this must be due to inadequate insulation to earth. If more than 10 to 30 mA escapes on the way, the circuit breakers are tripped.

If a live part of a device that is being supplied via a GFCI is touched and the current is conducted through the person's body to earth, the circuit breakers are tripped instantly and an electric shock is avoided.

GFCIs have one great disadvantage, however, in that all electric devices that are supplied with power via the same GFCI stop working when it trips. GFCIs used in domestic mains circuit boards have the inconvenience that the freezer and the refrigerator may stop working even if the electrical fault occurs somewhere else in the house. If the occupier is away from home at the time, this might not be discovered and the food will spoil.

In health care, GFCIs are seldom used, as a loss of power would constitute a safety hazard. Devices, such as ventilators and dialysis machines, for example, would not work. Therefore, **isolation transformers** are used instead. These consist of a transformer with outputs that are not earthed. Thus a person can touch either output wire and not receive a shock because a complete circuit is not formed to earth. The isolation transformer is also equipped with an integral test function, a line isolation monitor (LIM) so that its functionality can be checked. If an electric device with defective insulation is connected via an isolation transformer, the LIM triggers an alarm and lights a warning lamp as soon as an insulation fault is detected – the user will be alerted that something is wrong. The alarm can be turned off temporarily, so that the activity that was already started may be completed.

LEAKAGE CURRENTS

We have already established that the electrical conductivity of insulators is low. But unfortunately it is never nil, especially not for alternating currents. Some of the current will always leak through even the best insulator. This is a major problem when using devices in connection with investigations close to the heart. The leakage currents from any devices that are in one way or another connected to the patient must then be extremely low.

It is particularly important to limit such leakage currents. Having the patient electrically connected to earth is especially hazardous, as explained below.

One of the most common safety defects in electric appliances is a faulty earth circuit, and this occurs in old as well as in brand new devices of the best makes. Such an interruption is usually not noticed during ordinary daily use – until an accident happens.

In a device without any functioning protective grounding, various leakage currents will take other pathways to earth. If the patient is connected, for example, via ECG electrodes, there is a great risk that the leakage currents will travel through the patient. The greatest hazard arises when the patient is holding an earthed object, for example, the metal edge of an examination table. Unless the leakage currents were limited, life-threatening situations could result. For each investigation, the appropriate device type must be selected, Box 3:4.

Choosing the correct type of medical device is easy when only one device is needed. But if several devices must be used, for example, an ECG recorder, an electrosurgical generator and an electrical thermometer, it must be ensured that the combined leakage currents do not exceed the limit for the application in question. In order to assess the risks of electrical accidents from such device combinations, a clinical engineer must be consulted.

The power cords must be as short as possible, since leakage currents increase in proportion to the length, Figure 3:8. Thus extension cords must not be used; medical-technical devices should be connected directly to the wall outlets.

It is sometimes necessary to have several devices connected simulta-neously in a so-called **medical electrical system** (e.g. a personal computer, video player and other equipment that is not primarily designed for medical purposes). In such cases, the devices should be connected via an **isolation transformer** by a qualified clinical engineer. In an isolation transformer the primary and secondary coils are separated in a way that reduces leakage currents, Box 3:3 and Box 3:5. All the devices are placed on a special cart or in some other limiting fashion, and connected to the outlets of the isolation transformer. In this way, leakage currents to earth are limited even for such devices that do not meet the requirements for type B, BF or CF medical devices. Such device carts may neither be modified by unqualified personnel nor additional equipment connected – all such modifications must be carried out by a clinical engineer. In some countries changes must be recorded on the device card that accompanies the cart – the card serves the function of defining what devices are combined on the cart so that no additional device is added by a nonqualified person. Technical problems of medical electrical systems, including the use of isolation transformers, must be entrusted to clinical engineers.

Fundamentals · Box 3:4

Medical device types
Devices fall into three types, labelled with the following symbols:

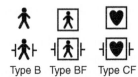

Type B   Type BF   Type CF

The symbols with the depicted defibrillation electrodes indicate that the device tolerates the high voltages generated during defibrillation.

Type B (body)
Devices that normally are electrically separated from the patient are, from a clinical engineering standpoint, seen as type B. Thus no conductive part of these devices is connected to the patient. Examples of such devices are X-ray machines, operating tables, and lung ventilators.

In certain cases, a type B device may be connected to the patient if the treatment so demands, for example, an operating table.

Type BF (body floating)
All devices that will be electrically connected to the patient via cables or liquid-filled catheters must normally be at least of type BF. Examples are endoscopes, blood warmers with patient-applied parts, electrosurgical devices, electrical pressure gauges and thermometers.

Type CF (cardiac floating)
These devices are required for any electrical connection close to the heart. Examples are devices for cardiac catheterization and intensive care monitoring, as well as defibrillators with internal cardiac electrodes.

Thanks to standards being applied and medical devices being well maintained, the risks during use are low. It is the simple errors that are treacherous, such as failing to keep track of loose power cords, especially when they are connected to the main power lines:

CASE 3:9 Patient connects her ECG leads to the power lines

A middle-aged woman had been admitted to the intensive care unit following stomach pumping, after she had swallowed 19 sleeping tablets. The next day she was completely conscious, was being monitored, and was later to be transferred to a regular ward. She was connected to an ECG monitor

Techniques • Box 3:5

Leakage currents

There is a distinction between resistive and capacitive leakage currents. The reason for the first type is that no insulation is perfect, and all insulators do conduct electricity to some degree. But this is not a medical-technical problem given modern materials. The difficulty lies in reducing the damaging effects of the capacitive leakage currents. These are caused by alternating currents passing through capacitances in transformers and between conductors, Boxes 3:2 and 3:3.

A simple case is shown in the top part of Figure 3:8, where an ECG machine is connected to the patient's arm, and the patient return electrode of a surgical diathermy generator is connected to the thigh. Leakage currents normally occur in the power cords and other components of both devices, and are conducted away through the earth wire and thus do not affect the patient.

Broken earth wires are among the most common electrical faults in hospitals. If we assume that the earth wire of the ECG machine is broken, as illustrated in the lower part of Figure 3:8, the leakage current is then conducted through the ECG machine – ECG lead – the patient's arm, trunk and thigh – the surgical diathermy return electrode – the surgical diathermy generator – earth; an obvious safety hazard.

Medical-technical devices must be designed with such features that prevent them from generating dangerous leakage currents and from propagating leakage currents from other faulty devices.

In type B medical devices, leakage currents are limited in normal situations to 100 µA. A leakage current of this size may pass through the patient since it is harmless. But if a patient is connected to a type B device and is exposed to 230 V through a contact with another faulty device, fatal currents might be conducted to earth via the type B device.

In type BF medical devices, leakage currents to the patient, as for type B, are limited in normal situations to a harmless 100 µA. But in order to protect the patient in the event of an unintended connection to 230 V, leakage currents to earth through type BF devices are limited to 5 mA. This prevents dangerous currents from being conducted through any part of the skin. However, this leakage current limitation is not sufficient when devices are connected close to the patient's heart.

In type CF medical devices, the patient-applied part must not be able to generate leakage currents in normal situations higher than 10 µA, and in this way dangerous currents are prevented from being generated during investigations near the heart. If the patient is unintentionally exposed to power voltage of 230 V, the leakage current through type CF devices is limited to a maximum 50 µA.

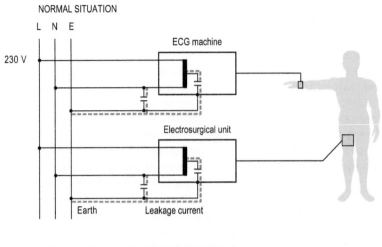

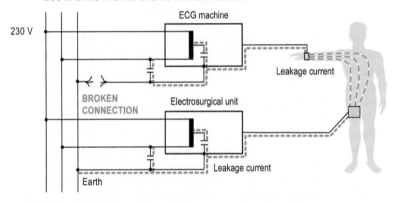

Figure 3:8 If the ground wire is broken, dangerous leakage currents can flow

for monitoring. As she turned in bed, the electrode leads were disconnected from the ECG monitor connecting cable.

So as not to trouble the ward personnel, she decided to reconnect the electrode leads herself. She found a cord on the floor with a three-contact female connector. Believing that it belonged to the cardioscope, she thought she would plug the three banana plugs of the ECG wires into this plug. When she inserted the second plug, she received an electric shock across her chest and lost consciousness.

An assistant nurse happened to notice that the patient was having contractions and convulsions and was unconscious. She called the doctor who connected the ECG and diagnosed ventricular fibrillation. The patient was defibrillated, but the fibrillation changed to asystole (the heart muscle stopped working). This condition was promptly reversed by giving adrenaline intravenously and heart massage.

Thanks to the rapid intervention, the patient did not suffer any brain damage. The cord to which she had connected the ECG leads was a loose power cord that was connected to a live outlet. The cord belonged to an infusion pump that was not being used.

 Keep track of all power cords. Never leave a loose power cord with the plug connected to an electric outlet.

BIOLOGICAL EFFECTS OF ELECTROMAGNETIC FIELDS

There is a distinction between **electric fields,** which are measured in volts per metre (V/m) and **magnetic fields,** which are measured in tesla (T), or more often microtesla (µT). Electric fields are easy to minimize with earth-connected shields; magnetic fields are much more difficult to eliminate. Both types of fields are intimately connected and originate from each other. It is therefore often hard to make out whether an effect is caused by one type or the other. Electromagnetic waves radiate, producing electro-magnetic fields. The biological effects depend on the frequency.

High-frequency electromagnetic fields

At high frequencies (e.g., 1 MHz), as mentioned earlier, a thermal effect on tissues is exerted depending on how much energy per tissue mass is released. This principle is utilized in surgical diathermy (Chapter 11). The risks are well known.

Whether high-frequency fields exert biological effects other than through heat is not known. It is reasonable to assume that the risk must be quite low, as appliances emitting such fields have been used for a hundred years without any obvious association being detected. The rapidly increasing popularity of mobile telephones, which when switched on emit high-frequency electromagnetic fields near the brain, has, however, once again rightly resulted in their safety being examined.

Low-frequency electromagnetic fields

It is also difficult to define the risks at the power-line frequency of 50 Hz. A distinction must be made between effects resulting from short-term versus long-term exposures. Several experiments have been performed on subjects with "electricity allergy", who have been placed in separate rooms and given **short-term exposures** to fields of known strengths. These persons have not been able to notice when the fields have been turned on or off. The symptoms of these patients (e.g., dizziness, concentration difficulties, tingling and itchy skin) are most probably caused by something other than allergy to electricity.

It has been suggested that **long-term exposure** to low-frequency fields could increase the risk of certain tumours in children. The reason for this suspicion is that a slightly increased number of leukaemia cases among children who have lived close to high-voltage transmission lines has been shown. This suspicion, however, has not been confirmed by carefully conducted studies. It is therefore believed that the effect on the children has not been caused by the electromagnetic fields around the power lines but by some environmental factor.

Engine drivers and electric welders are exposed to fields a thousand times greater than those that occur around high-voltage cables. We can safely conclude that there are no increased risks within health care compared to that of many other professional categories.

Electrostatic fields

Nonconducting objects, such as nylon clothes, often become charged with static electricity, especially when the air is dry. We see sparks when we pull the clothes over our head. Static electricity can also occur in connection with certain electric devices. A TV screen, for example, becomes dustier than the TV case, because the charged glass surface of the tube pulls dust towards it. Previously, when the glass on older computer screens had a different electric voltage than the person working in front of it, the pollution in the air was pulled towards the face (particles can travel in both directions depending on their charge). Problems such as irritated and itchy eyes and face could arise. Modern computer screens have to comply with stringent requirements with regard to the field strengths generated. Among other things the screens are now earthed to prevent electrostatic effects.

Magnetic fields

The very powerful magnetic fields that are generated around magnetic resonance imagers (Chapter 7) are not regarded as having any serious damaging effects. On the other hand, the risk increases greatly if a magnetic object is brought into the room, such as a key ring, tools or an oxygen tube. Such objects are attracted with great force and can fly like a cannon ball through the room and stick to the magnet. The patient should of course not have any surgically implanted parts, such as artificial joints, which can be attracted by the magnet.

Magnets can cause unexpected problems:

CASE 3:10 Health magnet causes heart attack

An elderly man with a pacemaker had been admitted to the cardiology department for an investigation. During several nights the patient experienced chest pains (angina) when lying on his left side. The nurse on duty noticed an increase in heart rate on the ECG monitor. The problems recurred for several nights. Eventually, the doctor solved the problem. He noticed that the patient had an unusual piece of jewellery hanging on a leather band around his neck.

The patient's granddaughter was very interested in natural medicine and had given her grandfather a magnet "to improve blood circulation". Every night when the patient turned on his left side, the magnet slid down so that it was lying on top of the pacemaker and triggered a test function of a hundred beats per minute.

Electromagnetic compatibility (EMC)

Electronics is becoming an ever more significant part of medical-technical devices. The risks of interference have therefore increased, as the devices suffer from an increased susceptibility to external fields. At the same time, the devices to an increasing degree also emit electromagnetic fields. For this reason, requirements for **electromagnetic compatibility (EMC)**, have been established.

The problems are greatest for old devices, which were constructed before the EMC standards were applied. A CE-labelling therefore does not automatically mean that the device does not cause or can tolerate interference.

Devices that can cause interference are, for example, mobile telephones, pagers, CD players, video cameras and microwave ovens. Even remote-controlled devices can interfere with other equipment. The most important of these groups are mobile telephones, as they can never be constructed so that they do not emit electromagnetic fields – their very purpose, after all, is to send out signals to a receiving station. The use of mobile phones were once prohibited in many hospitals, but recent designs emit lower field strengths and are now often allowed except in certain critical areas such as intensive care units.

Many devices of various makes have been demonstrated to possess susceptibility to interference. Infusion pumps are particularly sensitive. Other devices are blood pressure gauges, heart and respiration monitors, pace-makers, pulse oximeters, ventilators, incubators, surgical diathermy units, dialysis machines, blood warmers, older types of hearing aids and electric wheelchairs. Of these, infusion pumps constitute the greatest hazards.

Interference quickly decreases with distance. At short distances, less than about 20 cm, interference can never be avoided. Therefore, pace-maker patients should never carry switched-on mobile telephones in their breast pockets. But these risks exist even over much longer distances.

CASE 3:11   Runaway wheelchairs

A person in a wheelchair had a frightening journey. The wheelchair suddenly turned completely around and rolled away at high speed down a hill. The person suffered a fractured femur and several other injuries as well. The accident happened three blocks away from a very busy highway.

In another incident, a wheelchair-dependent patient was waiting for the light to turn green at a pedestrian crossing. While the light was still red, the wheelchair suddenly rolled out into the street. In both cases older-style nearby mobile phones were implicated.

CASE 3:12 Telephone call stops a ventilator

Another wheelchair-dependent patient was using a ventilator for breathing support. The patient bought a mobile telephone and had it mounted on the wheelchair. The first time the telephone rang, the ventilator stopped, set off the alarm and performed some very long expirations in various sequences.

Inside hospitals, the devices that have been affected most frequently are infusion pumps.

CASE 3:13 Infusion pumps stop

A patient was connected to three infusion pumps from two different manufacturers. Suddenly all three pumps came to a stop. In the next room the relative of a dying patient had used a mobile telephone.

The pumps were immediately started again. This was, however, an incorrect decision made by the personnel as other things could have gone wrong with the pumps due to the interference. The pumps should have been sent to the clinical engineering department for a check up and a functional test.

The incidents occurred with the old analogue-type mobile phones which were known to emit much higher intensity electric fields than modern digital types. Many other accidents and near accidents have been reported, where infusion pumps have both stopped and delivered incorrect volumes. It is important to note that on the whole, these events are rare. The situation will gradually improve as old devices are replaced by those that meet EMC requirements.

SUSCEPTIBILITY TO WATER

Normally, medical-technical devices must not be exposed to spills (e.g., infusion fluids, or urine). It has been necessary, however, to render some devices less sensitive to moisture. These usually carry some type of labelling; some old types still may be in use, Figure 3:9.

Instead of these symbols, a notation consisting of an ingress protection (IP) code, IPXN, is now used, where the letter X stands for a number

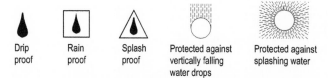

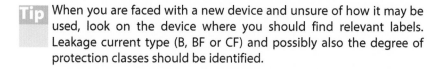

Figure 3:9 Old types of labelling to indicate device susceptibility to water

between 0 and 6 denoting the mechanical protection, and the letter N stands for a number between 0 and 8 denoting the protection against water. The higher the number, the better is the protection. The notations should be explained in the instructions for use.

Tip When you are faced with a new device and unsure of how it may be used, look on the device where you should find relevant labels. Leakage current type (B, BF or CF) and possibly also the degree of protection classes should be identified.

4

Gas, fire and heat

Even relatively simple technical devices can be potentially dangerous if people are unaware of how these should be handled. Everyone working within health care should note the precautions necessary when handling medical gases, which is why some important aspects of **gas technology** are summarized below. Many hospital fires could have been prevented, had people appreciated the various **fire hazards**. Numerous types of **thermal injuries** have occurred due to a lack of awareness of the possible causes of such injuries.

GAS TECHNOLOGY

Since **medical gases** possess various physical characteristics of importance for their handling, these characteristics, as well as the various **medical gas devices** in use, will be described.

Medical gases

In hospitals, certain medical gases are transported in pipelines from a **central source of supply**. Gases such as oxygen, nitrous oxide (laughing gas), medical air and medical air for driving medical devices are generally distributed in this fashion. There are emergency shut-off valves at the points where the gas lines enter the wards and also outside operating rooms, so that the supply can be shut off if necessary. In case of fire, it is important to be familiar with the location of these emergency valves. They are usually placed in a cabinet in a corridor where they can be easily accessed; however, as it turns out, sometimes too easily.

CASE 4:1 A gas valve is not a clothes hanger

In an intensive care unit, the oxygen supply from the central gas supply was suddenly interrupted. All patients immediately had to be ventilated manually with air, until oxygen could be furnished from gas cylinders nearby. The clinical engineering department was contacted, which was really not the proper procedure as the responsibility for hospital central gas installations fell on the hospital estate management, but the "contacts" were better with the clinical engineering department.

At first, no cause for the interrupted oxygen supply could be located, and the city gas distributor was contacted for emergency delivery of oxygen in cylinders.

However, after further investigations by joint staff from both the clinical engineering and the estates management departments, the cause was finally discovered: the ward central oxygen supply valve had simply been shut off.

The gas valve was located in a wall cabinet in the corridor. The ward personnel had noticed that this cabinet was empty except for some gas pipes, and had taken to using the apparently available space for storing handbags and clothes. Someone had even started hanging her coat on the oxygen valve. As this happened repeatedly, the valve had been gradually turned, little by little, until it had finally been completely shut off, thus causing the incident.

This example includes an important detail that might not seem relevant at first consideration. The delay in asking for help from the correct source, the estate management department, was caused by old unsolved personal conflicts. When carefully investigating the circumstances behind incidents, such contributing factors often appear.

Sometimes gas has to be supplied from **gas cylinders**, for example, during patient transport or if the medical gas supply system malfunctions. Gas cylinders are also used for oxygen treatment in the home. The most common medical gases can be supplied in gas cylinders at pressures presented in Table 4:1.

Oxygen

The pressure in an oxygen cylinder gradually decreases as the cylinder is emptied, and the amount that remains at atmospheric pressure can easily be calculated, Box 4:1. Oxygen is somewhat heavier than air and will therefore easily flow downwards and penetrate the bed linen, for example, if it leaks from a facemask. This poses a fire hazard as the risk of ignition increases rapidly with increasing oxygen levels. We will discuss the fire hazard later in this chapter; suffice it here just to point out that these fires easily become explosive. In order to understand how medical gas devices must be handled, it is vital to realize that practically any material will burn in pure oxygen. Contrary to general belief, even steel sheets will burn violently, as illustrated by the following example.

Table 4:1 Composition and colour codes for some medical gases according to the European EN 739 standard, with maximum gas cylinder pressures

Gas	Composition	Colour code	Cylinder pressure bar
Breathing Oxygen	O_2	White	200
Nitrous Oxide	N_2O	Blue	55 / fluid
Breathing Air	21% O_2 + 78% N_2	White and black	200
Air for driving tools	21% O_2 + 78% N_2	White and black	200
Mixed gas*	50% O_2 + 50% N_2O	White and blue	138
Carbon dioxide	CO_2	Grey	53.7
Carbogen	<7 % CO_2 in oxygen	White and grey	150
Nitrogen	N_2	Black	200 or fluid
Helium	He	Brown	200
Vacuum	(WAGs)	Yellow	< 1

*Of the two gases and concentrations indicated

WAGs = Waste anaesthetic gases

CASE 4:2 Patient dies during fire in operating room

An elderly woman was undergoing gall bladder surgery under general anaesthesia while attached to a ventilator. The ventilator in the operating room received its gas via a permanently installed supply console with gas and electric outlets. During the operation, a nurse tripped over an electric cord that was connected to an electric outlet mounted on the console. This caused certain electric components to contact – it was later found that these components had not been installed as per the current safety regulations. This contact resulted in a short-circuit and flying sparks. The gas line had been constructed of an unsuitable hose material, which had allowed oxygen to leak out into the console enclosure, and an extremely violent fire erupted. The steel sheet encasing the supply line rapidly caught fire, and molten steel dripped down onto the ventilator.

The personnel reacted quickly and shut off the oxygen supply. The fire was put out and none of the staff was hurt. However, in the midst of all the commotion during the fire, anaesthesia had not been administered correctly to the unconscious patient, who died.

Consequently, oxygen must be used with great caution. It is especially hazardous to allow pressurized oxygen to come into contact with grease and oils, which can **auto-ignite**. When installing gas pressure regulators,

Fundamentals • Box 4:1

Remaining gas in gas cylinders

For **oxygen**, the remaining gas is easily calculated by multiplying the cylinder volume V by the pressure P:

$$\text{Amount of oxygen} = V \times P$$

A 5 litre oxygen cylinder of 33 bar that can be emptied down to 3 bar (gas cylinders should never be completely emptied, for explanation see "Handling gas cylinders") thus contains $5 \times (33 - 3) = 5 \times 30 = 150$ litres of usable oxygen. At a consumption rate of 2 litres per minute, the remaining oxygen will thus last for a little over 1 hour.

For **nitrous oxide**, the gas cylinder must be weighed to determine the remaining amount of gas. Assume that the gas cylinder weighs M kg, and the empty weight (tare weight) is T kg. To determine the weight of the remaining gas, the difference between the cylinder weight and the tare weight is calculated. Each kilogram of nitrous oxide is equivalent to 550 litres of free gas at atmospheric pressure:

$$\text{Amount of nitrous oxide in litres} = 550 \times (M - T)$$

A 5 litre nitrous oxide cylinder, with empty weight 7.1 kg, weighs 7.9 kg. Thus, the amount of gas is $550 \times (7.9 - 7.1) = 550 \times 0.8 = 440$ litres. If the remaining gas pressure should be 3 bar, i.e., $3 \times 5 = 15$ litres, the usable amount of gas is $440 - 15 = 425$ litres.

Mixed gas is delivered at a gas cylinder pressure of 138 bar. The amount of this gas is derived by multiplying by a constant, 213, the volume V and the fraction of the remaining pressure P:

$$\text{Amount of mixed gas in litres} = 213 \times V \times (P/138)$$

A 5 litre gas cylinder contains $213 \times 5 = 1065$ litres at delivery. If after use the pressure has dropped to 70 bar, the remaining amount is $213 \times 5 \times 70/138 = 540$ litres. Using a remaining gas pressure of 3 bar and thus a remaining gas volume of $3 \times 5 = 15$ litres, the usable amount of mixed gas is $540 - 15 = 525$ litres.

for example, the washers must never be handled with greasy hands. Hands must be washed before installation.

Patients receiving oxygen should avoid using oily facial creams. But medically warranted care, such as for dry lips can be done without risk. Using oil-free moisturizing gels, or creams and lotions with low oil content, will reduce the fire hazard.

Nitrous oxide

Nitrous oxide becomes liquid when under high pressure. In a gas cylinder, nitrous oxide is thus in its liquid state, and the liquid gradually evaporates during use. A nitrous oxide cylinder must be used in the upright position – if placed upside down, liquid nitrous oxide would bypass the pressure regulator, which might be damaged by the very high pressures generated during evaporation.

The pressure in a nitrous oxide cylinder is constant while the cylinder is being emptied as long as any liquid remains, but then the pressure decreases rapidly. The pressure therefore cannot be used to calculate the remaining amount of gas, Box 4:1.

Just like oxygen, nitrous oxide will sustain rapid combustion, and both gases must be handled with equal caution.

Tip A nitrous oxide cylinder must always be used in the upright position.

Mixed gas

Mixed gas, consisting of 50% oxygen and 50% nitrous oxide, is marketed under names such as Entonox and Medimix. Under exceptionally cold conditions, such cylinders with mixed gases must be used in the position recommended by the manufacturer as indicated on the cylinder label.

Gas mixtures are used for pain relief during ambulance transport for fractures, kidney stones and heart attacks. Such gases may be given by the paramedics without prior permission from a doctor.

Carbogen

Carbogen consists of 6.5% carbon dioxide in breathing oxygen. This mixture is used to stimulate breathing during treatment for carbon monoxide poisoning and asthma; it is also used for neonates. The gas mixture must be handled with the same caution as pure oxygen.

Carbon dioxide

Carbon dioxide is used during endoscopic procedures to inflate body cavities for improved visualization (Chapter 7) and to stimulate neonates to breathe. In its liquid state, carbon dioxide is used to freeze tissues – when the gas evaporates, heat is consumed and the tissues freeze (Chapter 11).

The gas is supplied in two different cylinder types, depending on whether it is to be used in its gaseous or its liquid state – it is important that the cylinders be placed in the position indicated on the label. For endoscopy, carbon dioxide is supplied in special cylinders to avoid mix-ups with oxygen; cases are known where oxygen introduced in the abdominal cavity has led to explosions.

Tip Always read the mixed gas and carbon dioxide cylinder label carefully, and follow the instructions regarding positioning of the cylinder. Carbon dioxide cylinders must always be turned with the valve directed either upwards or downwards.

Nitrogen

Gaseous nitrogen is used to power surgical instruments. Liquid nitrogen, which is supplied at -196°C in thermos flasks, is used for cryosurgery and for freezing tissues, such as blood and virus for vaccines.

Argon and helium

Both of these are inert gases that do not react with other substances. Argon has therefore been used as a protective gas during diathermy (Chapter 11) to prevent the tissues from igniting. Argon also has been applied for tissue coagulation. Helium is used as a mixing gas for lung function measurements.

Medical gas devices

For safety it is vital that gas cylinders are **handled correctly** not just for the patients but also for the personnel using the equipment. It is also very important to know the **standards** to avoid any mix-ups and to some extent to know how **flow meters** work.

Handling gas cylinders

An inflated latex balloon when let loose will race around the room, driven by the air jet. The same might happen to a gas cylinder if dropped in such a way that the valve is damaged and the gas is allowed to flow freely. The kinetic energy of such a gas cylinder moving like a rocket is enormous after it has gained speed. It can fly straight through a wall. If spinning around – which may happen if the gas jet is directed in an oblique direction to the length of the cylinder – getting hit by the spinning cylinder is equivalent to getting hit by a helicopter rotor. And even if nothing is smashed but the gas just escapes freely, the effect may be astonishing:

CASE 4:3 Two changing one pressure regulator

A nurse was going to change a pressure regulator on a 2.5 litre oxygen cylinder. She was having trouble releasing the nut and a co-worker tried to help by holding the cylinder in place. While doing this, the other nurse grasped the cylinder valve with one hand and inadvertently opened the valve, resulting in gas flowing out of the cylinder. The gas cylinder was torn away from the hands of the nurses, spun around, and hit one nurse first on the knee and then on the ankle.

One of the nurses afterwards commented that it was too bad the cylinder had not been larger and heavier, "because then it would have been unable to spin around". Unfortunately she was completely wrong; if the gas pressure had been the same, a larger cylinder containing more gas would have resulted in much greater injuries.

CASE 4:4 A gas cylinder is not a handball

An anaesthetic nurse who was also a handball player was going to attach a regulator valve to a 2.5 litre oxygen cylinder. She did not get very far. In spite of probably possessing beyond-average muscle power and coordination, the cylinder was torn away from her hands when she opened the valve to flush it clean. The cylinder spun around and crashed to the floor with the shut-off valve first. The valve neck broke, and gas rushed out of the cylinder. The cylinder shot like a rocket through the entire corridor and smashed through the opposite brick wall, where it stuck half way through.

There were no personal injuries, but one nurse complained that her ears were still ringing two weeks after the impact.

To protect the valve from damage, gas cylinders must always be equipped with a **protective cap** during transportation. Some cylinders have a detachable protective cap, Figure 4:1, and others are furnished with permanently mounted caps, Figure 4:2.

Gas cylinders must be transported on **special gas carts,** and have to be secured when in use, for example, to the bed. The cylinders must be **secured with chains** while stored, to prevent them from being knocked over; even if they don't break, their weight is enough to crush a human foot.

A **pressure regulator (gas cylinder regulator, reducing valve,** Box 4:2), is mounted on the gas cylinder if the cylinder is not equipped with a permanently attached regulator. A **washer** is placed inside the yoke that connects the regulator to the cylinder to prevent gas leakage. Use only one single washer as fire can result due to the frictional heat generated when tightening two washers.

Modern regulators often have O-rings instead of metal washers for sealing. Then it is important to check that the O-ring is not worn or damaged; if it shows any sign of wear it should be replaced. The nut on the pressure regulator must only be tightened by hand force. Tools damage O-rings and then leaks can cause fires.

All components that will come into contact with the gas must be completely free of grease, oil and dirt. Tighten well before oxygen treatment is initiated.

It used to be considered necessary for the cylinder valve to be purged, by directing the gas outlet towards room air and opening the valve twice, very briefly. This was done to prevent dirt particles from auto-igniting after assembly. Because of accidents, this type of purge cleansing is no longer recommended.

Modern gas cylinders with a volume of 5 litres or less are designed with a **flow control valve** for prevention of excessive outflow rates, Figure 4:3. Older types of cylinders will, however, remain in use for many more years, as they are only replaced over time when they are pressure tested.

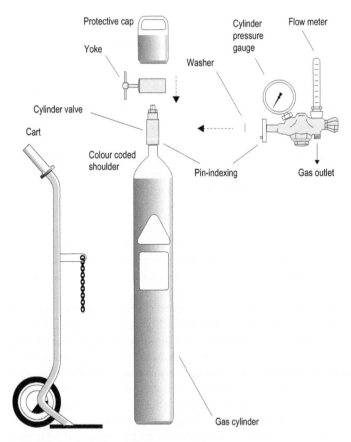

Figure 4:1 Gas cylinder and accessories

Anyone who has ever pumped a bike tyre will have noticed that the lower part of the pump gets hot because of the compression of the air. The same thing happens when the valve is opened and gas flows into an empty, shut-off regulator – compression heat is generated. If this happens rapidly, it can cause a fire, Box 4:3. Therefore, gas valves must always be opened with caution, so that the pressure increases gradually. Open the valve slowly with both hands, and use only moderate force when closing the valve.

Before using a gas cylinder with a replaced pressure regulator, it must be tested for tightness. To do this, first ensure that the regulator outlet is closed, and then open and close the cylinder valve. If the regulator cylinder pressure gauge indicates a constant pressure for a period of one minute, the connection is tight.

It has been considered that gas cylinders must be replaced before they are completely empty, when the pressure has decreased to a certain value, such as approximately 3 bar. There has to be a remaining pressure such

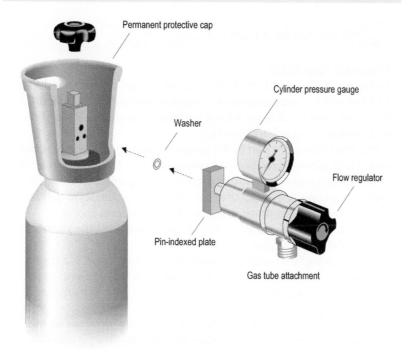

Permanent protective cap

Cylinder pressure gauge

Washer

Flow regulator

Pin-indexed plate

Gas tube attachment

Figure 4:2 Gas cylinder with permanent protective cap and pressure regulator. Yoke is not shown

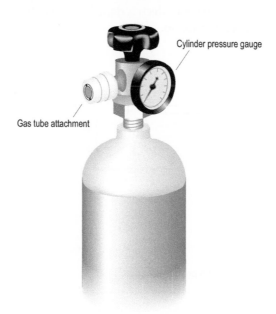

Cylinder pressure gauge

Gas tube attachment

Figure 4:3 Gas cylinder with integral valve and pressure regulator

Fundamentals • Box 4:2

Pressure regulator

As the gas is consumed, the high pressure in a gas cylinder is reduced to a low and constant pressure by means of the pressure regulator (this holds true for all gases except for those that are in a liquid state in a cylinder, such as nitrous oxide).

The most important part in the pressure regulator is the **valve cone**, which is displaced in relation to a **valve seat**. Two forces influence the valve cone, Figure 4:4. On the one hand, a spring exerts a force that pushes the cone away from the valve seat, causing the valve to open. On the other, the gas pressure pushes on a membrane that is connected to the valve cone, pushing the cone against the valve seat, causing the valve to close.

When the outflow pressure drops below a preset value, the spring load pushes the valve cone away from the valve seat allowing gas to flow into the space next to the valve seat, whereupon the pressure is automatically reset.

When the outflow of gas decreases, the pressure increases on the outflow side, pushing the membrane and thereby also the valve cone to the closed position. The spring load balances the gas pressure on the membrane, resulting in an outflow pressure that varies very little.

The pressure is factory set at a certain level (for example 4.5 bar) by adjusting the spring load, which is done by turning the threaded screw that supports the spring.

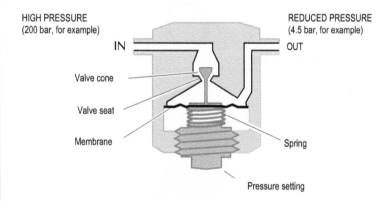

Figure 4:4 Cross-section of a pressure regulator

as at least 2 bar. In some countries no particular pressure is recommended, only that some positive pressure be left in the cylinder. This prevents corrosive moisture or dirt from entering the cylinder and later causing fire. In other countries the practice of leaving residual gas has been abandoned.

When the gas cylinder is empty, the sealing nut is screwed onto the valve outlet, it is verified that the valve is completely shut, and a protective cap may be mounted.

Any gas in a medical gas cylinder has a limited shelf life. An expiry date will be given on the cylinder labelling and this must be respected. This is not usually a problem as several years is normally given for safe use. Guidance is also given for the manufacturer to pressure test steel gas cylinders so that their mechanical durability is ensured, and this is normally done every 5 years. Newer cylinders manufactured from composite materials (plastics), which are preferable for transport because of their lower weight, must be pressure tested after three years. Even though the gas itself has a longer shelf life, it cannot be used after three years. But there is no need to reflect on the reason for the marking on the cylinder label – simply observe the expiry date.

 Techniques · Box 4:3

Adiabatic compression

The term adiabatic compression indicates that the gas will not release its thermal energy upon compression. (The opposite is isothermal compression, where there is enough time for the gas to release its thermal energy to the environment.) This does not concern the gas flowing out of the cylinder – this gas is indeed expanding – but it does for the small amount of gas in the pressure-reducing valve and also in the short part of the gas cylinder coupling outside the shut-off valve. This gas is at atmospheric pressure and room temperature. When the shut-off valve is opened, gas rushes out of the cylinder, and the gas in the reducing valve is momentarily compressed and thereby heated. If the gas consists of oxygen or nitrous oxide, this can cause a fire.

The explanation for such fires is probably that the gas stream carries small particles along with it, which gather such great kinetic energy that they are heated when they impact any part of the reducing valve. The temperature can increase to up to 1000°C, provided that the particles are of the "right size". If they are too small, the kinetic energy will be insufficient, and if they are too large their inertia will be too great.

Before using a gas cylinder, always check the expiry date.

Gas cylinders with siphon tubes

Cryosurgery (Chapter 11) is performed using carbon dioxide from a cylinder equipped with a siphon tube, Figure 4:5. These cylinders must of course be used in the upright position, so that the siphon tube reaches all the way down to the liquid carbon dioxide. The cylinder labelling in some countries states that "the medium will exit the valve as a liquid. Do not use a pressure regulator".

Gas cylinders must be handled with great respect for the potential risks:

CASE 4:5 Burns and splinters in the eye

A patient was being picked up by ambulance and the paramedics were going to give oxygen to the patient. When the cylinder valve was opened, a loud explosion was heard, sparks flew and caused a minor fire in the first-aid bag. During the explosion, the gas cylinder and the regulator became detached. The patient went into shock, but recovered. The paramedics suffered burns and one of them also received splinters in his eye and cheek.

The paramedics were in a great hurry to assist the patient and opened the valve too fast. Similar accidents have occurred during such emergency calls in the frenzy to save a life.

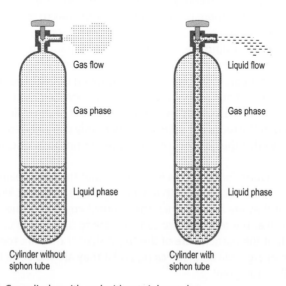

Figure 4:5 Gas cylinder with and without siphon tube

When replacing pressure regulators, remember the following:
- Avoid grease, oil or petroleum jelly on hands or device components – be sure to wash your hands before replacing a pressure regulator.
- When replacing a washer, always take a new original washer, and only one.
- When replacing an O-ring, check that it is not damaged, and do not use tools to tighten the nut.
- Tighten the nut or yoke slowly.
- Check for leakage.
- Open the valve cautiously using two hands; when fully open, turn knob back at least half a turn; when closing a valve use moderate force.
- If the protective cap is detachable, always attach it immediately after removing the pressure regulator.
- Secure all gas cylinders with chains whether they are full or empty.

Standards

Tragic accidents have happened because of mix-up of gases, and often more than one patient has been involved or killed. This has occurred both with gas from medical gas supply systems and with gas cylinders. The risks have decreased thanks to **non-interchangeable connections** and **colour codes**.

Connections are of two types. Non-interchangeable screw-threaded (NIST) connectors are based on different diameters and left- and right-hand screw threads, Figure 4:6. No wrong connections can be made. The other system in use is the pin-index system, Figure 4:7. The pin positions on the inlet connectors are unique to each gas and they only fit into correctly positioned holes on the valve faces. It has happened that the safety pins have deteriorated because of wear, or that irresponsible people have tampered with the safety pins or removed them, overriding the safety design.

Medical gases are delivered in cylinders with varying colour codes for easy identification. Unfortunately, no international or European standard has yet been generally applied. For example, oxygen is delivered in green

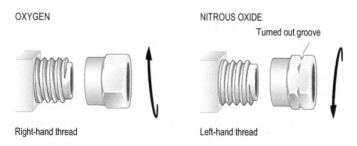

Figure 4:6 Non-interchangeable screw-threaded connectors

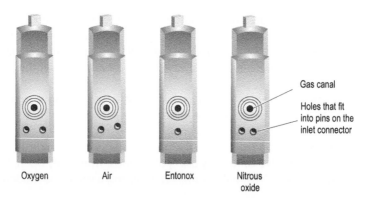

Oxygen   Air   Entonox   Nitrous
                                               oxide

Figure 4:7 Valve faces for four medical gases. Distances between holes are exaggerated to illustrate better the differences for the gases

cylinders in the USA, blue in Germany and in black cylinders with white shoulders (the upper rounded portion of the cylinder) in the UK.

The shoulders of cylinders are thus colour-coded to indicate the gas or combination of gases in a mixture. In Europe the EN 739 standard specifies the colour codes presented in Table 4:1. Even though standards exist, other colours are in use in Europe.

 Before you administer a **medical gas** from a gas cylinder to a patient, always check that the cylinder is labelled with the appropriate gas. The colour codes on cylinders might not be what you expect, and it has happened that irresponsible people have removed safety pins. The only safe way to convince yourself that a gas cylinder contains what you think is to read the label.

On several occasions it has occurred that more than one patient has died before a mix-up of gases was discovered:

CASE 4:6 Two fatal low-risk catheterizations

The heart of a 72-year-old female patient was catheterized at a hospital that annually carried out around 4000 such procedures. Because of her circulatory problems it was considered necessary to give oxygen. The patient died shortly after administering the gas. Her death was ascribed to her flagging health. Five days later another patient aged 69 died during similar circumstances in the same catheterization laboratory.

It was then realized that something was wrong. A pin in a nitrous oxide outlet was found to be broken, allowing an oxygen line connector to be plugged into the nitrous oxide gas outlet. The colour-coded outlets and connectors did not prevent the accidents.

It is not only the gases in a cylinder that can be deadly if mixed up; the pressure is in itself a risk independent of the type of gas.

CASE 4:7 Eight-month-old infant's lungs puncture

The infant was undergoing minor surgery and was connected to a ventilator via an endotracheal tube. At the end of the operation the infant's lungs suddenly punctured, causing death.

Immediately before the accident a tube from an oxygen cylinder had been connected to the endotracheal tube connected to the ventilator. When the valve on the oxygen cylinder was opened a sudden overpressure resulted in pneumothorax in both of the patient's lungs. No pressure release mechanism had been inserted to prevent the build-up of pressure between the cylinder and the tube to the patient.

Flow meters

To ensure that the proper amount of gas is delivered, pressure regulators are equipped with a measuring device, usually in the form of a floating body flow meter (**rotameter**), Figure 4:8. A common type consists of two concentrically placed pipes, of which the inner pipe is tapered and placed with the larger diameter facing upwards. The inner pipe contains the

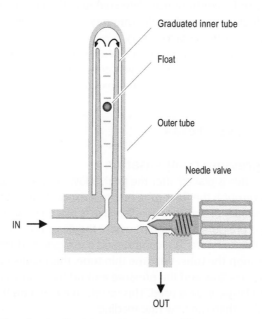

Figure 4:8 Design of a counter-pressure compensated float gauge

floating body, which may consist of a small ball. When the gas starts flowing, the ball is lifted to a height where the pressure drop at the space between the inner pipe wall and the floating body results in a lifting force that exactly balances the weight of the ball. This height is then a measure of the flow.

The gas flows down in the space between the inner and the outer pipe, and exits the flow meter through a needle valve and a threaded outlet used for attaching medical devices. For humidification, the gas is often fed through a container with water.

The function is simple. The gas flow is regulated by the needle valve, and the float rises as the gas flow increases. To avoid damaging the fine needle, the valve must be closed with **moderate force** only, the minimum force required to just shut off the flow.

Flow meters of this type are not very accurate. In order to ensure some degree of accuracy, the pipe must be mounted **vertically**. The accuracy is also dependent on whether the flow meter is of an old versus a new design, Box 4:4. In flow meters of old design, without **counter-pressure compensation**, the gas readings are highly dependent on the degree of resistance to the flow in the connecting tubing. If the inner diameter of the tube is small, the actual flow will be higher than what the gas reading indicates.

Oxygen concentrators

Chronically ill patients may be treated with oxygen in their own homes. If the gas were to be continuously delivered in cylinders, the costs would become very high, as considerable amounts are consumed, and several large cylinders must be replaced every week.

Since the handling of oxygen cylinders also poses safety hazards in the home setting, it is better to use oxygen concentrators. These consist of devices that can produce concentrated oxygen from air. Two types are

 Techniques · Box 4:4

Counter-pressure compensation

The needle valve is placed after the float, allowing the compressed gas to flow through the float tube before it expands after the needle valve. In the older design, the needle valve is placed before the float. Then the gas pressure at the point where the gas passes the float varies with the flow rate. The compressed gas expands during the passage through the tube. With the thin tube, this results in greater resistance to gas flow and the pressure around the float will be higher than when a larger tube is used. This results in a flow rate that is actually higher than the flow rate reading.

available: **molecular sieve concentrators**, which are capable of delivering 95% oxygen, and **membrane concentrators**, delivering 40%. The latter type has the advantage of also delivering a gas mixture saturated with water vapour. The principles of these two types are outlined in Box 4:5.

As a supplement to the oxygen concentrators, chilled liquid gas in specially insulated containers can be delivered when gas is needed during transport. Another alternative is to use gas supplied in specially designed, lightweight flasks made of composite materials.

Evacuation of waste anaesthetic gases

When gaseous anaesthetics escape in the work environment they are referred to as **waste anaesthetic gases** (**WAGs**). Such substances can produce adverse effects among health care personnel with long-term exposure at low levels. For example, both nitrous oxide and halogenated anaesthetics (halothane, enflurane and isoflurane) are suspected to increase the risk of reduced fertility, birth defects, miscarriages and neurological, renal and liver disease. Hence **recommendations for exposure limits** (**REL**) have been issued regarding gaseous anaesthetics.

To meet the safety demands, anaesthetic machines should include a **gas scavenging system** for the elimination of vented gas. Such a system

 Techniques · Box 4:5

Oxygen concentrators

In **molecular sieve concentrators** the nitrogen in the air is absorbed, yielding almost pure oxygen, which is stored in a tank. When used, the oxygen is mixed with air so that the desired concentration is achieved.

The devices consist of two cylinders filled with a porous silicate material that absorbs nitrogen. Air is alternately forced in and out of the cylinders. As the pressure increases, the nitrogen gas is absorbed and the remaining gas is oxygen enriched. When the system switches from one cylinder to the other, the level of absorbed nitrogen in the cylinder just used is high. The gas pressure in the cylinder is now lowered, and at the same time a small amount of oxygen is being flushed back through the cylinder, whereupon nitrogen gas is released from the silicate.

In **membrane concentrators**, the enriching is achieved by suctioning air through a membrane using a vacuum pump. As the nitrogen permeability of the membrane is lower, oxygen is concentrated. The water vapour permeability of the membrane is very high, resulting in the generated gas mixture being saturated, i.e., the relative humidity is 100% at the ambient temperature.

collects any WAGs from the breathing system and transports them to a special exhaust system in the building. Furthermore, when giving anaesthesia, the tightness of all connections between hoses and the anaesthetic machine should be checked before each operation. Note, however, that such local exhaust ventilation is effective only close to the leak. WAGs from a facemask, for example, can be evacuated only within a distance of about 10 cm or less.

Thus, local exhaust systems and gas scavenging systems cannot be replaced merely by improving the general ventilation system. Doing so would result in unacceptably high airflow rates, causing draughts, and also be very costly. But used correctly, modern anaesthetic systems result in only small amounts of WAGs, well below stated limit values.

The exhaled gas must be evacuated even after the surgical procedure has been completed. The elimination from the body is rapid – most of the nitrous oxide is eliminated after 5 to 10 minutes. Evacuation of this gas can be achieved by letting the patient breathe through the anaesthetic machine, or by attaching a **chin mask**, positioned below the mouth by means of a head strap. The chin mask is then attached to a local exhaust system.

In special situations, complying with the evacuation requirements may be more difficult. Examples are during anaesthesia via an open mask during deliveries, dental surgical procedures and ambulance transport. Another example is during anaesthesia to children with endotracheal tubes without cuffs, that is, tubes without an inflatable balloon-like part for achieving an airtight seal against the tracheal wall. In these cases, local scavenging systems are required. One solution is to use a double mask, Figure 4:9. The gas is delivered to the patient via the inner mask, and the gas leaking out is sucked away from the space between the inner and the outer mask.

Patient suction devices

It is often necessary to perform suctioning on patients in various situations, for example, for removing excess mucus from the airways. Principally, there are two different types of suction device: pneumatically powered **ejection suction** devices and electrically powered **vacuum suction** devices. The latter type is used in surgical departments, for removal of blood and secretions during surgery – the fluid is then sucked into a glass or plastic vacuum container. The ejector suction device, shown in Figure 4:10, is powered by the hospital pneumatic system. Pressurized air is released into a tapered inner pipe, which creates a very rapid airflow, dragging the nearby gas molecules into the surrounding outer space. The molecules of the gaseous anaesthetic are "blown along" with the molecules of the pressurized air, just as a person's hat will blow off in a storm.

Ejector suction devices are equipped with silencers with packed cotton. The cotton must not become dampened with the suctioned fluids, as this

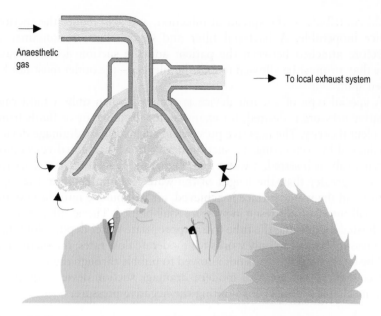

Figure 4:9 Double mask system for eliminating leaking anaesthetic gas

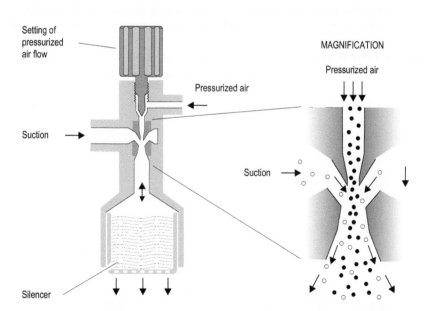

Figure 4:10 Ejector suction. To the right, the darker central part of the ejector suction device is shown. Black dots symbolize the gas molecules in the pressurized air, and white rings symbolize the molecules in the air being suctioned away

could contribute to the spread of infection, and also render the suction device inoperable. A bacterial filter and fluid collection container is therefore attached between the patient and the suction device. Please note that air must be allowed to exit the silencer – the outlet must not be taped shut.

A special type of suction device is required when only a moderate negative pressure is desired, for example, for draining air or fluids from the pleural cavity. The negative pressure in such a **Bülaw drainage device** is achieved by connecting the suction device to a water-filled vessel into which a tube is inserted, a **water seal**, Figure 4:11. As soon as a negative pressure greater than the height of the water column between the pipe orifice and the water surface is achieved, air will bubble into the system. This will automatically result in pressure equilibration. The negative pressure is adjusted by pushing the tube to an appropriate water depth. Note that the pressure limitation only works for moderate flow rates; the suctioning will be too great if the air is not allowed to bubble through the water seal fast enough. There are also modern drainage suction devices equipped with mechanical devices for limiting the negative pressure.

> **Tip** During intensive care, the multitude of tubes, which are often in a more or less intertwined mess, can easily become confusing. Examples of such devices often used simultaneously are ventilators and incubators, gas delivery and exhaust systems to and from wall outlets, and patient suction devices. If you are unable to make out how the tubes are connected, ask someone who knows. If you don't get a proper explanation – refuse to carry out the work.

It is very important to avoid administering pure oxygen to newborn babies, as this may cause eye damage, even leading to blindness:

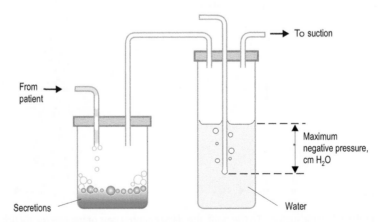

Figure 4:11 Drainage suction device. At moderate flow rates, the negative pressure can never exceed the pressure corresponding to the gauge water depth

CASE 4:8 Pure oxygen inadvertently given to premature baby

A premature baby girl was being treated with continuous positive airway pressure (CPAP) in an incubator (Chapter 8). As the baby had an oozing skin lesion in the groin, during the evening the nurse ordered the paediatric nurse assistant to apply 30% oxygen to the wound to promote healing. This gas mixture was to be obtained from a gas mixer connected to the wall outlets for oxygen and air.

The next day, the morning shift paediatric nurse noticed that the oxygen from the wall outlet was connected to the baby's nasal CPAP device via a flow meter and another device. This meant that the baby girl had inadvertently been administered 100% oxygen for ten hours during the night. The paediatric nurse assistant had asked the ward nurse how the tubes were supposed to be connected, but she had only received vague answers. In spite of this, she carried out the task and connected the tubes in the way she thought was right. She thereby connected the oxygen tubes to the CPAP system, which never should have been touched.

Oxygen treatment of skin lesions in this case should have been prescribed by a doctor. In spite of this, such treatment had at this hospital been regarded as "general care" and been prescribed by nurses. The investigation found that the assistant senior physician, the nurse and the paediatric nurse assistant all were responsible for the incorrect treatment.

FIRE

Hospital fires can be grouped into the following categories: ignition of **flammable gases and liquids,** ignition due to the effects of **oxidizing gases** (oxygen and nitrous oxide) and **common fires.**

For the first two types, ignition may be caused by **electrostatic discharges.** Such discharges can occur when two different, electrically nonconductive materials, which have been in contact with each other, are suddenly separated. Some examples of such materials are various plastics, rubber and synthetic fibres. Often electric potentials exceeding 2000 V are generated, and when discharged explosive and flammable substance can be ignited.

The likelihood of electrostatic discharges decreases as the humidity rises, and the relative humidity in the room should therefore be kept above 50%. This is, however, rarely achieved in countries with a cold climate, such as northern Europe or Canada, during the winter months when the indoor air usually is very dry.

Flammable gases and liquids

Gasoline products have occasionally been used for skin preparation; such a habit must, however, by all means be avoided. But there are many other flammable organic solutions, and whenever these are employed, the risk of ignition by open flame or electrostatic discharge must be eliminated.

Even when approved solutions are applied, such as alcohol for skin preparation, they must be allowed to dry whenever there is any risk of ignition. It is of course vital that all alcohol swabs are removed from the surgical area whenever diathermy or a laser is used.

CASE 4:9 Thighs and scrotum burned

A male patient was undergoing surgery for an inguinal hernia. After completion of the procedure, a small skin tumour was also going to be removed from the patient's buttock.

The patient was positioned in the leg supports and the skin cleaned with chlorhexidine alcohol. After removal of the tumour, there was bleeding from the incision. Diathermy was used to achieve haemostasis, whereupon a flame erupted from the patient's thigh and the lower side of the scrotum. The patient suffered second degree burns on both thighs and the scrotum.

The chlorhexidine alcohol should have been allowed to evaporate from the skin before diathermy was used.

There have been many similar accidents.

CASE 4:10 Defibrillation causes fire

A patient, who was being treated in the intensive care unit following thoracic surgery, went into ventricular fibrillation. Defibrillation was performed using external electrodes, whereupon it looked as if the electrodes had caught fire.

Pads saturated with saline, which are normally not flammable, were applied between the electrodes and the patient's skin. The electrodes had shortly beforehand been wiped with chlorhexidine alcohol for disinfection. At defibrillation, a spark shot out from one of the electrodes. The defibrillator had no technical malfunctions. The incident demonstrates the importance of always using water-based disinfectants in connection with defibrillation.

The stomach and intestines normally contain gases, which may ignite during diathermy procedures.

Diathermy also generates explosive gases. Thus when organic tissues are heated, gases such as hydrogen, acetylene, methane, ethane and propane are released. This is a well-known problem, and the collection of explosive gases in body cavities must be prevented:

CASE 4:11 Urinary bladder explodes

Men suffering from enlarged prostate glands often undergo surgery via a resectoscope inserted into the urethra, after which diathermy is used to plane off pieces of the enlarged gland. During one such operation, the gas produced was not being sucked away, and suddenly the urinary bladder exploded. The patient had to undergo open abdominal surgery for repair of the urinary bladder.

Oxidizing gases

In the preceding text, we have discussed the fact that oxygen dramatically increases the risk of fire, and that grease and oils can auto-ignite in an oxygen-rich atmosphere under pressure. Even at ambient pressure the risks are great. Textiles classified as being of low flammability will burn at a mere increase from the 21% oxygen in normal air to 28% oxygen.

Nitrous oxide fuels combustion just like oxygen. The fire hazard is, however, not as great, as nitrous oxide is mostly used with equipment designed with this risk in mind. For example, manufacturing critical components with low-conducting materials reduces the risk of electrostatic sparks by dissipating the charge.

Any therapeutic measure involving high temperatures, such as surgery using **diathermy** or **lasers** constitutes a risk when oxygen-enriched gases can come in contact with any heated tissue or instrument.

CASE 4:12 Hospital board fired

A 56-year-old male patient was going to have a tumour removed from his throat. He had no other health problems and was in excellent physical condition before the operation.

Immediately when the surgical team activated the laser, fire erupted out of the mouth of the patient. The cannula supplying oxygen to the patient's lungs caught fire, presumably because oxygen leaked out into the throat. The patient survived the operation but died two weeks later from the burn injuries. Autopsy showed that an explosion had occurred in the patient's throat.

The administrators at the hospital tried to cover up the incident. But relatives demanded an autopsy to establish the cause of death, and newspapers reported the accident. The hospital board was sacked.

 When surgical diathermy or laser surgery is going to be performed, stop all supplementary oxygen if at all possible at least one minute before using the unit.

Equally important is that all forms of **open flames** or **sparks** must be avoided whenever oxygen or nitrous oxide is being handled in any hospital area. There have been reports of several serious accidents with children in oxygen tents playing with toys intentionally designed for generating sparks, producing the same effect as a cigarette lighter. Merely smoking a cigarette can have devastating consequences:

CASE 4:13   Patient ignores no-smoking instructions

A patient suffering from emphysema and respirator insufficiency was being treated with oxygen in a double room. She had been told that smoking was not allowed while she was receiving oxygen, and was allowed to smoke only in the presence of the nursing staff, who first had to turn off the oxygen and remove the equipment for the oxygen treatment. Her relatives were forbidden to smuggle cigarettes to her; however, they ignored this.

One day, while receiving oxygen with no staff present, she lit a cigarette. An explosive fire erupted, which rapidly ignited the foam rubber mattress.

The sprinkler system was instantly activated, but in spite of this, the entire room filled with smoke, and the staff were unable to pull the patient or her room-mate out of the room. Instead they were forced to close the door and wait for the firefighters, who arrived promptly.

The cigarette-smoking patient suffered very severe and extensive burns, and the other patient suffered from smoke inhalation. Both patients had to be transferred to the intensive care unit.

CASE 4:14   Five dead in hospital fire

In a single-patient room at a hospital, a fire erupted very suddenly. After the fire had started, a ventilator exploded and oxygen escaped. The fire was contained, but in spite of this, patients in ten nearby rooms suffered smoke inhalation and four patients died.

In the room where the fire had started, remnants of matches and cigarettes were found next to the patient.

Smokers receiving oxygen treatment should remove lingering oxygen from their body by, for example, running a damp comb through their hair (a dry comb may be electrostatically charged and may therefore cause ignition). Oxygen-saturated textiles can also ignite without any open flame. Explosive fires may be caused by electrostatic discharges or faults in electric devices.

CASE 4:15   Two elderly patients killed in hospital fire

An 85-year-old woman was receiving oxygen treatment via a ventilator. A nurse was going to remove the ventilator from the patient, when an open flame erupted next to it, and an explosion followed. The nurse was thrown against the wall. Smoke quickly filled the entire corridor.

The woman died immediately, followed by another patient in an adjacent room. Two other patients and ten staff members suffered smoke inhalation. The room was so badly burned that reconstruction of the accident was impossible.

An electrical fault was suspected, as a physical therapist, who had treated the patient prior to the explosion, had reported getting an electric shock.

Underdeveloped babies in incubators are often given extra oxygen. Fortunately, fire caused by ignition is less common in incubators because of the high humidity. Whenever oxygen is given for treatment, staff must ensure that ignition cannot happen. Such fires are rare, but when they do happen, they are devastating. Oxygen is difficult to ventilate away, and an increased fire hazard may exist long after the oxygen flow has been shut off:

CASE 4:16   Infant burned on the operating table

A 15-day-old baby was to undergo surgery for a cardiac malformation. During diathermy, a pad ignited that had inadvertently become saturated with oxygen leaking from the anaesthetic machine. An explosive fire erupted and instantly spread to other oxygen-saturated textiles.

None of the staff was injured, but the baby suffered second-degree burns over 60% of its body surface. The baby died after little more than an hour.

 Never allow oxygen or nitrous oxide to flow out towards textiles. Open flames and smoking must be prohibited near gas outlets or gas cylinders.

Ordinary fires

Fires in hospitals are often caused by patients smoking in bed or by electric appliances left on, such as stoves or heating plates. Each hospital or other institution will have its own well-established rules for dealing with fires. Staff must ensure that they are familiar with the rules that can apply to them. It is vital that staff in any institution work together to deal with fire.

In case of fire, everyone is required to take action and try to get help. It would seem that such a rule – or law in certain countries – should not be necessary, but unfortunately this is not the case. The first author of this book observed people unable to react appropriately on two occasions.

The first instance occurred when over a dozen men were unable to help extinguish a fire that could have engulfed a whole forest. All were paralysed. The second occasion, not involving a fire, was when an old refrigerator suddenly leaked ammonium gas. Half a dozen men stood immobile while another without help from anyone pulled the heavy refrigerator to a nearby balcony. Thus people do not normally react.

Upon discovery of a fire, staff should act immediately, regardless of their position.

 By reacting and overcoming paralysis, you will be able to use sound judgement. You must legally follow the local instructions in your hospital, but you might save many lives by considering the following suggested tips – hospital fires out of control are totally devastating.

- Call for help by shouting if needed. If you know that someone has heard you, and if the fire is minor, immediately consider if you can handle the situation. For example, you might be able to grab the intact end of a burning item and pull it to the floor and smother the fire by covering it with a blanket. Another immediate action would be shutting off an oxygen valve close to a fire nourished by the gas.
- Ensure that someone has activated the fire alarm, and telephoned for help.
- Remove patients from danger if possible.
- If safe to do so, attack fire with extinguisher.

Further tips (in no order of priority):

- When calling the fire service, be sure to state the hospital, hospital building and department you are calling from.
- You should always know which extinguisher is to be used with which type of fire.
- When evacuating patients to a safe place you must avoid blocking exits. Pull bedridden patients down on to the floor on their mattresses and drag them to the emergency exit routes. Patients in traction or similar devices may be transported in their beds.
- Close the door to the room or space that is burning, so that you prevent smoke and fire from spreading. You can partly avoid the smoke by crawling along the floor (the hot smoke will rise upwards).
- If the smoke production is so great that you are unable to crawl along the floor and rescue the patients, you must close the doors even if there are still patients inside. You will have to leave the rescue to the fire service.
- Meet the firefighters or make sure someone else is meeting them where they will be expected to arrive.
- In some countries you must always alert the fire service even if the fire has been put out.

Many fires could have been avoided if the hospital staff had been prepared. They should therefore familiarize themselves with the emergency escape plan that must always be posted and where the locations of fire extinguishers are. Co-workers must decide who will do what, should a fire occur. They should also decide on a meeting place where everyone must go in case of evacuation – this is very important in order to be able to quickly assess whether anyone is missing.

THERMAL INJURIES

Thermal injuries within health care can be divided into three patient groups, depending on whether the patient (1) is **fully conscious**, (2) has **impaired perception of heat** or **impaired ability to communicate**, or (3) has had the **blood circulation shut off** during a surgical procedure. Injuries of the first group are rare, as the patients are able to react and call for help or prevent themselves from being injured.

Impaired states

Many burn injuries have been caused by heating pads being used on patients with impaired **perception of heat**, who were unable to sense that the skin was getting too hot. Another group are those who do sense the heat, but are unable to communicate, primarily senile patients and young children.

CASE 4:17 Senile patient scalded to death in bathtub

A brain-damaged patient was left alone in the bathtub. He then turned on the hot water tap, which produced scalding hot water at 60°C. When the patient was finally discovered, he had already suffered second- and third-degree burns over 80% of the skin.

Only special heating pads may be used within health care. These must be labelled "For medical use" and also labelled either BF or CF, depending on their compliance with electrical safety regulations. These types of heating pad have several temperature sensors, which limit the electric power output so as to prevent the pads from becoming overheated.

Accidents occur when nonapproved heating pads are used in health care. Pads with only one temperature regulating sensor, which shuts off the electric power when the pad gets too hot, are dangerous. If the pad area with the sensor is not placed in contact with the patient and is cooled, for example, by urine, the regulator then reacts as if the entire pad is too cool and switches on the power to the heating coil. The pad is then heated until the temperature sensor reaches the temperature setting, and this can mean that the part of the pad that actually does cover the patient becomes much hotter than 40°C. Heated waterbeds, although in general much safer than electrically heated sources, can also be hazardous:

CASE 4:18 Child suffers third-degree burns during surgery

A one-month-old baby was undergoing a 12–15 minute surgical procedure, while lying on a heated mattress. After 10 minutes, the mattress felt unusually hot, and was switched off. After the operation, burns were detected on the baby's back. The baby contracted third-degree burns where the skin had been in contact with the mattress ridges containing the heating coils.

The heated mattress was designed to be used with circulating water and had been connected to a water bath. Due to a handling error, the water bath thermostat had been set to 60°C. The water bath had no technical defects.

CASE 4:19 Burns caused by a water mattress at 42°C

A patient was operated on while lying on his back for 5 hours on a water mattress with the heating element set at 45°C. Because of heat losses in the tubes from the separate heating unit, the mattress temperature reading was only 42°C. After surgery, large pressure ulcers (10 × 10 cm) and burns were discovered on both buttocks.

It is not just heating pads and heated water mattresses that can be hazardous. When routines are changed, even a simple cast application can become dangerous:

CASE 4:20 Incompetent doctor

A boy had fractured both the tibia and the fibula. When applying the cast, the doctor used hot water when soaking the plaster bandages. Contrary to the manufacturer's recommendation, to reinforce the cast he applied twice the recommended amount of bandages around the leg. He then placed the leg on a pillow covered in plastic. The boy complained several times of severe pain, and he received two injections for the pain. It was discovered too late that the boy had contracted extensive thermal injuries.

The boy was flown to an orthopaedic clinic where his fractures were treated. But the permanent damage to the skin and nerves of the lower leg could not be prevented.

Using hot water, twice the amount of plaster bandages and placing the leg on plastic thereby preventing water from evaporating were all wrong. The doctor did not know that heat is generated when plaster bandages set.

"Cold light" lamps, that is, illumination devices equipped with special heat-absorbing filters, can cause burns and even fires during surgery.

CASE 4:21 Fibre-optic device caused burns

A newborn baby was the subject of a clinical demonstration, where a lower arm artery was to be localized for blood sampling, using illumination. For this purpose, a 150 W cold light device was being used, from which the light was transmitted to the lower arm via a fibre-optic light cable. To avoid thermal injuries, a paper sleeve 13 mm long had been attached to the cable end to prevent it from touching the skin.

After an hour, burns were noted where the light had been illuminating the skin. In spite of the heat-absorbing filter, the cold light device and the paper sleeve, the temperature had still been too high.

Blood circulation shut off

A healthy individual without facial protection can without harm be exposed to -30°C, and sit in a sauna at 90°C. Thanks to the great capacity of the blood circulation, heat is rapidly transported both to and away from the skin. But when the blood circulation is shut off, the skin has neither protection from cold nor from heat.

During surgery, in order to achieve a bloodless field, the blood circulation in an extremity is often shut off, for example, by means of a blood pressure cuff. Vascular surgery is possible only after the blood circulation has been temporarily shut off.

With hands kept close to the patient's skin or organ, it is not possible to physically sense whether a patient, whose blood circulation has been shut off, is being exposed to a risk. A temperature that is very agreeable to a normal person can still cause severe burns to a body part that has no blood circulation. The only sure way is to measure the patient's skin temperature with a special thermometer.

Remember that the risk of injuries when the blood circulation has been shut off does not just apply to heat. The skin is also much more sensitive than normal to other effects such as from chemical disinfectants.

> **Tip** Be very careful not to subject the extremity to **heat or chemicals** during **surgery in a bloodless field**. Check the temperature.

5

Measurement techniques

". . . when you can measure what you are speaking about,
and express it in numbers, you know something about it; but when
you cannot measure it, when you cannot express it in numbers,
your knowledge is of a meagre and unsatisfactory kind . . ."

(Lord Kelvin, 1883)

The above quote has often been repeated in order to emphasize the importance of using good measurement methods in science and technology. The quote is equally applicable to modern health care, which to a large extent is based on using measurements to describe a patient's condition. Often the correct treatment can be given only when the results of an investigation can be expressed in numbers.

But numbers also possess a "magic" that may mislead. If the "accuracy" of an instrument is expressed to many significant figures, we believe the instrument to be very accurate even if we have no information as to what the numbers are actually based on. If the statistical significance of a study is expressed in p-values with many zeros, we are lulled into thinking that the results are convincing even if the investigation is of questionable design. Numbers have a mysterious intrinsic property that can numb our powers of judgement.

There are examples of reports and studies on which medical decisions are based that do not comply with even the most basic technical requirements for the specification of accuracy. The authors (and even the reviewers), it seems, are satisfied with the measurement uncertainty being expressed as a certain percentage, without further information on how the percentage was derived. It is enough that the uncertainty is given, even if no one can understand its meaning.

Both instrument manufacturers and users within health care often treat the specifications of measurement uncertainty too lightly. Note that the term "accuracy", which has a qualitative meaning, should not be used when **measurement uncertainty** is expressed in numbers. The correct term in that case is really **inaccuracy**.

CASE 5:1 Inaccuracy of infusion pumps

One of the larger manufacturers once specified the "accuracy" of one of their infusion pumps as 5%. This was linguistically incorrect, as the intent had been to specify that the pump measurement uncertainty was 5%. There was no information as to what the percentage was based on, or under what conditions the determination had been made. Most people would assume that the 5% value represents the maximum error, under all possible circumstances. How had the manufacturer determined this, and was this really the maximum error and not some average? Was the specified percentage error of 5% (whatever this may signify) calculated for the measured value or for the maximum value of the measurement range?

The measurement uncertainty in the example above should have been specified more clearly without ambiguity. This could have been as the average error or as the maximum error encountered in clinical use. Information about the infusion time during which the error had been calculated was also missing, which is another flaw, as the measurement uncertainty as a percentage of the infused volume is many times greater for short infusion times.

CASE 5:2 Low accuracy still preferred

Measurement accuracy is vital for any medical device, yet confusion with device error is still all too common. In 2005, a published international standard referring to the importance of accuracy in pulse oximetry measurements stated that the ideal accuracy would be less than 1%, with practical accuracy less than 4% over the working range. Thankfully the calculation provided in the document clearly indicated that these values referred to errors.

Many clinicians have, no doubt through their own experience, developed a healthy scepticism with regard to measurements. But a certain degree of blind faith in lab results may still exist. In everyday health care, clinicians do not have time to worry about the technical characteristics of the instruments. It is the clinical engineering staff that must make sure that the instruments fulfil the performance requirements.

Good health care naturally requires that the measurement results received are reliable. This presumes that the instruments comply with certain specifications regarding maximum allowable inaccuracies. Such data must therefore be defined accurately when procuring the device. If the requirements are met, then we know to what extent the measurements obtained can be trusted.

For this assumption to be valid, however, the instrument must be calibrated with a **standard**. For blood pressure measurement the standard may be a pressure meter from a biomedical testing equipment company or a mercury manometer, and for a chemical analyser the standard may be a standard solution. Chemical standards should be analysed together with and undergo the exact same procedures as the patient samples. If a deviant result is obtained for the standard, then the instrument can be calibrated and the results of the analysis corrected.

ACCURACY AND PRECISION

Accuracy is not the same as precision. The **accuracy** of a measurement is the degree of agreement between a recorded value and the true value. If the body temperature is measured repeatedly with the right technique and with a thermometer that has recently been checked and approved with regard to measurement errors, and very similar results are obtained with each repeat measurement, then it is likely that the accuracy is high.

The **precision** is the degree of agreement between repeated measurements with the same instrument. If the temperature is recorded repeatedly and very similar results are obtained with each measurement, then the thermometer precision is probably high; the accuracy can, however, still be low if the thermometer is defective and, for example, always shows values that are systematically too high.

High accuracy presumes high precision, but the accuracy can be low even when the precision is high. Target hits are often used to illustrate this difference, Figure 5:1. The marksman hit the left target shot with great accuracy; he not only aimed his rifle carefully but he also used a very good rifle with a correctly calibrated gun sight. The bullets hit the bull's-eye. The marksman, who hit the middle target, aimed his rifle with equal care and skill towards the centre and the bullets hit within a similarly confined area. But the gun sight was incorrectly calibrated and the bullets ended up at the upper right of the target. The precision of both marksmen was equally high, but the one that shot at the left target also had a high accuracy, thanks to a good rifle with a good sight. The marksman shooting at the right target shot with both low accuracy and low precision.

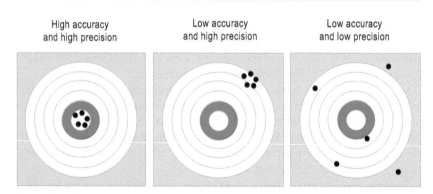

Figure 5:1 A common way to illustrate the difference between accuracy and precision

MEASUREMENT UNCERTAINTY

One of the most important characteristics of a measurement system is the accuracy that can be expected. The difference between a measured value and the true value is called the **measurement error**. If obvious **user errors** are disregarded, such as reading a value of 39.3°C when the temperature is actually 38.3°C, then there are two different types of errors, **random** and **systematic** measurement errors.

The **random errors** vary each time a reading is made. One example of random errors is the reading obtained when blood pressure is measured with a blood pressure cuff (Chapter 6). The blood pressure reading differs somewhat for each measurement (even if the patient's blood pressure is unchanged). When the air is released from the cuff and the systolic pressure value is read, measurement error would be reduced if the cuff pressure for each sequential measurement was exactly the same as the artery pressure just as the blood pulse was being transmitted below the cuff. Similar logic would apply to the diastolic pressure. But this is not possible, as the release of the air cannot be controlled to such an extent. Therefore slightly different values are obtained at each measurement, and that contributes to measurement uncertainty.

The random errors can be expressed as a standard deviation, and are called **standard errors** when applied to measurement techniques. If the measurement uncertainty is low, the standard deviation is small, and the instrument or measurement method has a high precision. Precision is thus a measure of the agreement between repeated measurements. But even if the precision is high, as previously described, the accuracy may be low due to systematic errors – something that must be avoided in health care.

Systematic errors always produce values that deviate in a particular direction, so that the measured value is always either greater or smaller than the true value. The error may be constant throughout the measurement range, and is then referred to as **bias**, or may be a function of the measured value. One example of bias is when an instrument dial has been twisted around its axis. If the blood pressure cuff dial is not set exactly at zero before the pressure is pumped up, a systematic error will occur, and all blood pressure readings will be either consistently too high or consistently too low every time the defective device is used, depending on the direction to which the dial is wrongly set. This is an **absolute error**.

An example of a systematic error with a magnitude proportional to the measured value is measuring time with a stopwatch that runs too fast. This is a **relative error**.

The error is often expressed as a percentage. Thus for a measuring device, it is usual to express the error as a percentage of the full scale. A thermometer that reads temperatures in the range 0–300°C with a manufacturer-specified measurement uncertainty of ±5% of full scale, will at 70°C have a measurement uncertainty range of between 55 and 85°C. The measurement uncertainty range of ±15°C is the same throughout the measurement range.

If the error range is a fixed value, the error range as a percentage of the measured value can be calculated, as shown in Figure 5:2 for the above thermometer example. Such a diagram is called a trumpet curve.

The same types of curves may be used to describe the accuracy of an infusion pump, for example, by drawing a diagram of the error as the ratio of the error in the actual volume infused to the volume set. The uncertainty is a very large percentage at small infusion volumes. These low volumes

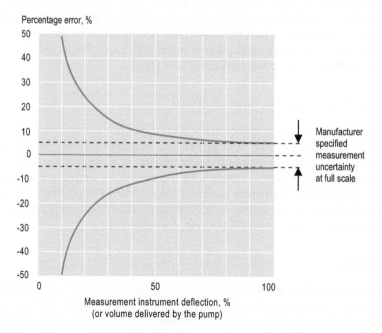

Figure 5:2 The magnitude of the percentage error at various values on a measuring device

constitute a very small fraction of the volume at which the measurement uncertainty was specified, and the magnitude of the percentage error is correspondingly many times greater. Infusions delivered during short time periods result in large percentage errors.

The measurement error of a measuring device is determined by **calibrating** the device with a standard, such as a mercury manometer for blood pressure. The measurement uncertainty of an instrument or a method is the sum of the random and systematic errors.

 Avoid using the lower third of the scale of the measuring device, if this is possible, by changing the measuring range of the instrument.

CHARACTERISTICS OF MEASURING DEVICES

Measurement range

The measurement range specifies the interval within which a measuring instrument can be used. A common measurement range for fever thermometers is 35–42°C, which covers the clinical requirements well.

Sensitivity

Every instrument has a limit as to how small a change in the input signal it can detect, and this sensitivity to some extent is independent of the measurement range. Thus, the sensitivity is a measure of the resolution of the instrument. For a digital thermometer able to display to one decimal place, such as 37.3°C, the resolution is 0.1°C.

Frequency-response characteristic

At a certain chosen amplification, the output amplitude should not change with the frequency of the input signal. This requirement may be difficult to fulfil. The frequency-response characteristic of an instrument specifies how the output amplitude varies with frequency. An ordinary telephone has a rather small frequency range of about 350 to 3500 Hz, which is enough to convey normal speech. A good music system amplifier has a much greater range, 20 to 20,000 Hz, for example.

Stability

When the input to a device is constant, the output must not vary over time; but if it exists such variation is called **drift**. Normally, the baseline is checked for any drift when the instrument is turned on. The stability can be expressed as the maximum change in output over time for a constant input, for example, millivolts per hour.

Signal-to-noise ratio

Noise occurs as variations in the output signal, without any change in the input signal. The noise can be caused by properties within the measuring instrument itself (which is not a significant problem within health care), or by some interference transmitted from the power lines to the patient's body or to the instrument cables. Interference is common during ECG recordings. The actual signal must of course be as large as possible compared to the noise.

The user of, for example, patient-monitoring equipment can often facilitate a high signal-to-noise ratio by fastening the electrodes according to the instructions – first and foremost by ensuring as good a contact between the skin and the electrode as possible.

The signal-to-noise ratio is expressed as a ratio, for example, 10:1, which means that the signal amplitude is ten times that of the noise.

Electrical isolation

Patients must be protected against electric shock and the instruments against interference from other devices. For mains-power-operated devices, it is most important that the electrical separation between the power transformer coils is adequate. Special circuits can also be employed to electrically isolate the patient from the measuring device, for example, when the measurement signal is transferred via optical components. The patient circuit then has a barrier that separates the patient from the rest of the measuring device. Telemetry – signal transfer via radio waves – provides excellent isolation.

As discussed in Chapter 3, medical devices are categorized into three classes, B, BF and CF, depending on the leakage currents that may be conducted to the patient. This classification is dependent on the degree of isolation that can be achieved.

Devices must also be protected from damage. For example, an ECG unit for monitoring patients with myocardial infarction must tolerate the high voltage used during defibrillation. It has special protection circuits that prevent damage to the device.

6

Measurement methods and values

This chapter describes technical perspectives on some common investigative methods, as well as on the data being measured. We begin by discussing **temperature, pressure, sound** and **blood flow**, and then continue with **electrophysiological measurements** and **monitoring**.

TEMPERATURE

Body temperature is regulated from a centre in the hypothalamus. Blood flows to both the brain and the eardrum via the internal carotid artery, and the temperature in this blood vessel corresponds well to that in the brain centre. We would therefore think that reliable measurement of body temperature would be obtained from the **eardrum**. But this temperature has been shown to fluctuate rapidly, and for this reason the suitability of measuring the temperature at the eardrum has been questioned. A momentary measurement is not entirely relevant, despite the fact that the temperature reading does correspond well to that of the temperature centre of the brain. The most stable and accurate measurements are instead obtained from the **oesophagus**, Figure 6:1, a method sometimes used during anaesthesia and in intensive care. Measurements obtained from the **rectum** are also very accurate. Rectal measurements are more reliable than **oral** temperature readings, which can be 0.3–0.7°C lower, and furthermore vary much more and in an irregular manner from the true value. Oral measurements thus have greater uncertainty, because of their lower precision (Chapter 5). The oral temperature also displays local

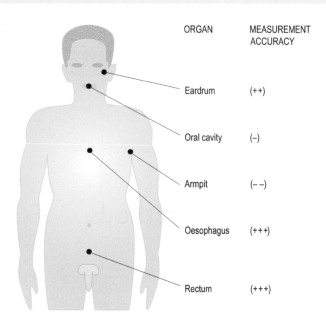

	ORGAN	MEASUREMENT ACCURACY
	Eardrum	(++)
	Oral cavity	(–)
	Armpit	(– –)
	Oesophagus	(+++)
	Rectum	(+++)

Figure 6:1 Temperature measurements at different sites have varying accuracy (+++ is best)

variations, and the best readings are obtained from under the tongue far back in the oral cavity. The temperature accuracy from the armpit is even lower.

Clinical requirements

In principle, the body temperature is measured for two different reasons. If the body temperature regulation system is functioning correctly, the body temperature can often serve as a simple indication of whether the patient is healthy or sick, and measurements may need to be performed only twice daily. But if the body temperature regulation system is malfunctioning, as, for example, during deep anaesthesia, readings are taken more frequently to ensure that the patient does not become too cold. A body temperature reduction of up to 2°C is not unusual under such conditions. A lowered body temperature increases the risk of complications.

Thermometers

Within health care, **electronic thermometers** are applied widely for measuring body temperature. Mercury thermometers are banned because of environmental concerns. The electronic ones usually consist of a thermistor, the electrical resistance of which decreases with increasing temperature, a circuit for determining the resistance, and a digital display.

Some electronic thermometers have single-use thermistors that are replaced between each reading. However, most are designed to be reused, and require only a protective sheath to be replaced between uses to prevent the transfer of infection.

To determine the eardrum temperature, an instrument is used that detects the infrared radiation from the blood vessels. The reading is taken without actually touching the eardrum, but it is important to direct the instrument so that it "sees" the eardrum. Also in these instances a disposable protection cap is used to prevent the spread of infection. The measurement, which is made with an instrument about the size of a telephone handset, takes only a few seconds.

CASE 6:1 Medical thermometer delays treatment

A child with a viral infection suffered a febrile convulsion at home, and required urgent hospital attention. It was discovered that the parents had been using an infra-red ear thermometer, and the temperature readings had falsely reassured the parents.

A subsequent investigation showed that a dirty lens or incorrect placement of the device probe in the ear canal could have caused the problem.

Incubators

Relative to its weight, a newborn baby has a much larger body surface area than an adult, and a much thinner skin and fat layer. This explains why a baby easily loses body heat; it is even more pronounced for underdeveloped babies.

Newborn babies often suffer from **respiratory distress syndrome (RDS)** because their lungs are not fully developed. The fluid balance in an underdeveloped baby is also unstable, and as a result the air passages can easily dry out. Such cases are treated by placing the baby in an incubator. Chapter 8 describes ventilation during incubator treatment; here we will just describe how body temperature is maintained.

The objective is to achieve a **thermoneutral ambient temperature** in the incubator. This is defined as "the thermal environment in which the body temperature is normal, the oxygen uptake lowest and the body temperature remains constant through changes in the peripheral circulation or degree of perspiration". If stimulated by a cold environment, a normal newborn baby is capable of doubling his oxygen uptake to increase his metabolism and thus also his body temperature. The baby can quadruple his cooling through perspiration, so that the body temperature is lowered. But underdeveloped babies born more than approximately 8 weeks too early do not perspire. The risk of the baby getting overheated with incubator temperatures that are too high therefore increases with the degree of underdevelopment. Thus incubators need to be equipped with good temperature regulation.

The thermoneutral ambient temperature in the incubator is determined by the baby's weight and the room temperature, typically 25°C. Babies weighing more than 3500 g require a temperature of 29–33°C. The smaller the baby, the higher the temperature, and at weights less than 1000 g, the temperature should be 35–37°C.

Measuring the baby's temperature rectally is a poor method for determining whether the incubator temperature is right. The rectal temperature decreases only when the baby's regulatory mechanisms for maintaining the body temperature have been pushed to the limit, which can mean a two- to three-fold increased metabolism. The skin temperature is actually a better indicator of whether the ambient temperature is correct.

Types of incubators

Different types of incubators have been developed depending on the various requirements. The simplest are **open incubators** that warm the baby but do not provide any other controlled environment. The baby lies in a box, open at the top and lighted from above with a warming lamp. The advantage is the simple construction and the easy access to the baby, including for some therapeutic measures. Open incubators are not used for long-term treatment.

Generally, **closed incubators** are used. In these, temperature, which in the majority of cases is the most important feature, as well as oxygen supply and humidity, are regulated by modern technology. The temperature is controlled either by manually selecting the desired air temperature or by **skin temperature control**. A thermal sensor (also called a **probe** or **transducer**) is placed on the baby's skin, usually in the armpit, to allow the adjustment of heat to keep the baby's skin at the desired temperature. Skin temperature control carries certain risks:

CASE 6:2 Baby dies through overheating in incubator

An underdeveloped baby was being treated in an incubator with skin temperature control. When the baby was being washed, the skin sensor was removed and left hanging outside the incubator after the washing. Thus the sensor started measuring the room temperature (approx. 25°C). The control circuits therefore increased the heat to maximum level, and the temperature in the incubator rose to more than 45°C. The baby died.

For increased safety, incubators must be constructed with an extra control circuit that prevents overheating in case the skin sensor is misplaced. The incubator in question was indeed equipped with such a safety circuit, but the circuit was defective.

Skin-controlled regulation of temperature is highly superior to manual temperature setting. But one disadvantage is that if the baby has a fever, the incubator temperature is decreased automatically, which increases the baby's heat loss. To detect this, the incubator temperature should be monitored continuously. If the temperature decreases, this might be an indication that the baby has a fever.

In closed incubators, the humidity is also controlled in order to optimize the baby's ambient environment. Since the incubator is warmer than the room temperature, the air inside the incubator would become very dry if water vapour was not supplied. A high humidity is desirable, as this prevents the baby from losing fluid due to evaporation. On the other hand, more than 50% humidity is not desirable as this would increase the risk of infection due to bacterial growth. Another disadvantage with high humidity is that moisture then condenses on the walls making it difficult to watch the infant.

To facilitate monitoring, modern incubators are equipped with alarms for air temperature, skin temperature, oxygen concentration and humidity. The alarms are both visual (red warning lamps) and audible (beep signals). These warn when measured values exceed permitted limits, as well as when faults occur in sensors and in cases of mechanical faults. Examples of such faults are a fan that has stopped or a humidifier that has run out of water. In some incubators the audible alarm may be silenced, but resumes after 10 min if the fault remains.

Underdeveloped babies may need to be transported from delivery wards to neonatal wards in other hospitals. Therefore, **transport incubators**, which are a type of closed incubator, have been developed. For transport within the hospital, batteries are used for heating. During ambulance transport, energy is taken from the battery in the transportation vehicle.

A disadvantage with certain incubators is the unnecessarily high fan noise level. The designers have assumed that a newborn can stand noise levels that would be totally unacceptable to adults.

SOUND

The hearing of the examiner is used both to listen to sounds created when tapping on a patient, **percussion**, and to sounds that are spontaneously emitted by the patient, **auscultation**. Advanced instruments are rarely needed for auscultation; an ordinary stethoscope suffices. Occasionally, the sounds from the heart are analysed by **phonocardiography**.

Characteristics of sound

Sound is generated when a medium is made to vibrate, as when beating on a drum, and the sound waves then travel through the air to our ears. Sound has four characteristics. **Intensity** or **amplitude** is a measure of the sound strength – the harder the drum is hit the better it is heard. The **pitch** or **frequency** of the sound describes the number of oscillations per second, and this is determined by the size of the cavity or the object where the vibrations originate – a large bass produces tones of lower frequency than an ordinary violin. **Tone quality** describes the purity of the tone, the number of overtones and their relative intensity, inclusion of noise, and mix of all frequencies – tones from a flute are pure and clear with few overtones, while a hoarse saxophone is richer in overtones. **Damping** describes how quickly the tones reduce in intensity – the pianist presses a pedal when the music requires the tones to be heard longer and releases it when tones are to cease more quickly, and be damped.

If the source of the sound is placed against the wall of an air-filled cavity, the sound is amplified – a guitar string stretched between two nails on a board can barely be heard, but when mounted on a guitar it produces a tone that can fill an entire hall. The vibrations of the string cause the air in the cavity and the cavity walls to oscillate through **resonance** resulting in a louder sound – the intensity, or amplitude, increases.

To be able to interpret the findings when examining a patient, it is also important to realize that sound is strongly reflected at interfaces between air and solid or liquid media (a window made of thick glass keeps noise out). Interfaces between media with very different densities act as a wall. They stop the sound.

Percussion

The principle of percussion is simple. A person practices it unknowingly when they tap on a door. From the sound produced they can determine whether it is made of solid wood or just two plywood sheets with air in between.

The use of percussion in medicine is based more on personal experience of evaluating the sounds and on using the tactile sensitivity in the fingers, rather than on knowledge of physical principles. But knowledge of the principles can enable the beginner to create in their mind a three-dimensional image of the patient's organs.

Percussion is done by placing one hand with the fingers slightly apart on the patient, and tapping on the middle finger with the middle finger of the other hand, thus causing the organs to vibrate. By assessing the sound and tactile sensations in the hand, it is often possible to determine whether the internal organs are diseased, especially in the chest and abdomen. The sounds that are generated can be described by the four physical characteristics defined above.

Examples of extremes in various types of sound can be found by percussing below the rib cage anteriorly on both sides of the abdomen, Figure 6:2. Over the stomach on the left side of a supine patient, a sound known as tympanic is generated, a sound of high intensity and predominantly of a single frequency, which is caused by the ever-present air in the stomach. The air keeps the stomach and the abdominal walls stretched,

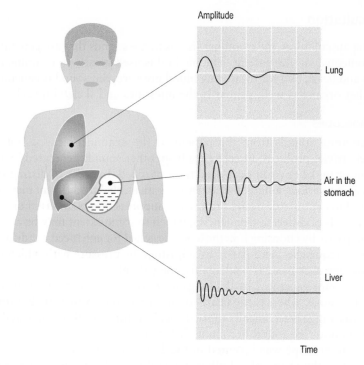

Amplitude

Lung

Air in the stomach

Liver

Time

Figure 6:2 Three types of percussion tones. Only fundamental frequencies are shown

enabling the abdomen to vibrate like a drum. On the right abdominal side over the liver, the sound generated is of much lower intensity and has a highly dampened, dull character, as there are no air-filled spaces nearby.

Over the lungs, the percussion sound is of an intermediate intensity, pitch, tone quality and dullness, which vary due to a number of factors. When the lungs of a large, thin, adult man are percussed, a sound with lower pitch and higher intensity is obtained than when percussing the lungs of a child. This is because the oscillations generated in the large air-filled chest of the man are of lower frequency and greater intensity, similar in some way to a large bass drum. But if the man is obese, the percussion tone is suppressed and thus duller, since the walls of the chest cannot as easily be made to vibrate.

The presence of fluid in the pleural space can easily be demonstrated. The fluid produces a very dull sound in the lower parts where it accumulates; the tone is very different from that generated more superiorly, where the air-filled lung lies adjacent to the chest wall. If the patient changes position, the position of the fluid–lung interface also changes and as a result, so do the percussion findings. The size of the liver can to some extent be assessed through percussion.

Auscultation

During auscultation, the examiner listens to the sounds that are generated spontaneously in the patient. The method is used mostly to examine the lungs and heart, and for measuring blood pressure. But sound is generated by other organs as well, primarily the intestines and skeletal muscles.

Stethoscopes

Transmitting sounds from the patient to the examiner's ear is not an entirely trivial problem. Interference from other sounds generated by the patient or in the environment need to be avoided. In order to distinguish between the various sounds emitted by the patient, slightly different methods are used to capture the desired tones and suppress others. Internal organs emit sounds of different frequencies, which to some extent may be accentuated, partly by choosing a stethoscope designed for enhanced conduction of these frequencies, and partly by adjusting the pressure with which the stethoscope chestpiece is held against the patient.

The sounds generated by the lungs have frequencies within the 100 to 2000 Hz range, whereas the heart sounds are in the 25 to 100 Hz range. The latter range is technically more difficult to transmit through a stethoscope without the sound becoming distorted.

The stethoscope was invented in the 1810s, and was originally made of wood in the shape of a hollow tapered tube, Figure 6:3. The same design is still used today, in obstetric stethoscopes. Its great advantage is that it allows very little noise to be transmitted since it is held firmly in place by being pressed between the mother's abdomen and the examiner's ear. The transmission of the foetal heartbeat frequencies is also relatively good – in other words, the frequency characteristic (Chapter 5) of the obstetric stethoscope is suitable for its intended use.

The chestpiece of an ordinary stethoscope, which is held against the patient, has two different sound channels. Either can be selected by using a dial or by twisting the chestpiece, Figures 6:4 and 6:5. One channel consists

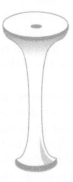

Figure 6:3 Fetal wooden stethoscope

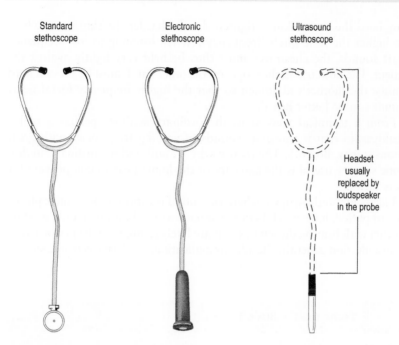

Figure 6:4 Different types of stethoscopes. The standard and electronic stethoscopes are used for auscultation, while the ultrasound stethoscope based on the Doppler principle is used to indicate blood flow

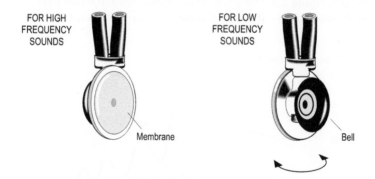

Figure 6:5 Stethoscope chestpiece of standard type

of an open bell about 2 cm in diameter, and is best for low-frequency sounds, such as heart sounds. The other channel has a membrane approximately 4 cm in diameter, and is intended for higher frequencies, such as the lung sounds.

When the bell is used, the patient's own skin serves as a membrane. By pressing the bell against the skin with varying pressure, the skin is stretched to varying degrees in the same way that the pitch of a drum depends on how hard the drum skin is tightened – the harder the skin is stretched, the higher the tone pitch (frequency). When listening to low-frequency heart sounds, the chestpiece must thus be held very lightly against the patient. The obstetric stethoscope, on the other hand, must be pressed hard against the mother's abdomen so that the higher-frequency foetal heart sounds can be better heard.

From a technical viewpoint, the ordinary stethoscope has a major weakness in that it transmits sounds of varying frequencies with great inconsistency, Box 6:1. The reason why we still find the ordinary stethoscope so very useful is the capacity of the human ear to compensate for these flaws.

Electronic stethoscopes, where the sound is captured by a microphone and amplified, have much better characteristics. These are mainly used by doctors with hearing difficulties, but are likely to improve the performance of auscultation generally. Besides amplification, modern electronic stetho-

 Techniques · Box 6:1

Stethoscopes

The acoustic connection between the body surface of the patient and the ear of the investigator is very poor. Standing waves arise in the air column enclosed between the stethoscope chest piece and the eardrum, Figure 6:6. There is a certain improvement when the membrane is used – the lowest tones are somewhat suppressed.

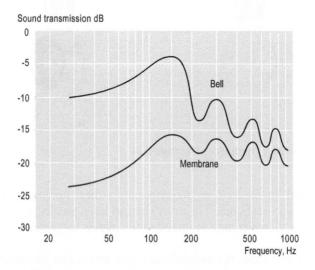

Figure 6:6 Frequency characteristic of a standard stethoscope

scopes have several other useful properties, such as the possibility to record, store and replay sounds. Some also have an output permitting a second person, another doctor, nurse or medical student, to hear the sounds. This has an obvious advantage for training purposes.

In a patient with a pneumothorax, no lung sounds can be heard due to reflections at the lung–pleural air interface. But if the lung is instead filled with fluid and in contact with the chest wall, the sound conduction is better than normal and the intensity higher due to fewer reflections in the air-free lung. Breathing sounds from the bronchial tubes can be heard more clearly on the diseased side than on the normal side.

Phonocardiography

To display the heart sounds as waveforms, the sounds are recorded by a microphone placed on the chest, amplified, filtered into one or more frequency bands and then printed out along with the electrocardiogram. From the waveforms it is then possible to determine exactly where during the cardiac cycle each sound occurs. The importance of phonocardiography has diminished since the development of ultrasound technology, which gives images where the blood flow can be displayed visually in real-time (Chapter 7).

PRESSURE

The pressure within the organs of the body must stay within certain limits. Some organs are more sensitive than others. The intracranial pressure, for example, must not exceed 30 mmHg. An elevated pressure following a head injury or brain surgery is a condition that in itself can lead to irreversible damage and death. When the intracranial pressure exceeds the systolic pressure, blood circulation in the brain ceases and the patient becomes brain-dead.

Within science and technology, SI units are generally accepted as units for pressure, but despite efforts on the part of the clinical engineers, this conversion has not been achieved within medicine.

Pressure can be measured in two principally different ways. For an **indirect pressure reading**, the organ does not need to be punctured. A prerequisite for this method is that the organ must have soft walls that can be subjected to an external pressure of varying magnitude, and that it is possible in some way to observe when the wall gives way. The indirect method is routinely used for measuring the pressure in the blood circulation and the eyes, and to detect uterine contractions during labour.

For a **direct pressure measurement**, a catheter or sensor must be introduced into the organ. This has the advantage of a higher measurement accuracy than can be achieved with the indirect method. Some of the practical problems in measuring blood pressure and intraocular pressure are described below.

Blood pressure

Indirect blood pressure measurement

The common principle for blood-pressure measurement was described by Riva-Rocci in 1896, Figure 6:7. A cuff, consisting of a flat rubber bladder with an outer restraining collar, is placed around the upper arm and pumped up to a pressure that is higher than the systolic pressure. The cuff pressure, which is read from a pressure gauge, is then slowly deflated, and the pressure at which blood is again flowing under the cuff is recorded. The flow can be detected by placing a stethoscope over the elbow crease and listening to the sound produced when the artery wall partly occludes the flow during each heart cycle. This pressure reading represents the systolic blood pressure. By reducing the cuff pressure further, the cardiac cycle interval during which the blood is able to flow is extended. During this period, a Korotkoff sound can be heard, and it is produced by the turbulence in the blood. The cuff pressure at which the blood flow becomes continuous, when turbulence can no longer be heard, corresponds to the diastolic pressure.

Pressure determined in this way is called **auscultatory blood pressure**. For a quick check of a patient's condition a simpler method is often applied

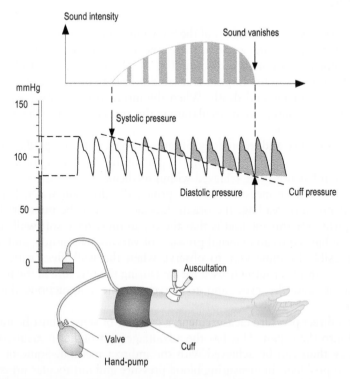

Figure 6:7 Principle for blood pressure measurement with a cuff

by just feeling the pulse over the radial artery, **palpatory blood pressure**. Then only the systolic pressure can be read. An electronic instrument can perform an **automatic blood pressure** measurement, which is common during intensive care and surgery.

Carelessness in performing indirect blood pressure measurements can lead to incorrect diagnoses, called "cuff hypertension". As a result, people are unnecessarily treated with blood-pressure-lowering drugs, even though their blood pressure is actually perfectly normal. Therefore, even if the measurement principle is simple, it must be done with care. The patient should ideally rest for at least 5 min before the blood pressure is taken, and should stay away from coffee and tobacco for at least 30 min before the measurement.

The cuff must be of the correct size, with the length of the bladder being at least 80% of the extremity circumference for the measured pressure to equal the arterial pressure. Too small a size will result in too high a pressure reading, since the resulting pressure on the arterial wall will then be lower than that in the cuff. Different patients therefore require cuffs of different sizes, and a range of cuffs should be available. Adjustable cuffs can also be used.

CASE 6:3 Blind faith in numbers – unnecessary treatment

A young woman was being treated for bulimia. Because of her emaciation, her arms were very thin. When her blood pressure was checked, an abnormally low value was found and she was therefore started on blood-pressure-increasing drugs.

A normal-size cuff for adults had been used for the measurement, but for this particular patient the cuff was much too large, resulting in an overlap.

The patient's upper arm must be **bare**, with no tight clothing either above or below the cuff. If the patient is lying down during the measurement, a pillow must be placed under the arm, so that the cuff is brought to the same level as the heart, Figure 6:8. Should the arm with the cuff be placed, for example, 14 cm below the level of the heart, the resulting blood pressure reading would be 10 mmHg too high. This is an example of a systematic error, or bias (Chapter 5).

The patient, when sitting, should lean against a chair backrest since, on average, the recorded blood pressure is about 6 mmHg too high without a backrest.

Lowering the cuff pressure must not be done too quickly, since it can result in too low a measured systolic and too high a diastolic pressure. If different blood pressures are measured in the two arms, which can occur for patients with among other conditions arteriosclerosis, the one with the highest pressure should be used.

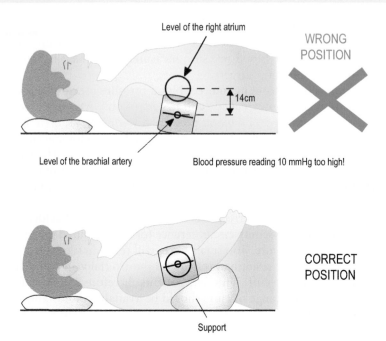

Figure 6:8 The blood pressure cuff must be at the same height as the right atrium

Tip For small children, where an auscultatory measurement can be difficult, the systolic blood pressure can be estimated by slowly inflating the cuff until the waveform from a pulse oximeter disappears (Chapter 8).

During an **automatic blood pressure measurement,** where the measurement is done electronically, an arm cuff similar to the one used for manual measurements is used. There are various ways of determining when the cuff pressure is equal to the systolic and diastolic pressures. The most common method uses the small, pulse-synchronous variations in cuff pressure, using so-called **oscillometry.**

These types of systems have also been miniaturized, allowing the pressure to be measured in the lower arm, near the wrist. A cuff is fastened around the arm just like a large wristwatch, and a small battery-powered box, Figure 6:9, controls the entire process. The blood pressure is shown on a digital display. The advantage of this method is that it enables patients to easily measure their own blood pressure. The risk of erroneous measurements with these designs is, however, greater than with an upper arm cuff, including when the patient easily forgets to keep the wrist at the level of the heart.

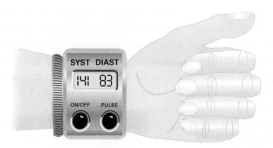

Figure 6:9 Device for automatic blood pressure measurement at the wrist

---

CASE 6:4 Nerve damaged after pressure measurement

A woman in labour needed to have her blood pressure continuously monitored, and an automatic blood pressure monitor with an arm cuff was therefore used. The monitor was of a sophisticated type, and on several occasions repeated the measurements many times, as it seemingly was unable to obtain acceptable values with a small spread. The monitor alarm was activated several times and indicated that the measurement data were unreliable. Since the staff felt the alarm was disturbing, the measurement intervals were changed first to every 5 min and later to every 8 min.

After the delivery, the patient complained of a feeling of discomfort in the arm, and the next day it was found that the patient's radial nerve had become paralysed.

No defects were found in the monitor. It was subsequently assumed that the cuff had ended up too far down on the upper arm and this had resulted in the radial nerve being subjected to much higher pressures than normally exerted when the cuff is placed higher up on the arm.

Another possible cause could have been that automatic blood pressure monitors have an inbuilt function that evaluates the probability that each measured value is correct and when in doubt takes a new measurement with higher pressure. Many discarded values lead to many extra high-pressure compressions of the arm.

Another contributing cause could have been noise causing the automatic blood pressure monitor to measure with higher pressure. Automatic devices often simplify the work within health care, but it cannot be assumed therefore that they are always safe.

Direct blood pressure measurement

Continuous measurements may be necessary during surgery and in intensive care. A catheter is inserted into a blood vessel and connected to a pressure sensor. Miniaturized sensors placed at the tip of a catheter may also be employed.

It is common to measure the pressure at the entrance to the right atrium, the **central venous pressure** (**CVP**). It determines the **preload** on the right side of the heart, which affects cardiac output. Cardiac output is also dependent on the **afterload**, the resistance to ventricular ejection, and arterial blood pressure. The CVP gives an indication of the volume of blood pooling in the veins. During intensive care, CVP is sometimes measured to avoid overhydration when intravenous fluids are given – if the pressure is about 5 mmHg administration of fluids can be done safely, but not if the pressure exceeds 15 mmHg.

When the venous pressure is measured with an external electronic pressure sensor, the sensor must be placed at the same height as the right atrium, Figure 6:10. In a supine patient, the right atrium is located approximately at the intersection between a vertical line through the fourth intercostal space at the sternum and a horizontal line through half the thorax height. As the central venous pressure normally varies between 2 and 6 mmHg, it is easy to see the importance of an exact height adjustment.

A catheter that is used to connect an electronic pressure sensor must have the right length and inner diameter in order to be able to display the pulse waveform. The catheter must also be completely free of air bubbles. A bubble can distort the waveform in entirely different ways, depending on where it is located. If the bubble sits near the sensor, the measured pressure may be too high due to resonance, and if it is near the catheter tip, the measured pressure may be too low due to attenuation.

The pressure in the radial artery is often measured with a catheter inserted into the artery. This method gives accurate values for systolic and diastolic pressure as well as information on the pulse waveform. The set-up for an arterial catheter inserted into the arm is illustrated in Figure 6:11. Blood samples may be obtained via a three-way stopcock. To prevent the blood from clotting inside the catheter, normal saline solution is slowly and continuously infused through the catheter. It is also important to increase momentarily the flow immediately after taking a blood sample via the catheter, so that the blood is flushed away before clots can form.

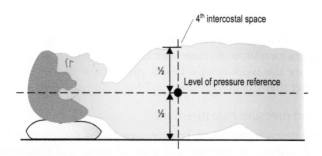

Figure 6:10 The blood pressure is related to the pressure at a reference point located at half the thorax height

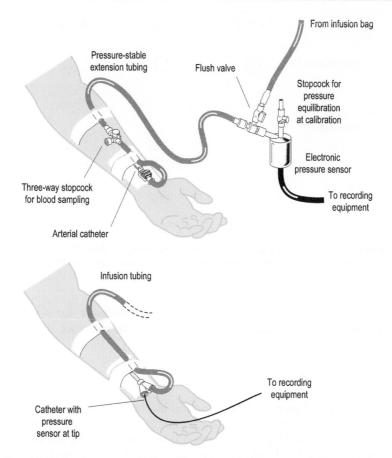

Figure 6:11 Blood pressure measurement using separate sensor (top) and catheter tip sensor (bottom)

Indirect measurement of intraocular pressure

The eyeball is kept distended by a positive pressure that normally should not exceed about 22 mmHg. In glaucoma, the pressure is often too high, and it is therefore considered important that this pressure be measured in elderly patients, so that treatment may be initiated before any damage to the optic nerve occurs.

The eye pressure is determined by measuring how much of a depression is created by mechanical force. This force is usually applied to the cornea. Many pressure-measuring instruments operate on the principle of applying a force sufficient to flatten the cornea into a ring-shaped surface of a specific diameter – these are called **applanation tonometers**, Figure 6:12. The force that the cornea is exposed to is a function of the intraocular pressure.

Many different types of tonometers have been developed. Some have been designed to permit measurement without the need to first anaes-

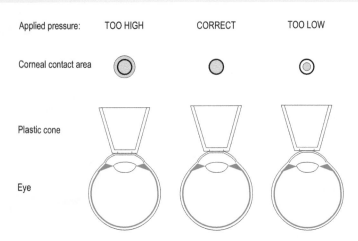

Figure 6:12 Principle of an applanation tonometer. The figure shows how to set the applied pressure to ensure that the recorded value corresponds to the intraocular pressure

thetize the cornea with eye drops, which is necessary for the types applying the pressure with a plunger. One modern type uses an air puff to apply the pressure.

BLOOD FLOW

Even if increased pressure often produces increased flow, a good estimate of the circulation cannot be obtained from blood-pressure measurements. This is because the blood flow is much more determined by the width of the blood vessel than by the pressure. Some blood-flow methods measure the average flow during a certain period of time, whereas others measure the momentary flow, the flow variations from heartbeat to heartbeat.

A distinction is made between measurements of the **central** and the **peripheral circulation**. The central circulation consists of the flow through the heart (**cardiac output**), and the peripheral circulation of the flow through the other parts of the body, via **arteries, capillaries** and **veins**.

Central circulation

If someone standing by a stream pours a carton of milk into it, the concentration of milk in the water will depend on the rate of the water flow. If the stream flows slowly, the concentration will be high and the water will become white, but if the stream flows swiftly, the milk will dilute fast. The degree of dilution of the white milk is an indication of the flow.

This is the principle used when determining the cardiac output with the **indicator dilution method**. Another similar method is **Fick's principle**. Both are indirect methods, in that they are based on calculating a mean blood flow over a period of many heartbeats.

Indicator dilution method

An indicator whose concentration can be measured easily is injected into the blood stream. This is most often done through a catheter placed in the right atrium. The concentration in the pulmonary arterial blood is measured during the period after the injection. The lower the concentration, the higher the flow. The cardiac output is derived by a simple calculation, Box 6:2.

If dyes or electrolytes are used as indicators, the measurements cannot be repeated too often, as these tend to accumulate in the blood. It is therefore more beneficial to use cold, which is called **thermodilution**. A cold saline solution is injected, such as 10 ml at a temperature of 0°C, and the decrease in temperature downstream after dilution in the blood is measured. The smaller the temperature decrease, the higher the cardiac output.

The advantage of the thermodilution method is that the indicator quickly disappears, thanks to the temperature equilibration that takes place when blood flows through the tissues. The method has been widely used for physiological measurements during cardiac investigation, during surgery, and for monitoring during intensive care.

The method does, however, have the disadvantage of being invasive. Efforts are being made at replacing such invasive flow measurement methods with ultrasound.

Fick's principle

The patient inhales oxygen from a bag containing a known volume for a certain amount of time, and the oxygen uptake per minute is calculated.

 Techniques · Box 6:2

Calculation of blood flow

In the **indicator dilution method**, the flow Q is given by dividing the quantity of injected indicator A by the average of the varying concentration C times the measurement time t:

$$Q = \frac{A}{\text{area under } C.t \text{ curve}}$$

As per **Fick's principle**, the flow Q is derived from the quantity of the measured substance uptake V per unit of time. For thermodilution we divide the cold content of the injectate by the area under the temperature versus time waveform. When oxygen is consumed by the lung, we divide millilitres of oxygen per minute by the arterio-venous concentration difference $C_a - C_v$:

$$Q = \frac{V}{C_a - C_v}$$

The difference in oxygen concentration between the venous and the arterial blood is determined – this is the **arterial–venous oxygen concentration difference**. The cardiac output is obtained by dividing the oxygen uptake by the arterial–venous oxygen concentration difference. The higher the oxygen uptake and the lower the arterial–venous oxygen difference, the greater the cardiac output, Box 6:2.

Fick's principle for determining the cardiac output with oxygen as the indicator is regarded as the best method, and is the reference for other methods. One disadvantage with this method is, as commonly applied, that the patient must undergo cardiac catheterization to obtain mixed venous blood.

Peripheral circulation

There is no simple, general method for measuring the peripheral circulation, and the techniques therefore have to be adapted to the special problem being investigated. Different methods are generally used for measurements in **arteries, capillaries** and veins. It is often only possible to arrive at a qualitative assessment of the flow, since quantitative measurement may actually be impossible to carry out.

Arterial blood flow

When arteriosclerotic changes are suspected, the arterial blood flow needs to be measured so that the degree of dysfunction and the exact location of the stenoses are known before any surgical treatment.

The best way to obtain information about the state of the arterial system is to take an X-ray, an **arteriogram** (Chapter 7). The contrast agent is injected proximally and images obtained as the contrast agent goes by, which yields very detailed images of the stenoses and anomalies. The disadvantage is that an arterial puncture must be done, and that the method requires expensive equipment, as well as access to a radiologist.

It is much simpler to use **Doppler ultrasound** to measure the flow. A high-frequency ultrasound beam, for example, 1 MHz (1,000,000 Hz), is directed towards the blood vessel, Figure 6:13. The ultrasound is reflected by the blood cells and is then captured by a receiver. During the reflection, the frequency is slightly changed, in the same way as sound from a passing ambulance has a higher tone when it is approaching than when it is going away. If the blood flow is directed towards the ultrasound receiver, the reflected sound thus has a slightly higher frequency, 1,000,500 Hz. An electronic circuit generates a signal that has a frequency equal to the difference between the transmitted and reflected signals. This results in a 500 Hz signal, which is within the audible range. Just using our own hearing, it is possible to gain a very good assessment of the flow. The instrument, which can be as small as a pen, is very easy to use. The instrument can also be shaped like a stethoscope, Figure 6:4.

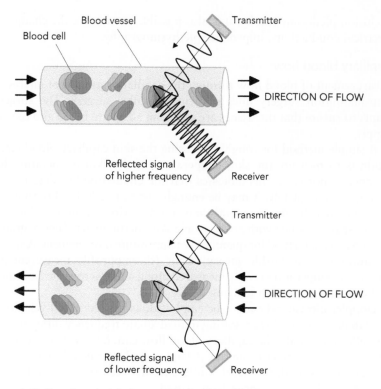

Figure 6:13 Doppler principle for measuring of blood flow

Doppler ultrasound is often used for fetal monitoring, and it is easy to differentiate between the maternal and fetal blood flow signals thanks to the different heart rates.

Flow measurements with ultrasound have low accuracy. The reason is that the flow profile (the flow rate variation over the cross-section of the vessel), and the ultrasound direction relative to the axis of the blood vessel, affect the values obtained.

Another qualitative method that has been used for many years is **oscillometry**, where the pulse synchronous volume changes in an extremity are measured. A cuff similar to a blood pressure cuff (see Figure 6:7) is placed around the extremity and the volume changes observed at different cuff pressures. Oscillometry is thus an objective method of measuring what is subjectively assessed when palpating the pulse.

Plethysmography is a similar method, where rapid changes in an extremity are measured after sudden stopping of the venous circulation. The venous occlusion is achieved by placing a blood-pressure cuff proximally around the extremity and inflating it so that only the arterial blood may pass. Immediately thereafter, measurements are made of the extremity volume or circumference increase over time, and this is known as **venous**

occlusion plethysmography. It is also possible to measure the changes in electrical conductivity, impedance plethysmography.

Capillary blood flow

Measurement of blood flow through the capillary system is of interest in transplantation surgery and following vascular surgery. The surgeon wants to ensure that the tissues are receiving adequate blood and oxygen supply.

A simple method for roughly assessing the skin capillary blood circulation is to measure the skin temperature. If the skin temperature has dropped abnormally, this indicates that the circulation has deteriorated or stopped completely. It may be enough just to touch the skin to determine whether the skin temperature is normal. More accurate values can of course be obtained with an electronic skin thermometer. Thermography (Chapter 7) is a method for quantitative temperature measurement. A special variation is heat profile measurement (thermoprofile measurement), where the temperature is only measured along a line across the extremity, and does not require an imaging device.

Doppler ultrasound cannot be employed, as the blood cell velocity in the capillaries is too low, resulting in inadequate frequency differences in the reflected sound. The capillary blood flow can, however, be measured with the laser Doppler technique (Chapter 7). The principle is similar to Doppler ultrasound, that is, the difference between the transmitted and the received light frequencies is measured.

Veins

Measuring the venous blood flow is important in the case of venous thrombosis, especially in the lower legs. The surest method is to perform a phlebography, an X-ray investigation following injection of contrast distally to the diseased section of the vein. But this method is uncomfortable for the patient, cumbersome to execute and sometimes the foot is so swollen that it is impossible to find an accessible blood vessel for the injection.

With thermography, or even simpler by thermoprofile measurement, the temperature difference between the two legs can be determined, which can be useful when a deep venous thrombosis is suspected (Chapter 7, Figure 7:17). The venous return flow is forced through more superficial veins, raising the temperature in the diseased leg.

Scintigraphy involves injecting a radioactive element (such as technetium), which chemically binds to a carrier absorbed by a blood clot. The resulting radioactivity in the clot can be measured with a gamma camera (Chapter 7).

ELECTROPHYSIOLOGY

When muscle fibres contract and nerve cells are excited, ions are displaced across the cell membranes. This results in action potentials and electric currents being conducted to the surrounding tissues. These potentials can be recorded by electrodes placed on the skin or inserted into the body.

Several important methods are based on such measurements. **Electrocardiography (ECG)** is by far the most important. Other examples are **electroencephalography (EEG), electromyography (EMG)** and **motor conduction velocity (MCV)**. For all these methods, it is important for the electrodes to be applied to the skin with great care. Electrical interference from the patient or the environment must also be avoided. These types of problems are discussed below, along with some of the important things to remember when taking an ECG – the same principles apply to all types of electrophysiological measurements.

Electrocardiography

The cardiac muscle fibres are bundled in a similar fashion in all people. As a result, action potentials from all muscle fibres in all individuals are added together in the same fashion and conducted to the skin, where they cause similar variations in electric voltages in all individuals. The potentials change rapidly during each heartbeat and they vary depending where on the body they are measured. The amplitude is about 1 mV.

During ECG recordings, muscular activity may generate electric potentials that are superimposed on the ECG signal. The patient must therefore remain as still and relaxed as possible. Sometimes a **stress ECG** is done, where the patient performs physical exercise on a stationary bike or treadmill, and computer signal processing is then used to minimize the muscle interference. Electrical interference, which is sometimes unavoidable when ECGs are recorded at the bedside, can to some extent be eliminated by connecting an electric filter. But this has the effect of flattening the curve, and as a result the finer signal details may not be observable.

ECG leads

The electrodes are attached to the extremities, Figure 6:14, and to the chest, Figure 6:15. Normally 12 separate leads are recorded. The three original leads are the **bipolar extremity leads,** which measure the voltage between both arms, between the right arm and left leg, and between the left arm and left leg respectively. From these three leads, the three **augmented unipolar extremity leads** are derived, via an electrical calculation of the voltage between each electrode and the mean voltage of the two other electrodes. Finally, the voltages from six **chest leads** are recorded.

Electrode technology

The electrodes, which may be disposable or reusable, must be in good electrical contact with the skin. An electrically conducting gel is used as a conduction medium. In some single-use electrodes, the electrode gel is pre-applied in a thin foam disc. This is a pre-gelled electrode, which is

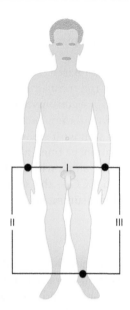

Figure 6:14 Standard ECG leads

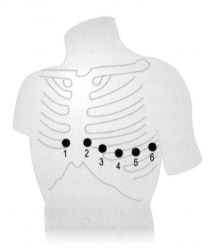

Figure 6:15 Chest leads

held in place by a self-adhesive outer ring. Reusable electrodes are often attached with suction, which simplifies the investigation, especially when many chest electrodes are used.

Mechanical movements in the skin or between the electrode gel and the metal electrode can cause undesired electric voltages, or **artefacts**.

Electrical interference is transmitted from the power lines in various ways. **Capacitive interference** can be reduced in two ways. First of all, cables from the electric wall outlets must be kept away from the patient and the electrode cables. The cables should be separated by a distance of at least 1.5 m. Secondly, such interference can be reduced by ensuring optimal electrode-to-skin contact. Removing all oil from the skin, abrading and removing the uppermost corneal layer of the epidermis, and moistening the skin with electrode gel achieve this.

Inductive interference can be diminished by keeping all the electrode cables bundled together, Figure 6:16. Heating pads and other nonessential electric devices can be removed, and fluorescent lights switched off when it is essential to minimize all interfering electric fields.

ECG recording devices

Various methods are used for ECG recording. The most common are **Electrocardiographs**, often referred to as **ECG Machines**, which print out a paper strip with several leads recorded from different sites on the body. During surgery and in intensive care it is more practical to show the ECG on an ECG monitor, a special monitor where the waveforms are continuously displayed.

Many cardiac arrhythmias occur only sporadically, and in such cases storing the ECG on a small portable recorder can be helpful. The ECG signals, or at least the interesting parts of the signals, are recorded and stored during a period of 24 hours. The entire recording is then scanned and interpreted using a special analyser. This method is called the **Holter technique** after its inventor.

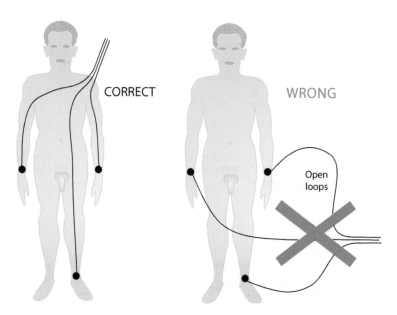

Figure 6:16 During electrophysiological measurements the electrode cables must be kept close together

ECG waveforms

ECG recordings are primarily used to check if the **cardiac rhythm** is normal or abnormal, if the **oxygen supply** to the **cardiac muscle** is sufficient and whether any part of the cardiac muscle is damaged, for example, due to an **infarction**. These three areas of application are all based on analysing the ECG waveform.

Figure 6:17 shows a normal ECG complex. It also shows an example of interference at the power-line frequency from the power line, and the improvement achieved when using a filter. Interference is also often caused by muscle activity, producing muscle artefacts, which produce an even noisier signal – these can also be partially suppressed by using a filter.

In the electrocardiogram, the P-wave (atrial depolarization) corresponds to atrial contraction, the QRS complex (ventricular depolarization) to ventricular contraction and the T-wave (repolarization) following the end of the ventricular contraction. Since it is possible to distinguish between the atrial and the ventricular contraction, it is easy to detect rhythm disturbances, such as when ventricular contractions do not occur after a normal delay (corresponding to the time required for the depolarization to travel from the atrium to the ventricle). If this **conduction time** is prolonged, when the P–Q interval is longer than the upper normal limit of 0.22 s, then the patient has **first-degree heart block**, Figure 6:17. If some atrial impulses are not conducted to the ventricle, then there is **second-**

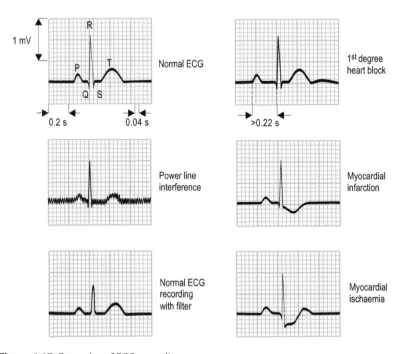

Figure 6:17 Examples of ECG recordings

degree heart block, and when no atrial impulses get through to the ventricles, resulting in the atria and ventricles beating entirely independently of each other, the condition is called **complete heart block.** Heart block can be treated with a pacemaker.

When the oxygen supply to the myocardium is compromised due to coronary insufficiency, typical changes called **ST segment depression** are seen in the ECG waveforms, Figure 6:17.

The shape of the ECG waveform during a myocardial infarction is entirely dependent on where in the heart muscle the infarction is located. When the infarction is located in the posterior wall of the heart there are sometimes no visible ECG changes. Figure 6:17 shows typical changes after an acute myocardial infarction.

The sensitivity of the heart to electric shocks varies during the cardiac cycle. The greatest risk of inducing a ventricular fibrillation is when the current goes through the heart during the **vulnerable interval** (Latin: *vulnus* = wound). This interval occurs during the T-wave.

Computerized ECG analysis

Electronic circuits that can trigger an alarm in the event of ventricular fibrillation have existed for a long time. These became necessary when continuous monitoring was introduced in intensive care units, as it was impossible to observe continuously the ECG display. The technology can be used for **arrhythmia detection,** for example, to trigger an alarm in the event of such ventricular rhythms that may lead to fibrillation. Another important function is **trend analysis,** measuring changes in a patient's condition, such as an increased number of ventricular extrasystoles. Computers are also used for **averaging** of several ECG waveforms in order to reduce the effects of muscle artefact when recording a stress ECG.

Modern ECG machines even produce a suggested medical diagnosis. The diagnoses are on average more accurate than those made by a doctor without specialization in cardiology or clinical physiology. In doubtful cases, some degree of overdiagnosis can be employed on purpose with some false-positive diagnoses allowed. This can be preferable to having false negatives for clinically important conditions, and actually failing to identify a patient requiring treatment. However, not all conditions are diagnosed error-free. Arrhythmias must be evaluated by a cardiologist, and electrical interference can cause the machine to incorrectly report that the patient has a pacemaker.

Electroencephalography

The electroencephalogram (EEG) records electric signals from the brain by means of an array of 21 surface electrodes, Figure 6:18. The electrodes are held together with elastic straps and placed on the head like a cap. The technical problems are similar to the ones discussed in the section on ECG. But an even better methodology is required, since the amplitude of

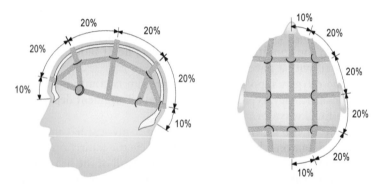

Figure 6:18 EEG electrode placement

the signals is just a tenth of the ECG signal, approximately 100 μV. Frequencies range from less than 1 Hz to 50 Hz. The EEG record is a sensitive indicator of the degree of alertness and is used to measure changes in the degree of alertness during natural sleep or in the case of brain disease.

Diagnosing epilepsy is another important application. Milder forms of epileptic attacks can only be diagnosed by the demonstration of typical EEG changes. These can occur sporadically, but may also be triggered by hyperventilation, light and sleep. When epilepsy is suspected, the patient may therefore be asked to hyperventilate or be subjected to short light flashes, or be requested to come to the test without having slept the previous night.

A similar method used for investigating pathways to the central nervous system is **evoked potentials (EP)**. When examining the visual sense, the patient is asked to look at a checkerboard pattern, and is stimulated by alternating the black and white fields. The signals are recorded between two electrodes, one of which is placed on the forehead and the other over the visual cortex at the back of the head, Figure 6:19. In multiple sclerosis, the signals are delayed due to diseased conducting pathways in the optic nerve. Auditory evoked potentials are also utilized, for objective assessments of hearing defects. Here, sound of different frequencies is used as the stimulus.

Magnetic encephalography is a development of the EEG methodology. Instead of measuring the electric potentials with electrodes, the very weak magnetic fields that are generated around the electric currents of the brain are measured without wires. The device involved is very complicated – it requires specially designed, shielded rooms and cooling of the detectors to -269°C in liquid helium. Few hospitals have such devices. With this method, a more precise localization of functional defects in the brain can be obtained, such as in preparation for surgical or radiation treatment of epilepsy.

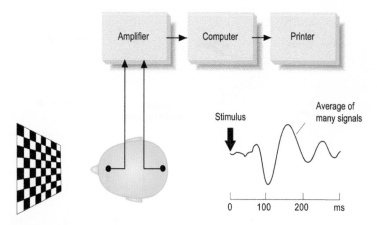

Figure 6:19 Example of evoked potentials in investigation of optical conducting pathways

Electromyography

In EMG, the degree of activity in skeletal muscles can be measured via skin electrodes. The method is often used to record signals from single motor units, that is, groups of muscle cells that are activated simultaneously via one single nerve cell in the spinal cord. This is done by inserting thin needle electrodes into the muscle, Figure 6:20. In addition to the printer recording, it is helpful also to connect a loudspeaker, so that the needle position during insertion may be tracked by listening to the captured signals.

The recorded action potentials, which thus represent the motor unit, have a repetition frequency of up to 50 Hz, an amplitude of 50 µV to 2 mV, and a duration of 2 to 10 ms.

EMG plays a central part in the investigations of neuromuscular diseases, for example, in order to determine whether the nerves to the muscle are damaged. If this is indeed the case, certain motor units will be absent while others function normally, provided the nerve is not completely damaged. If the disease is instead located in the muscles and certain muscle fibres are nonfunctional, the action potential waveforms will be split. In myasthenia gravis, the action potentials diminish during muscle contraction, and this is caused by the depletion of the synapses between the nerve and muscle cell. The process can be tracked with **single-fibre electromyography** (**SFEMG**), where very thin electrodes with a very small contact area are used to record the activity from individual muscle fibres.

Motor conduction velocity

To treat a traumatic nerve injury, the exact location of the injury must be identified. This can be done by measuring the **motor conduction velocity** (**MCV**) of motor nerves. The nerve is stimulated with a brief electric

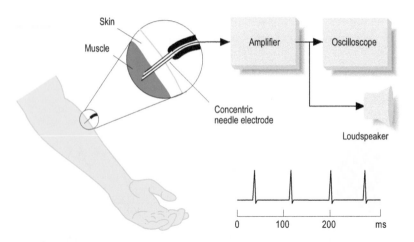

Figure 6:20 Electromyography

shock via an electrode placed on the skin above the nerve, Figure 6:21. The stimulus produces impulses in the nerve fibres and when the impulses reach the muscle, it contracts with a quick jerk. The muscle action potential is recorded together with the stimulating impulse.

The time delay, or **latency** between the stimulation and the muscle action potential, consists of the time needed for the nerve impulse propagation, and for the conduction of the impulse to the muscle.

To measure just the nerve conduction velocity in a nerve section with suspected injury, the latency after stimulation on two points of the section is recorded. The conduction velocity of the section can then be derived from the ratio of the distance between the stimulation points divided by the difference in latency. In Figure 6:21 the distance is 310 - 60 = 250 mm and the difference in latency is 9 - 4 = 5 ms, which yields a conduction velocity of 50 m/s.

INTENSIVE CARE MONITORING

Intensive care is based largely on our capacity to follow continuously the patient's condition and obtain an overview of how the condition changes over time. Such observation is often called **monitoring,** and the display unit on which the data are presented is called a **monitor.** The monitor is often connected to a central computer. The data are measured with various types of **sensors (transducers)**, which are attached to the patient. One example is the electronic blood pressure sensor in Figure 6:11, which must be connected to some device that can display the blood pressure. Nowadays, this is usually achieved by a computer that compiles data from several measurements and produces a blood pressure curve for display on a monitor (Chapter 12). An ECG is often recorded at the same time.

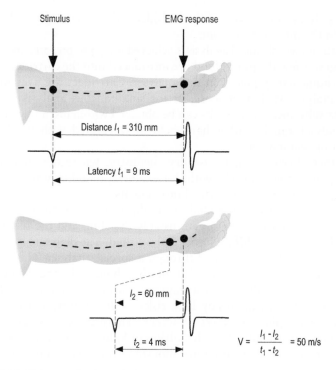

Figure 6:21 Motor conduction velocity

Sensors and analytical instruments

A medical sensor is a device that produces an electric signal that can be measured when it is placed on or inside a patient. Sensors can be **invasive** or **noninvasive**. Sometimes the term **minimally invasive** is also used, to emphasize the importance of avoiding subjecting the patient to unnecessarily extensive procedures. One example of such a sensor is a **temperature sensor,** which, when inserted into a body opening (such as the mouth or rectum) produces an electric current that is proportional to the patient's body temperature. On the other hand, a **pressure sensor,** which is inserted into a blood vessel for measuring the venous pressure, is invasive. Some of the most common sensors used in intensive care have already been described, and others will be described in the following chapters.

Chemical analyses form an important part of intensive care. Among the parameters measured are blood gases, oxygen and carbon dioxide, as well as the blood pH. They provide immediate information about the patient's respiratory status. Information regarding other ions, such as potassium, calcium and sodium, is also important. Such analyses can be done in several different ways. Previously, blood samples were collected and sent to the hospital clinical laboratory for standard **wet chemistry** analyses, and the results were sent back to the ward after some time. Nowadays, many analyses can be done at the bedside, with special analytical instruments in the intensive care unit.

Sometimes wet chemical analysis is achieved using pre-prepared **measuring cartridges**. A few drops of blood are introduced into the cartridge, which is then immediately placed in the analyser. Cartridges are available for single analysis, such as glucose, or for simultaneous analysis of many different substances. The results can be obtained within just a few minutes. The analyser can be either hand-held or integrated with the bedside monitoring equipment.

Another alternative is to use **dry chemistry**, where the analyses are done by preparing dipsticks with, for example, blood or urine and then reading them in special analytical instruments.

A third possibility is **microdialysis**. In this method, an "artificial blood vessel" is inserted into the organ, usually the skin, and the tissue fluid molecules allowed to diffuse into a dialysis fluid. The dialysate is pumped through a circuit that is routed through a special analyser. This method yields a continuous measurement of the changes in the tissue fluid composition. Microdialysis is a minimally invasive method, as it does not subject the patient to any high risks or discomfort, and it enables continuous sampling for days or weeks. The method is sometimes of value in the care of patients with diabetes or kidney failure, and following plastic surgery for monitoring metabolism in transplanted tissues.

Monitored functions

Various methods are combined, depending on existing needs. After a heart attack, for example, in addition to ECG monitoring it is also important to monitor the blood oxygen saturation, which is conveniently done with a pulse oximeter (Chapter 8). More accurate determinations can be made by measuring the blood gases. Blood pressure can be monitored continuously with automated blood-pressure devices.

Table 6:1 lists some of the most common monitored functions. Intensive care is used in various conditions, for example:

- Heart failure, most often due to myocardial infarction.

- Postoperative care of high-risk patients, such as post-cardiac surgery patients, and neonates in respiratory distress.

- Patients with multiple traumas, e.g. traffic accident victims.

- Newborn infants with respiratory distress syndrome.

- Suicide attempts with brain drug effects.

Monitors and entire intensive care equipment are now so miniaturized that they can comfortably be transported on the patient's bed during patient transport. It is also possible to reconnect the equipment to the ward or

Table 6:1   Examples of commonly registered parameters in intensive care

Function	Measured parameters	Instrument
Circulation	Oxygen saturation, Pulse rate	Pulse oximeter
	Blood pressure	Blood pressure cuff
		Intravascular catheter
	Cardiac electrical activity	ECG machine
	Blood flow	Ultrasound machine
Respiration	Oxygen saturation, Pulse rate	Pulse oximetry
	End tidal carbon dioxide	Capnograph
	Respiration frequency	Impedance plethysmograph
	Lactate level in blood	Wet chemistry analyzer
Renal function	Urine volume	Volume meter
	Serum creatinine, Serum urea	Wet chemistry analyzer
Brain function	Consciousness	Clinical observation
	EEG, Evoked potentials	EEG equipment

hospital network (Chapter 12) after transport is completed, for central collection of the data.

FETAL MONITORING

During labour, the baby runs a certain risk of **asphyxia**, or oxygen shortage. One possible cause may, for example, be umbilical cord constriction with resulting obstruction of blood flow. The purpose of monitoring is to be able to detect any asphyxia early so that the delivery can be speeded up or completed by emergency caesarean section or vacuum extraction.

Immediately after delivery, the baby's condition can be rated by calculating an **Apgar score**. Points are awarded for skin colour, muscle tone, excitability, breathing and pulse rate. The score assumes a maximum value of 10 if the child is in perfect condition, and lower values at different degrees of reduced vitality, which can be due not only to ongoing asphyxia, but also to asphyxia that occurred earlier.

Of course, direct measurements cannot be obtained until the foetal membranes have ruptured and a blood sample has been taken. Before that, the only possibility is for indirect evaluation. Normally the **fetal heart rate (FHR)** is recorded – it should display characteristic changes following each uterine contraction. This monitoring can be carried out by a midwife listening to the heart beats with a stethoscope, or with the help of electronic devices.

Electronic monitoring of the fetal heart rate and the uterine contractions is performed using **cardiotocography**. In cases where the mother does not wish the baby to be exposed to ultrasound during delivery (there is general agreement that ultrasound is not harmful) the foetal heart rate can instead be obtained by recording a **fetal ECG**. A **scalp blood sample** can be taken for direct determination of the blood pH, lactate value and oxygen saturation; a more gentle method is to use a special **pulse oximeter.** Combining cardiotocography with telemetry has a great advantage, in that it enables the mother to walk and move around freely during the labour.

Cardiotocography

A cardiotocograph (Greek: *tokos* = childbirth) or **CTG machine,** consists of at least two parts, one for measuring the foetal heart rate with **Doppler ultrasound** and one for measuring the **uterine contractions.**

Doppler ultrasound

Earlier we described how Doppler ultrasound can be used to measure blood flow and cardiac movement. In CTG, the ultrasound transducer is placed on the mother's abdomen and echoes are received primarily from the baby, Figure 6:22. The frequency used is 1 to 2 MHz and the sound intensity only reaches a few mW/cm^2, which is a very weak level. The change in the frequency of the reflected ultrasound is a measure of all the movements of the tissue parts that reflect the beam.

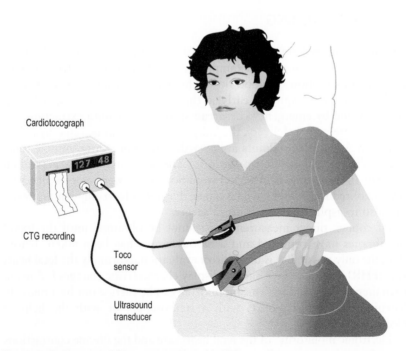

Cardiotocograph

CTG recording

Toco sensor

Ultrasound transducer

Figure 6:22 Electronic labour monitoring with CTG

Through advanced microprocessor signal processing, it is normally possible to measure the fetal heart rate, which is printed out and compared with the uterine contractions.

Fetal ECG

An alternative method for measuring the baby's heart rate is through a fetal ECG recording, where an electrode is placed on the baby's scalp, which can be done when the membranes have ruptured. Such an electrode has one or two spiral-formed, corkscrew-like metallic fasteners that are screwed superficially into the baby's scalp.

The appropriateness of attaching such a scalp electrode to the baby without anaesthesia has been questioned – the baby feels pain, as the heart rate increases dramatically during the attachment.

In addition to the fetal heart rate, some indication of possible asphyxia can also be obtained from the fetal ECG through demonstration of ST segment depression.

Measuring the uterine contractions

During labour, the muscle tissue contracts causing a pressure increase in the uterus. This can be felt by placing a hand on the mother's abdomen; during a contraction the abdominal wall cannot be pushed inwards with a finger as easily as between contractions, when the uterus is relaxed.

A tocograph works in the same fashion. A box with a spring-loaded piston is tightly fitted around the stomach with a belt, Figure 6:23. Between contractions, the piston pushes somewhat into the abdominal wall as the uterus is soft, and then retracts back into the box when the uterus hardens during a contraction. This is normally how each contraction is recorded on the CTG printer along with the fetal heart rate.

A more accurate measurement of labour contractions is obtained by measuring the intrauterine pressure (IUP). This can be done once the foetal membranes have ruptured, by inserting a liquid-filled catheter connected to an external pressure sensor into the uterus. There are even miniaturized sensors that can be directly inserted into the uterus.

CTG Interpretation

The fetal heart rate should normally be between 120 and 160 beats per minute. The rate should vary in a typical fashion, with some acceleration

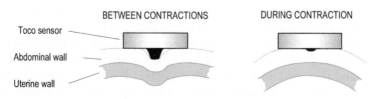

Figure 6:23 Sensor for registration of uterine contractions

immediately after the beginning of a contraction and a deceleration following the contraction. The absence of such typical variations is called a **silent pattern**, and may be an indication that the fetus is receiving too little oxygen, and has asphyxia. A high increase in fetal heart rate can also indicate this condition. Interpreting CTG recordings requires extensive experience as well as knowledge of neonatal physiology.

Scalp blood samples and pulse oximetry

During asphyxia, the blood pH decreases and the lactate level increases. A measurement of pH or lactate on a capillary blood sample taken from the baby's scalp can give an accurate indication of the baby's condition.

The oxygen saturation can also be determined in a blood sample taken from the baby's scalp. But such blood samples provide only information on the baby's condition at the time when the sample was taken. Continuous monitoring can be achieved using **pulse oximetry**. The sensor is especially designed to be placed between the uterine wall and the baby's scalp. This method has the added advantage of not subjecting the baby to the stress experienced when scalp blood samples are taken.

Telemetry monitoring

In standard CTG monitoring, the mother is forced to stay in bed because of the cables attached to the monitoring equipment. This means that she is essentially strapped to the bed or delivery table. The supine position prolongs the labour and makes it more difficult, and also increases the risk of vena cava compression, which reduces blood flow through the uterus and other organs.

Wireless transmission of the measurements to a receiver in the delivery ward enables the mother to walk and move around freely, Figure 6:24. She can also assume positions that are tolerated best. The labour is facilitated, as the increased gravity increases the pressure exerted by the fetus on the birth canal and thus promotes the dilatation of the canal. In one study, it was found that labour became on average three hours shorter, the need for analgesia was cut in half and when analgesia was given, the doses could be reduced. The need for assisted delivery of the baby by vacuum or forceps was also reduced.

The value of labour monitoring

Several studies have shown that there is no statistical evidence that electronic monitoring is superior to monitoring with a stethoscope. The reason could be that although asphyxia can be detected earlier, this does not counterbalance other disadvantages. In one international study, it was thus found that the number of stillborn babies because of asphyxia had possibly decreased, but that an increased number of babies had died due to mechanical trauma in connection with forceps deliveries.

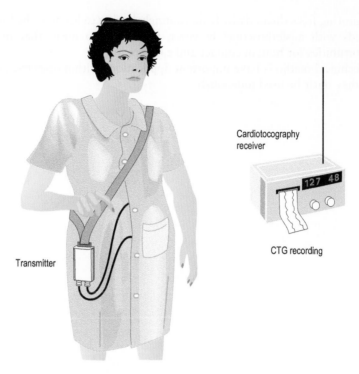

Cardiotocography receiver

127 48

CTG recording

Transmitter

Figure 6:24 Telemetric labour monitoring

CASE 6:5 Fatal error in fetal monitoring

A fetal monitor using an ultrasound transducer showed an apparently normal foetal heart beat. But when the infant was delivered, it was stillborn.

Analysis of the CTG trace showed that the monitor had locked onto the mother's heart beat. A confidential enquiry into similar incidents identified that midwives and medical staff lacked knowledge and training in the interpretation of CTG recordings.

The use of technical methods to monitor labour is therefore somewhat controversial. One disadvantage of electronic monitoring is that the numbers of caesarean sections and instrument-aided deliveries have increased due to CTG data having been misinterpreted.

Most mothers do, however, perceive electronic monitoring as an added security, as the CTG graphs clearly show that the baby is alive. Other mothers worry that the scalp electrode may hurt the baby. Electronic monitoring frees the midwife from routinely having to listen to the foetal sounds with a stethoscope; however, this can also mean that many opportunities for human contact and care are lost.

Technical methods have important applications within obstetric care, but they must be used judiciously.

7

Medical images

Human vision is highly developed. We are able to distinguish between faces without necessarily being able to verbally describe the differences in the features, and without knowing how visual impressions are actually being processed. We can instantly distinguish a donkey from a horse, even if all we see is the head of one and the tail of the other. A computer cannot be programmed to perform the same feat, and still cannot replace the radiologist.

The visual sense, however, has certain limitations that can be compensated for by various technical methods. Cavities that would otherwise be inaccessible may be visually inspected and internal organs operated on via an **endoscope**. Lesions in the organs that cannot be directly examined can sometimes be visualized by **special optical methods**. The technologies of **X-ray** and **nuclear medicine** employ electromagnetic radiation outside the visual spectrum, and thus offer even further possibilities. A highly advanced method is **magnetic resonance imaging**, which uses strong magnetic fields and radio waves. **Ultrasound imaging** utilizes the differences in the physical properties of tissues.

Types of images

Medical images are produced in two principally different ways: by **central projection** and **tomography**.

Central projection images
The eye receives information by the image being directly projected onto the retina. An ordinary X-ray image is produced in the same fashion – a

shadow of the organs is projected onto the image plane from a centre, which is the focal spot of the X-ray tube, Figure 7:1.

Central projection nearly always gives a distorted image of reality due to the effects of distance. The farther away the item, the smaller is its projection on the retina. The same type of image distortion occurs in an endoscope. On an ordinary X-ray image, the corresponding distortion results in the organs **closer to the X-ray tube** appearing **larger** (not smaller) than the organs that are closer to the imaging plane, which can be a film, an image intensifier or an image detector.

Centrally projected images are produced by **photography** (visual light), **endoscopy, thermography** and **standard X-ray imaging.**

Tomography

In the various forms for tomography (Greek: *tomos* = section), sections of the body may be viewed as if the body had been sliced apart into two sections, and the cross-sectional areas viewed, Figure 7:2. Such images can be generated by X-rays in **computer tomography (CT)**, in **magnetic resonance imaging (MRI)**, in the **imaging methods of nuclear medicine (scintigraphy)** and in **ultrasound tomography**. The way these tomographic images are produced varies from method to method, but all are based on advanced computer processing.

ENDOSCOPY

The interior of body cavities can be visualized with endoscopes. The method is widely applied, both as a purely diagnostic tool and for different surgical procedures with instruments that are introduced via

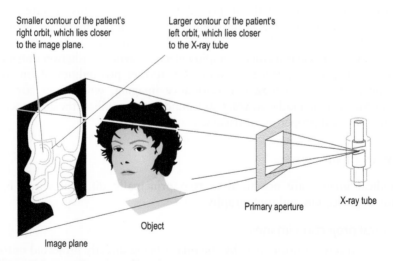

Figure 7:1 Centrally projected X-ray image

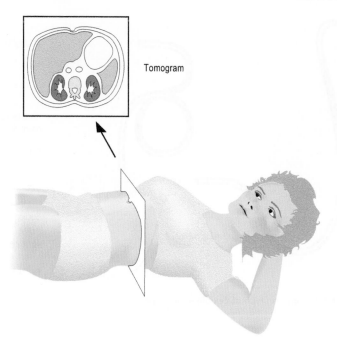

Tomogram

Figure 7:2 Tomographic image

the endoscope working channels. Such instruments are, for example, **brushes** to scrape up cells for microscopic examinations (brush biopsy), **forceps** also for tissue sampling, **wire snares** for removal of polyps, electrodes for **surgical diathermy** for achieving haemostasis and removing tumours, and **fibre optics** for directing laser-light treatment of tumours. Endoscopes are mostly flexible and the tip may be oriented in various directions so that the desired part of the cavity can be visualized.

Principle

An endoscope consists of three principal parts: a device that illuminates the cavity to be inspected, an optical system that transfers the image from the cavity interior, and a working channel, Figure 7:3. Nowadays, illumination is almost always done using an external cold light source, from which the light is transferred by means of flexible light fibres. Special types of endoscopes have been developed for various organs. The image may be transferred via ordinary lens systems or light fibres, or electronically in the form of a TV image, a video technique, Box 7:1.

There are **rigid** and **flexible** endoscopes. The flexible ones can be introduced far into the body, for example, all the way down to the small intestines.

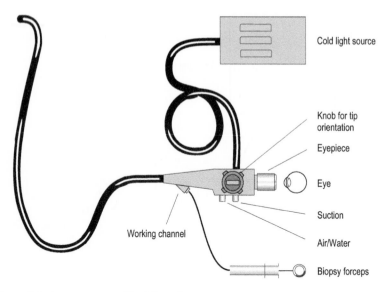

Cold light source

Knob for tip orientation

Eyepiece

Eye

Suction

Air/Water

Working channel

Biopsy forceps

Figure 7:3 Common type of flexible endoscope

![gear icon] Techniques • Box 7:1

Endoscope designs

Endoscopes originally consisted of straight, rigid tubes with simple lamps for illumination, and the same design is still valid today in, for example, laryngoscopes and rectoscopes. With the development of flexible instruments, endoscopy has become more widely applied. This development has occurred thanks to two technical innovations based on fibre optics and video technology.

Fibre endoscopy uses optical fibres both for illumination and image transmission. The illuminating fibres conduct the light from an external light source of high intensity to the inner tip of the endoscope. Two advantages are gained by the external light source: higher light intensity can be achieved than with just a small lamp placed at the inner end of the endoscope, and the heat emission can be reduced by placing special filters between the light source and the illumination fibre bundle.

The fibre bundle transmitting the image faithfully reproduces the image at the other end, as the position of each fibre at one end corresponds exactly to the position of the same fibre at the other end. This way, an image projected by a lens onto the optical fibre bundle inside the body can be seen at the external end of the bundle,

Techniques • Box 7:1—Continued

Figure 7:4. The number of fibres limits the optical resolution, that is, the picture becomes grainy, since each fibre is seen. But since the fibre diameter is only about 10 μm, there is room for many fibres, and good optical resolution can still be achieved.

Image transmission in the **video-endoscope** is based on the same principle as that of television, i.e., the image is broken up into a number of lines of varying intensity and colour. The picture is projected with a lens onto a small **charge-coupled device (CCD)** at the tip of the endoscope, and the CCD is then scanned electrically, producing a video signal that is transmitted to the monitor.

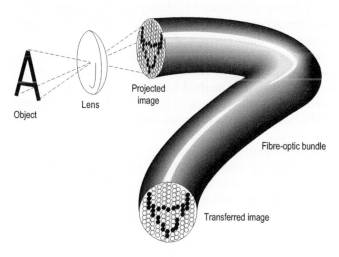

Figure 7:4 Principle of fibre-optic endoscopy

Use

Endoscopes have two major applications, **diagnostic procedures** and **endoscopic surgery**. The inspected body cavity is distended with gas (air or carbon dioxide) or fluids (water or saline or mannitol solutions) for enhanced visibility. The medium is selected based on the organ to be examined and taking into consideration the potential risk of gas embolism among other factors. Carbon dioxide is the preferred medium due to its high blood solubility, which enables a gas bubble to quickly disappear. Air bubbles dislodged in the capillaries, on the other hand, can result in a complete obstruction of blood flow potentially leading to infarction, for example, in the brain.

Gastrointestinal endoscopy

Gastroduodenoscopes, colonoscopes, sigmoidoscopes, rectoscopes and **proctoscopes** are the instruments most commonly used to investigate and treat the stomach and intestines. Inflammations, tumours and bleeding ulcers are common findings. Foreign bodies may also be retrieved and bleeding oesophageal varices treated.

The **mother–baby endoscope** has a special design. This instrument consists of a wide-calibre "mother" endoscope and an additional "baby" endoscope with a diameter of only about 5 mm. The baby endoscope may be introduced via the mother endoscope working channel, and used for examining the bile duct, for example. The baby endoscope working channel, which has a diameter of about 1.7 mm, enables the operator to introduce an instrument which electrically generates mechanical shock waves, capable of crushing stones obstructing the bile duct. The method is similar to lithotripsy (Chapter 11). This procedure requires the cooperation of two physicians – one operating the mother endoscope and the other operating the baby endoscope.

Gastroscopy is a relatively simple method, which is often preferred for the primary investigation in cases of vague symptoms from the upper gastrointestinal tract. The method has a high diagnostic sensitivity and has replaced X-ray investigations of the stomach and duodenum, which do not yield as unequivocal a diagnosis and in addition expose the patient to a certain amount of radiation.

A rectoscope consists of a straight, rigid tube, which can be introduced all the way up to the sigmoideum. For inspecting the entire colon, a flexible colonoscope is needed – this instrument resembles the gastroscope in its design in that the image is transmitted via fibre optics or video technology. These instruments are most often used to diagnose tumours or inflammatory processes.

Laparoscopy

In laparoscopy, it is the abdominal cavity that is examined. First, the cavity is filled with 2 to 4 litres of carbon dioxide, and then the laparoscope is inserted through a small incision above or just below the navel. Today, some surgical operations can be performed with endoscopic techniques.

Fetoscopy

For diagnosing certain hereditary diseases, the foetus may be examined through a fibre-optic fetoscope inserted through a small incision in the abdominal wall and the uterus. By puncturing an umbilical blood vessel, fetal blood samples may also be collected. The procedure is not risk free as it can lead to a miscarriage, and is avoided in early pregnancy. But the method makes it possible to diagnose several hereditary diseases that cannot be diagnosed as early by any other means.

Bronchoscopy

Bronchoscopy is performed in cases of suspected lung cancer and enables cytological samples to be taken with biopsy forceps or a brush inserted through the working channel. In infectious cases (pneumonia and bronchitis) there may also be an indication for performing bronchoscopy, for diagnostic sampling and evacuation of excess mucus. A foreign body stuck in the airways, such as a peanut, can also be removed with the aid of bronchoscopy.

The flexible design of the bronchoscope enables visualization of the bronchial tree down to its branches. The examination, which is relatively harmless for the patient, can be performed after administration of a local anaesthetic to the airways. This is also possible for intubated patients after insertion of a special type of cannula.

Cystoscopy

Cystoscopy is the common method for examining the urinary bladder for stones, tumours and inflammation, and for locating the source of bleeding in haematuria. A cystoscope also enables the insertion of catheters into the ureters and all the way up to the renal pelvis in order to fill these with contrast media in an investigation called **retrograde pyelography**. Removal of tissue from the prostate gland is achieved with a special endoscope called a **resectoscope**, which burns off slices of the prostate gland with an electrosurgical wire loop.

Arthroscopy

The interior of joints, most commonly the knee joint, can be examined through an arthroscope. Loose fragments can be retrieved, damaged cartilage on the patellae removed ("shaving"), adhesions removed and meniscal tears repaired. The procedure is performed either under general anaesthesia or with the joint region anaesthetized by injection of a local anaesthetic. The arthroscope is introduced through an opening lateral to the patellar tendon or in the suprapatellar bursa. Surgical instruments can be introduced through a second opening in what is called a second puncture technique.

Endoscopy in otolaryngology and ophthalmology

Until recently, the laryngoscope, otoscope and ophthalmoscope have been of relatively simple designs, as the target organs are easy to reach. But with the increasing demands for improved image quality the designs have become technically more advanced.

Endoscopic surgery

Conventional surgery can often be replaced by **endoscopic surgery**. This method is becoming more important, as it results in significantly shorter hospital stays. But the surgical procedure itself often lasts longer than for the same type of surgery performed in the conventional way.

The principle of abdominal endoscopic surgical procedures is illustrated in Figure 7:5. Several holes are made in the abdominal wall by means of a sharp instrument, a **trocar**, Figure 7:6, and an introducer sheath is left in place. This also functions as a gas seal, so that the abdominal cavity may be distended with gas, most often carbon dioxide. The endoscope and surgical instruments are introduced through the sheaths,

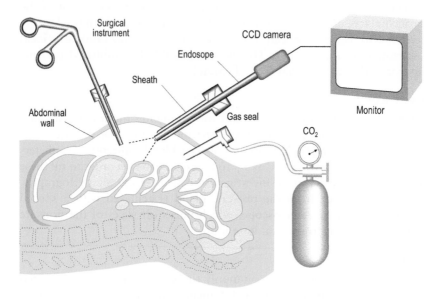

Figure 7:5 Principle outline for endoscopic surgery

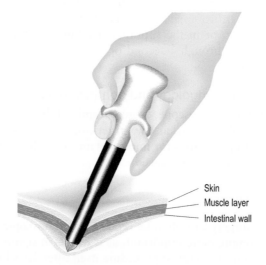

Figure 7:6 Trocar during insertion through abdominal wall

as well as other special devices as needed, such as ultrasound transducers for visualization of the organs from within the abdominal cavity.

Examples of common endoscopic operations are gall bladder surgery and various gynaecological procedures, such as ligation or coagulation of the fallopian tubes for contraceptive purposes, or retrieval of eggs for in vitro fertilization. Appendectomies and inguinal hernia repairs are also sometimes done endoscopically.

Other procedures, such as the removal of polyps, are performed in the gastrointestinal tract where the endoscope is introduced through the natural orifices of the mouth or the rectum.

Risks

For several reasons, there are greater risks associated with endoscopic surgery than with conventional surgery. It is much more difficult to understand the anatomy by observing a screen than when directly looking down into the open surgical field. Furthermore, the operator does not have an immediate tactile feel for the amount of force exerted on the organs, which can easily result in tissue damage. The risk is especially great if an artery is punctured with ensuing haemorrhage. The surgical teams must therefore be prepared for possible conversion to open surgery to immediately stop such haemorrhages.

There have been several fatal accidents in cases where such preparedness was not at hand.

CASE 7:1 Woman dies during surgery for hand sweat

A 37-year-old woman was undergoing a procedure called transthoracic sympathectomy for excessive palmar perspiration (hand sweat). An endoscope was introduced into the pleural cavity and the sympathetic nerves to the hand transected at the point where they pass through the thoracic wall at the level of the second, third and fourth rib.

During the procedure, a blood vessel was damaged with ensuing haemorrhage into the pleural cavity. Since the anaesthetist used the arm with the automatic blood pressure cuff for the infusion of blood and intravenous solutions, blood pressure could not be monitored during the infusion. The patient was placed in a recumbent position for half an hour, with no possibility for blood pressure monitoring during most of this time.

The woman was transferred to the intensive care unit, having contracted irreversible brain damage. Nine days later she was declared brain-dead.

Several serious errors had been made. The necessary skills and resources for performing open surgery had been missing. Using the same arm for both infusions and blood pressure measurements was entirely wrong, and made it impossible to monitor the blood pressure. When the haemorrhage occurred, the patient should have been placed in the head-down position, which would have increased the blood flow to the brain.

With appropriate planning and surgical competence even the worst scenarios need not be fatal:

CASE 7:2 Aorta punctured during laparoscopic surgery

A 53-year-old man was going to be operated on for an inguinal hernia. When the trocar was inserted the aorta was punctured. Blood immediately filled the abdominal cavity. The abdomen was opened by traditional surgery and the bleeding finally stopped after great difficulties. The blood loss amounted to about 10 litres, and the patient had to be given 4.5 litres of erythrocyte concentrate and 2.2 litres of plasma.

After the operation the patient developed a pneumothorax on the right side, which was discovered three days after the operation. The patient recovered completely.

The gas pressure is kept constant by means of an automatic insufflator, which compensates for gas losses during the procedure. It is vital that the correct gas is used. Oxygen during endoscopy should by all means be avoided since it involves a grave risk of explosive fire if surgical diathermy is used.

 Before initiating an endoscopic procedure, **always check the gas cylinder**. It must have a label specifying the correct content and that the gas is intended for medical use.

The insufflation of gas for facilitating visualization constitutes an ever-present danger of gas embolism, especially when carbon dioxide is not used:

CASE 7:3 Patient dies during cholecystectomy

During an endoscopic gall bladder operation, bleeding in the liver bed following the removal of the gall bladder was stopped with argon plasma coagulation (Chapter 11). Immediately following the coagulation, the patient developed symptoms of gas embolism, which was confirmed at autopsy.

But even carbon dioxide can pose a risk if large quantities are instilled, but quick action may save the patient:

CASE 7:4 No blood pressure for two minutes

A 60-year-old man was undergoing laparoscopic cholecystectomy. The insufflation pressure was set at 12 mmHg, and this level was not exceeded during the operation.

When over two-thirds of the gall bladder had been freed from the liver bed, venous bleeding occurred. The heart rate increased to 125/min and the blood pressure dropped to zero. A distinct murmur was auscultated over the heart, and could even be palpated on the chest surface. The insufflation was immediately stopped and the gas let out. The patient was placed in the head-down position and attempts were made at evacuating the gas by inserting a central venous catheter. But no bloody foam could be aspirated.

Laparotomy (abdominal incision) was immediately performed and the bleeding stopped by means of compression. The blood pressure was normalized and the patient suffered no sequelae from the incident.

A special risk associated with endoscopic procedures is the spread of tumour cells to the tissues surrounding the trocar port. For this reason, endoscopic surgery for malignant tumours is not recommended.

Other risks associated with endoscopic procedures are associated with the difficulty in sterilizing these instruments. It has been shown that the lubricant on movable mechanical components can contain bacteria and viruses that are not eliminated by standard sterilization media. Approved solutions for sterilization must be used – many instruments have been ruined because of incompatible solutions resulting in optical glass lenses falling out. This has even happened during operations. Endoscopic equipment is expensive, and must be carefully maintained.

Special optical methods

Soft tissues are somewhat translucent. A person's fingers placed in front of a light source will shine slightly red. The reason why the skeletal parts in the fingers cannot be seen is that the light is scattered in all directions. However, with special methods it is possible to produce images by transilluminating the tissues using visible light. This method is called **diaphanography**. It has been tried for diagnosing tumours of the breast, the scrotum and the neonate brain. Tumours give off darker shadows, as opposed to liquid-filled cysts, which appear bright, and fibroadenomas, which appear cherry red. The drawbacks in performing diaphanography with a simple light bulb are the difficulty in distinguishing tumours from haematomas and inflammation, as well as the poor resolution due to the light scattering, which results in blurred images.

The resolution can be enhanced greatly by intermittent transillumination, with very short bursts of laser light. Only the first pulses that emerge from the tissues are captured; the ones delayed by the criss-cross course from the light scattering are blocked. Another possibility is to collimate the light in the same fashion as in isotope studies (see below). None of these methods has yet found applications to any great extent, but they are of interest since they do not expose the patient to any potentially harmful radiation.

For special purposes, organ imaging may be undertaken by **scanning** along parallel lines. The image is compiled in a computer and presented on a monitor, in the same fashion as a TV image. The image is most often presented in colour, which yields more information.

Scanning often works with a wavelength range that cannot be captured by the human eye, such as heat radiation in **thermography**, Figure 7:19 in Box 7:6. Thermography has, for example, been used for detecting temperature abnormalities in Reynaud's disease and for diagnosing thrombi in the deep veins of the lower leg. When a thrombus is formed in the deep lower leg veins, the venous return is redirected through the superficial veins, which increases the skin temperature in the affected leg. A simpler method is **thermoprofile measurement** (Chapter 6) and it can have almost the same diagnostic accuracy. The exact thrombus location cannot be determined with thermography, since the method demonstrates only the redistribution of the blood flow in the leg.

Another similar method, the **laser Doppler technique**, measures the capillary blood flow, Box 7:6. The laser beam scans the tissue surface and measures the Doppler shift.

X-RAY DIAGNOSTICS

There are basically two different methods for examining a patient using X-rays: **radiography** and **fluoroscopy**. In radiography, Figure 7:1, the image, a radiogram, is obtained in the form of an exposed film or an image stored in a computer. Evaluation of the radiogram is done after being developed or from the stored image in the computer, and it can thereafter be archived. In fluoroscopy, the diagnostic evaluation of the patient is done using an image intensifier. The images are viewed directly on a screen, Figure 7:7. **Computer tomography** is a special type of radiographic investigation.

Radiography produces highly detailed images thanks to its superior geometrical resolution. The images can be evaluated at a later convenient time, without the need to expose the patient to additional doses of X-ray radiation. Most of the time, radiography exposes the patient to relatively small doses of radiation, with none to the examiner, who leaves the room during the exposure. Another advantage is the objective documentation of the patient's condition that is obtained, which can be compared with later findings during the course of the disease. A disadvantage with radiography is that the interpretation is complicated by the fact that the images of all organs in the radiation beam are superimposed on one another.

With **fluoroscopy**, an overview can quickly be obtained. The patient can be turned for optimal direction of the beam to project the various organs separate from one another. Organ movements can also be visualized and the position of catheters inserted into the organs can be adjusted. Fractures can be repositioned under fluoroscopic visualization

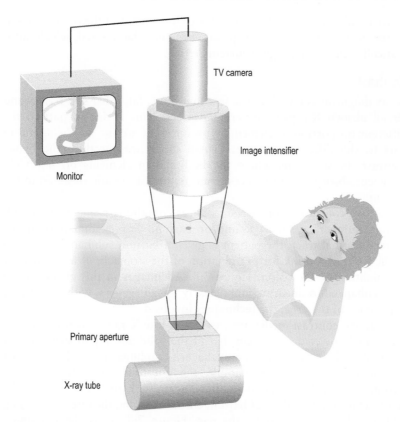

Figure 7:7 Fluoroscopy with image intensifier

with an image intensifier. A disadvantage with fluoroscopy is that unless the usage time is kept within limits, the patient may be exposed to considerably high doses of radiation. Fluoroscopy has become less distinct as a separate method with the development of computerized techniques allowing digital storage of images for later retrieval.

Principle

X-rays are generated when electrons are accelerated by a high voltage and decelerated in an anode, which most often consists of tungsten. The principle of the X-ray machine is quite simple. Two parameters are set: the **kilovoltage** (kV), which is the voltage for the X-ray tube, and the **mAs** value, which is the product of the current in milliamperes and the time in seconds. The exposure of the film increases rapidly with increasing voltage, and is directly proportional to the mAs setting. These values are adjusted based on the organ examined – the kilovoltage is set for optimal image contrast, and the mAs for appropriate film exposure.

To avoid blurring of the image due to movement of the organs caused by the heartbeats, a shorter exposure time may be selected, which automatically results in a higher current setting.

Contrast

X-ray diagnosis is based on the fact that bone, fat, other soft tissues and air all absorb X-rays to different degrees. This is due in part to the different proportion of elements with different atomic numbers, and in part to the different densities. These differences produce the image **contrast**. In situations where the body's own elements do not yield sufficient absorption differences, contrast media are administered to the patient.

Positive contrast media are substances containing elements with high atomic numbers, such as iodine or barium. For examination of the gastrointestinal tract, the patient is given a barium sulphate suspension in the form of a drink for examination of the stomach, or an enema for examination of the colon, Figure 7:8. All images in this chapter have been enhanced to illustrate more clearly for all readers, with or without experience in the area, the techniques involved.

Negative contrast media are gases with low X-ray absorption due to their much lower density than that of the solid and liquid structures of the body. These two types of media are combined in **double contrast** examinations, where, for example, the intestine is first filled with a barium enema, then emptied and filled again with air or carbon dioxide, resulting in some residual of barium enema covering the intestinal lining, which is kept distended by the gas, Figure 7:8. Thus the remaining barium contrast produces an image of the intestinal contour.

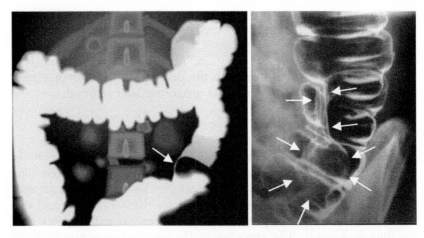

Figure 7:8 Illustration of the radiological double contrast method. To the left, the colon has been filled with barium contrast. A suspected lesion can be seen at the small arrow. The image on the right is obtained with double contrast, by emptying the intestine of the barium enema and filling it with air. A pedunculated polyp is clearly seen

Injection of contrast media consisting of water-soluble organic iodine compounds is often used for vascular imaging. The method is called **arteriography** when arteries are examined and **phlebography** when veins are examined.

By adjusting the kilovoltage, it is to some extent possible to choose whether or not to visualize the bones. The skeleton causes a higher contrast at low kilovoltage settings, and a lower contrast at high settings. When examining the lungs, depiction of the ribs is undesired, and therefore a high voltage is selected, approximately 150 kV. But after a chest trauma it is important to examine the patient for any rib fractures, and in this situation a low voltage is selected, approximately 70 kV, which gives a better image of the ribs.

In **mammography**, the mammary glands are visualized using radiation generated by a special X-ray tube operated at extremely low voltages. This improves the possibilities for detecting tumours in the soft tissue. To detect very small tumours that cannot be palpated, the examiner looks for microcalcifications, calcium deposits less than a millimetre in size, which may constitute the first sign of a malignant tumour. But repeatedly exposing women to X-rays also constitutes a risk for the development of cancer. The balance of potential benefit and harm of **mammography screening** varies with age. Because of a lower risk of breast cancer, the benefit of regular mammography of women younger than 40 to 50 is smaller, and the balance of benefit and harm is closer. The practice for women between 40 and 50 varies among countries. For women over 70 it is not usually deemed justified to perform routine mammography since, among other reasons, tumours in older women can grow more slowly.

Digital X-ray technology

The photographic film is often replaced by **digital X-ray technology**. The word digital, which means numerical, refers to the fact that the image is divided into small picture elements, called **pixels**, that are processed in a computer. The image can be captured by various techniques, for example, using a selenium plate in the same way as in an ordinary copy machine. The electric charges of the selenium plate are transferred to a computer, where they are stored on various types of memory media in a **radiology information system (RIS)**, Box 7:2.

Digital X-ray techniques have many advantages. The traditional film development using aqueous solutions is eliminated, and the images are more easily accessible than when stored in large X-ray film archives. The images can rapidly be transmitted to other departments within the same hospital, and even to other hospitals.

The stored images may also be computer processed and enhanced afterwards, as opposed to the unchangeable nature of the film image. Fine details can be enhanced with **spatial filtering**, while larger unimportant parts are subdued. Contrast enhancement is thus obtained.

Techniques • Box 7:2

Radiology information systems

Digital technology has contributed more than just the possibility for improved image quality. Most of all, this technology can reduce the risk of mix-up, prevent the loss of images in archives, speed up the entire examination procedure and reduce the staffing need. A fully deployed **radiology information system (RIS)**, which also has to include a **picture archiving and communication system (PACS)**, can comprise the following elements.

Prior to a planned examination, the system uses the patient personal identification number to retrieve the patient's demographic data from the population file, with the correct name and spelling. A selection of images from previous examinations of the patient is brought from the image archive.

When the patient arrives at the X-ray department, a photograph of the patient's face can be taken and stored in the system. This photograph and the images selected from the archive are sent to the radiology assistant who will carry out the new examination. Using the old X-ray images, the radiology assistant can plan the examination procedure beforehand. Thanks to the photograph, the assistant will recognize the patient at their very first meeting.

During the examination, the images are displayed for a few seconds following the exposure. When the examination is completed, the images are immediately available to the radiologist at the workstation in the evaluation room. Nobody needs to carry cassettes to a developing machine and no delays occur.

During the X-ray clinical conferences, the examination images can be presented on large monitors, where they are easier to evaluate in detail than when hung on antiquated light cabinets. High-resolution paper copies can be printed out immediately, and, for example, handed to surgeons, who can then use them to plan an operation at their convenience.

After completion of the examination, all images are transmitted to digital image archives where they are retrievable for a certain period depending on the time elapsed since first recorded.

Since personnel costs constitute the largest expense within health care, the high investment costs for a RIS/PACS system can quickly be regained.

With **time filtering** it is possible to visualize selectively only those details that have moved at a certain speed, such as the passage of the contrast medium through the coronary vessels during angiography. Other parts of the image which are either stationary or moving very rapidly due to the heart beats, can be eliminated. By gating image collection to the ECG, it is also possible to avoid the effect of rapid movements from heart beats.

It is further possible to compare two images taken right after one another – this technique is called **digital subtraction angiography**. The blood vessels can be visualized more clearly by subtracting an image obtained without contrast from an image taken with contrast, Figure 7:9. Blood vessels in the extremities are often examined using this method.

Digitally stored X-ray images are reviewed at a radiographic **workstation**, which may be equipped with several screens for easy comparison of different images. At the workstations it is possible to modify the images by adjusting the contrast, brightness and filtering. As there are

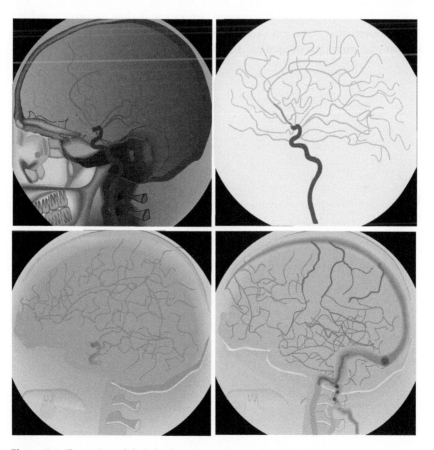

Figure 7:9 Illustration of digital subtraction angiography of the cerebral arteries. Normal radiogram top left; subtraction images show the contrast medium passage at different times after the injection

numerous settings available, it can sometimes be difficult to recreate a certain imaging situation afterwards. This may also have legal consequences, as one physician may have been unable to observe something that a colleague notices later sometimes with the hindsight of additional clinical information.

Computer tomography

An important method, for which the developers were awarded the Nobel Prize in medicine, is **computer tomography** (**CT**). As the name suggests, this method produces tomograms, cross-sectional images. Instead of irradiating the patient with a cone-shaped beam of X-rays to project an image of the entire organ, the patient is scanned with a number of thin X-ray beams. The intensity of each beam traversing the patient is measured, Figure 7:10. This procedure is repeated for a great number of beam directions, or projections, while the tube and detector array are rotated full circle around the patient. An image is then reconstructed by a computer of the section of the body studied, Figure 7:11. This figure shows the simplest procedure for visualizing a section of the body, a

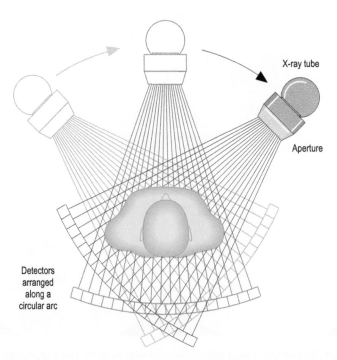

Figure 7:10 In computer tomography a section of the patient is scanned by a fan-shaped X-ray beam

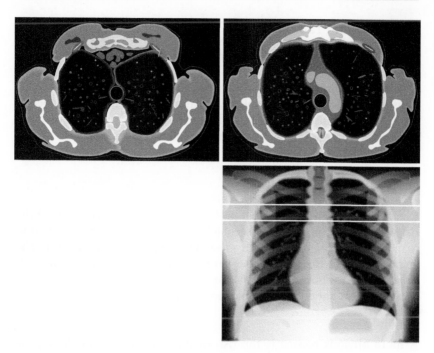

Figure 7:11 Illustration of computer tomography of the thorax. Bottom image displays positions of the two CT sections shown at the top. The machine has been set to display the skeleton in white. The air in the lungs and the trachea is black. Pleura, bronchi and cross-sectioned vessels are in grey

tomogram. Images of adjacent sections are obtained by repeating the procedure.

This investigation is often done by scanning the patient in a helical fashion, **spiral tomography**, which enables **volume rendering**. In this volume, it is not only possible to select any desired section after the investigation is completed, but also to display certain textures while suppressing others. It is possible to start by displaying the skin, which gives a photo-like image of the patient, and then successively remove the soft tissues until only the skeleton remains. A disadvantage of this method is that the patient may receive a fairly high radiation dose if many sections are scanned.

Computer tomography yields a significantly higher resolution of small contrast differences than conventional radiography. As a result, the imaging of various soft-tissue types is much better – a tumour can, for example, be clearly distinguished from normal tissue, and coagulated blood from fresh blood. The images also show the organs in their correct size relative to one another, which makes this method well suited for dose planning in preparation for radiation treatment.

Interventional radiology

In **interventional radiology**, therapeutic procedures are performed in combination with diagnostic X-ray investigations. A common treatment is balloon dilatation of stenotic coronary vessels, PTCA (percutaneous transluminal coronary angioplasty, Chapter 11). Another therapeutic technique is the insertion of a vascular prosthesis (Chapter 10) in arterial aneurysms for wall ballooning that could otherwise rupture if left untreated.

Risks

Every examination or treatment puts the patient at some risk, even if the risk might be so small as to be negligible. For X-rays, the risk evaluation is more complicated than with most other types of investigation. The greatest risk for the patient is often that the diagnosis may be missed, either due to technical deficiencies or by misinterpretation of the images. Such mistakes happen many times each year.

General risks

A more obvious hazard is the risk of injuring the patient during the investigation. Contrast injections for examination of blood vessels have sometimes resulted in allergic, or anaphylactic shock. Patients have suffered rib fractures caused by the compression during an abdominal X-ray investigation. Patients have even been injured, for example, by falling equipment parts, such as aperture plates and entire image intensifiers (Cases 2:2, 2:5 and 2:7). Crushing injuries are also common, especially when examination tables are power driven.

Risks of ionizing radiation

The problems most discussed with regard to X-ray investigations are the risks associated with the radiation exposure. Radiation injuries are of three types: **somatic**, that is those that affect the somatic cells, **genetic**, those affecting the germ cells, and **teratogenic**, injuries to the foetus. The somatic cell injuries cause a slightly increased risk of cancer. It has been estimated that about 10 cancer cases per million inhabitants yearly are caused by medical X-ray examinations. This can, however, be compared with some 60 cases that are caused by radon in dwellings, 13 cases caused by natural background radiation, and 0.4 cases (50-year average) caused in Sweden by the Chernobyl accident, which was one of the first countries to be reached by the radioactivity beyond the former Soviet countries.

The problem of radon in dwellings illustrates the irrational attitude to risk management on the part of our society. Radon in dwellings kills in the same order of magnitude as the number killed in traffic accidents. Even the risk of cancer from exposure to electric fields, the existence of which has not even been scientifically verified, attracts more public attention.

Some methods involve a particularly large risk because of exceptionally high radiation levels. In particular, computer tomography can result in excessive doses when large regions of the body are imaged. A full scan of the whole body results in almost as high a radiation level as the Hiroshima victims received 2 kilometres from the blast epicentre. Infants are particularly sensitive and imaging merely the skull involves a clearly established risk for impaired intellectual development.

Some injuries are unfortunately caused by technically faulty X-ray machine designs or by malfunctioning X-ray machines. There have been several cases of undesired radiation exposure to both patients and staff.

CASE 7:5   Two children and staff exposed to radiation

Two patients were to undergo X-ray examinations at the dental department of a central hospital. In connection with the examinations, it was discovered that the X-ray tube was very hot. This had been caused by a short-circuit in the control circuit. This resulted in the X-ray tube receiving the full voltage so that it was continuously generating X-rays. The audible alarm that was supposed to warn of exposure was not working, and the yellow light indicator on the tube arm that was supposed to fulfil the same warning function could not be observed due to strong sunlight.

As a result, two children were exposed to direct irradiation and two others, as well as the dentist and dental nurse, were most likely exposed to secondary radiation (scattered radiation within the room). Even if greater vigilance could have prevented the accident, the primary cause was a technically faulty design, which does happen.

Sometimes, there is unfortunately also insufficient knowledge of the operation of X-ray machines. The following incident serves as a tragic example:

CASE 7:6   Excessive radiation exposure

A child was to have an X-ray examination of the lungs with a mobile X-ray machine. After adjusting the X-ray tube settings, one of the radiology assistants left the room to fetch lead aprons prior to the exposure. When ready to perform the exposure, it was discovered that the fluoroscopy function had been switched on during the entire tube setting procedure, for about 10 min. The film beneath the child was so overexposed that it was completely black after it was developed.

During the ensuing investigation, it was found that the child had probably been lying in the primary X-ray beam for 4 to 5 min, and had received a radiation dose of 25 to 30 mGy (Chapter 11) over a major part of the body. The radiology assistant probably received a 2 to 3 times higher dose on arms and hands.

The film dosimeter worn on the chest by the affected radiology assistant, which had not even been in the direct X-ray beam, registered a dose corresponding to a tenth of the yearly limit for radiology personnel.

There is rarely any reason to perform fluoroscopy using mobile X-ray machines; in fact, this function could be permanently disconnected in this type of machine.

Dosimetry

All personnel working in departments where ionizing radiation occurs must carry a dosimeter. The dosimeter is personal and a log must be kept to make it possible to check whether anyone has been exposed to high radiation doses, and if so where and when.

All ionizing radiation blackens photographic film, which is the basis for the common **film dosimeter**. The film badge is worn outside of the clothing and sent in for development after a certain period of time, usually one month. The dosimeter must be worn at all times. The advantage of the film dosimeter is that it is cheap, sturdy, easy to handle and can be sent by mail. The disadvantage is that the reading is only obtained after a delay of perhaps a couple of weeks after development.

In some workplaces, personnel are equipped with **thermoluminescent dosimeters**. These are also worn outside of the clothes, just like the standard film dosimeter. The dose is measured by inserting the dosimeter into a special device that heats the thermoluminescent substance so that light is emitted. The amount of emitted light is a measure of the dose received.

The radiation dose administered during radiation therapy sessions can be monitored by **semiconductor technology**. This enables continuous dose monitoring during the treatment procedure. A computer measures the readings during the ongoing therapy session, which provides for very reliable monitoring.

Use

The risk of radiation injuries is not great enough to prevent X-ray examinations of nonpregnant women, provided there is a clear diagnostic indication and a reasonable chance that a conclusive answer will be obtained. But when the indication is unclear, investigations should be avoided; an X-ray investigation should never be undertaken simply for the lack of a rationally based decision.

It should be noted that a referral for X-ray is not the same as ordering a certain type of X-ray image; it is a consultation of a radiologist. The radiologist may suggest an alternative method, such as gastroscopy instead of an X-ray of the stomach.

Many X-ray investigations require patient preparation, such as a special diet and a laxative prior to an abdominal X-ray examination. By emptying the bowel, images of improved quality can be obtained; with insufficient preparation, investigations may not be very successful. The colon must be completely empty in order to avoid, for example, mis-diagnosing remaining intestinal content as a tumour.

A large number of diseases can be diagnosed by X-ray techniques. **Skeletal fractures** can be seen directly, and following repositioning, the result can be checked and the healing process monitored. **Pulmonary atelectases** and infiltrations as well as **pleural fluids** can be demonstrated. The entire **circulatory system**, including any narrowed segments of the blood vessels can be studied, and a measurement of the total heart volume obtained. The **digestive organs** can be examined to diagnose tumours, ulcers and gallstones. X-ray investigations of the **excretory organs** provide a measure of the kidney function, and urinary stones may be detected. For examining disorders of the **central nervous system**, computer tomography is the method of choice. As already mentioned, mammography is an important method for early detection of **breast cancer**.

Bone mineral densitometry

In spite of the fact that bone absorbs X-rays much more efficiently than the soft tissues, it is not possible to determine the degree of osteoporosis, or "porous bone" just by looking at an X-ray image. It is only in very advanced stages of the disease that a somewhat fainter skeletal image than normal may be discerned.

Osteoporosis is often discovered after the patient has suffered a fracture. Fragile bones afflict a great part of the female population – it is estimated that approximately 25% of the women in European countries will suffer a hip fracture at some point during their lives. The health care costs are staggering, and preventive treatment is therefore highly cost-effective.

In order to quantify the degree of osteoporosis, the difference in absorption of two X-ray beams with different energies is measured. A special device, a **bone densitometer**, is required. A carefully selected measurement site is scanned, and a profile of the amount of the **bone mineral density (BMD)** is obtained. The vertebrae of the lower back, the femoral neck and the heel bone are common measurement sites. It is important not to limit the measurements to just one site, as the bone mineral levels often vary from region to region in the body.

MAGNETIC RESONANCE IMAGING

By placing the patient in a strong magnetic field, various soft tissue structures can be imaged using radio waves. This method is called **magnetic resonance imaging** (**MRI** or **MR**). The investigation is carried out using a very complex device that is often simply called an **MRI** or **MR machine**.

Principle

Magnetic resonance imaging visualizes the protons (hydrogen atoms) in the tissues, and how "loosely" the protons are bound to the chemical compounds of which they are part, Box 7:3. By detecting the amount and "mobility" of these protons, various types of soft tissues can be

---

 Techniques • Box 7:3

Principle of MRI

Many of us will have played with toy tops (gyros) when we were children. When the top was spinning at full speed it stood straight up, but then it began to lean more and more while simultaneously spinning around the vertical axis until it finally toppled over. The physical term for this type of rotation, where the rotation axis describes a cone-shaped motion around the vertical axis with the tips of both axes centred together on the floor, is **precession**.

The protons in the body tissues also rotate like a gyro. If the body is placed in a powerful magnetic field, all the protons will be oriented with their axes of rotation nearly parallel to the magnetic field. At the same time, the rotation axes will describe a cone-shaped orbit, i.e. precession. The precession speed, the so-called **Larmor frequency**, is determined by the strength of the magnetic field. At 1 T (tesla), it is 42 MHz.

When a short external radio-frequency (RF) pulse at the Larmor frequency is added, the protons absorb the energy. Immediately afterwards, the protons again release the energy at a certain speed, depending on how tightly bound they are to the tissue chemical compounds. This can be measured by the **relaxation times**, **T1** and **T2**.

To achieve this, the strength of the radio signal returned from the tissue, and the signal decay over time, must both be measured. This must be determined for every individual partial volume of the body, called a **voxel**, so that an image can be constructed from a number of picture elements, **pixels**, each representing a voxel.

Techniques • Box 7:3—Continued

In order to distinguish the different voxels, the magnetic field is rendered inhomogeneous, so that the protons acquire the right Larmor frequency in just one single line of voxels at a time. As shown in Figure 7:12, this inhomogeneity is achieved by using gradient coils which affect the magnetic field in three directions, x, y and z.

The images are reconstructed in a manner similar to that for CT, using detected signals that are proportionate to the proton concentration as well as to the relaxation times, T1 and T2. Different structures in the soft tissues can be shown in either light or dark colour, Figure 7:13.

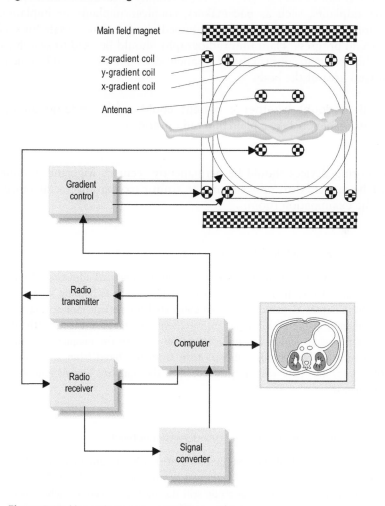

Figure 7:12 Magnetic resonance imaging machine

depicted. Bone tissue cannot be imaged directly, as the protons in bone are virtually immobile, but the skeleton forms a negative image, an absence of structures, compared with the surrounding soft tissues.

Risks

There are no known risks due to any effects of the magnetic field on the body. However, metal objects can be "sucked" into the very strong magnetic field and cause mechanical injuries. This is the **missile effect**. Patients with metallic prostheses or who have had metal clips attached to blood vessels during surgery must not be examined if there is any risk that the material might possess magnetic properties. Also patients with metallic foreign bodies such as bullets and shrapnel must not be scanned if a movement of the foreign body is potentially hazardous. Patients with active implants, such as pacemakers, cochlear implants or implanted infusion pumps must also not be examined; designs that are safe for such use are in progress. Plain film radiography should be used to search for metallic objects to confirm that the patient does not have metal fragments in a vital area of the body.

 If in doubt whether a patient could safely undergo an MRI examination, take a **plain film radiograph**.

Monitoring devices should be permanently secured. Rigorous routines must be exercised to prevent anyone from carrying any metal objects into the examination room.

CASE 7:7   Capnograph torn from nurse's hand

During an MRI examination, the patient position needed adjusting. While carrying out this manoeuvre, an anaesthetic nurse was holding a capnograph (Chapter 8), which had been connected for patient monitoring. As the imaging pallet with the patient re-entered the magnet, the anaesthetic nurse followed, and ended up coming too close to the magnet with the capnograph. The capnograph was torn from her hand from a distance of 1.5 m, and flew with great force into the magnet. The patient was unharmed.

CASE 7:8   Child killed after oxygen cylinder smashes head

A 6-year-old boy had successfully had a benign brain tumour removed by surgery and was going to be examined postoperatively by MRI. The boy was anaesthetized to be able to lie still during the procedure, which was expected to take half an hour or more. The anaesthetist noticed a problem with the piped oxygen flow, and he knocked on the partition window to the technologist but could not draw attention to his problem. A nurse about to leave the MRI suite noticed the anaesthetist's dilemma and grabbed a nearby 2 kg oxygen cylinder and handed it over to him. The cylinder was immediately pulled out of the anaesthetist's hand and shot through the air towards the 10 ton magnet gantry. The cylinder hit the boy on the head.

The boy died of the blunt trauma two days after the accident from his fractured skull and brain haemorrhage.

The accidents illustrate that professionals, who are not by their daily work familiar with MRI technology, face a risk of causing accidents. Both the nurse and the anaesthetist attempted to help the patient. Many similar nonfatal accidents involving oxygen cylinders have occurred in many countries.

Tip During MRI examinations only **nonferrous** oxygen cylinders, fire extinguishers and other supplies are allowed. Devices where magnetic materials have been replaced by aluminium are safe.

Monitoring of critically ill patients has been a problem since non-magnetic devices have not been available. Standard pulse oximeters (Chapter 8) have been employed during MRI examinations, but even this practice has clearly been unsafe. Special monitoring devices have now been developed.

CASE 7:9 Patient badly burned during MRI examination

A 59-year-old woman was to be examined for back problems. As she was unable to hold still during the procedure, she was put to sleep. A standard type pulse oximeter was attached to her finger.

After the examination, when the patient was coming to, she complained of severe pain in the finger where the pulse oximeter had been attached. A third degree burn was discovered, which later required reconstruction with plastic surgery and tissue transplantation.

The pulse oximeter was investigated after the accident, but no defects were found. It was concluded that the pulse oximeter cables had been placed in a loop, enabling the magnetic field to induce an electric current. (Figure 6:16 illustrates open electric loops.)

Tip Avoid standard medical devices such as pulse oximeters if they have electric cables that might pick up electromagnetic fields. If monitoring devices with electric cables have to be used, ensure that all cables going to the patient in the MRI machine are laid close together and never in open loops.

Even if there is no evidence of any harmful effects, examinations of pregnant women during the first few pregnancy weeks are considered undesirable. There is always the possibility of unknown risks. But examinations during late pregnancy are generally considered safe.

Use

Administration of contrast media to the patient is not necessary, but some types of images are enhanced and captured faster when organic compounds containing a heavy metal are given.

The examination takes at least 10 min, and often longer. A disadvantage with magnetic resonance imaging is that very sick patients cannot be monitored in the usual fashion during the examination, as no metallic parts that are magnetic to any degree are allowed in the magnetic field, close to the patient.

A variety of diagnostic problems involving soft tissues of the body can be solved – examples of the excellent imaging of these are shown in Figure 7:13. **Tumours** and **metastases** can be distinguished from surrounding normal tissues. **Fat tissue** can be distinguished from muscle, and white **brain matter** from grey. It is also possible to image **ligaments**, **menisci** and tears in these, as well as **haemorrhages** and **infarctions** in various organs. With a special technique to visualize **flowing blood**, the vessel system in the body can be seen. Changes in the brain caused by dementia, alcoholism and psychoses can be studied.

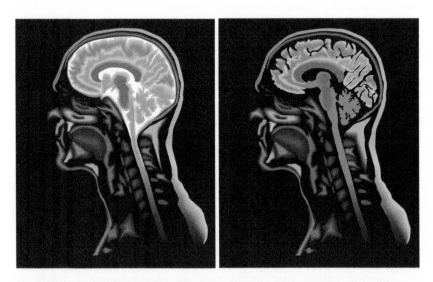

Figure 7:13 Illustration of types of MR images. By adjusting the settings on the MRI machine, different tissue structures can be displayed with different levels of optical density. Thus the cerebral spinal fluid is displayed in light shades in the left, and in dark shades in the right image

Special MRI machines have been developed for **intraoperative** imaging. These allow the surgeon to image during the operation. The surgeon can then observe the position of the instruments relative to the organs on a screen.

NUCLEAR MEDICINE IMAGING

Organs can be imaged and their functions studied by administering radioactively labelled substances taken up by the organ, and then measuring the ensuing radiation emission from the organ.

Principle

Imaging can use nuclear medicine methods, which in general is called **scintigraphy**. When several radiation detectors are combined, and computerized techniques are employed for obtaining two-dimensional images of the distribution of a radioactive substance within the body, **gamma cameras** can be used, Box 7:4. Radiation going toward the camera can be "seen", but the depth from which it emanates cannot be determined.

This can, however, be achieved with two different tomographic methods, **SPECT** (single photon emission computed tomography) and **PET**, Box 7:4. For all three methods the images are constructed in a computer following measurement of the ionizing radiation.

Risks

The risk evaluation for nuclear medicine examinations is the same as that for radiological methods. It is necessary to weigh up the risk of exposing the patient to ionizing radiation with the risk of not reaching a correct diagnosis. Whenever there is a clear diagnostic indication, the investigation is usually performed.

Use

The radionuclide is selected depending on the organ to be examined. The short half-life of only 6 hours of technetium 99m makes it suitable for many scans, including **bone scans**. A phosphate compound labelled with the isotope is taken up in skeletal regions where new bone formation is taking place. The uptake is therefore increased in such areas as well as in areas with increased blood flow. The method is highly sensitive for the detection of skeletal tumours, Figure 7:15.

Technetium 99m is also preferable for measuring the blood flow through the lungs in **perfusion scintigraphy**. The patient is given an intravenous injection of an emulsion of particles labelled with the radionuclide. The particles are large enough to stick in the lung capillaries

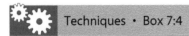

Techniques • Box 7:4

Gamma cameras

The three most important parts of a gamma camera are (1) a collimator that restricts the radiation beam, (2) a large NaI crystal in which light flashes (scintillations) occur when gamma photons are absorbed, and (3) a number of photomultipliers that record the scintillations from each incoming gamma photon and convert them to electric pulses.

The collimator is made of lead and usually has a large number of parallel channels aimed towards the scintillator crystal. Only the photons that are parallel to the hole hit the crystal; all nonparallel gamma photons are absorbed by the lead. This results in a scintillation distribution over the crystal surface corresponding to the radionuclide distribution in the organ, Figure 7:14.

Each scintillation position can be determined by simultaneously measuring the intensity in all photomultipliers, and comparing the light intensity with that in adjacent photomultipliers. The position of each scintillation can thus be calculated, since the intensity will of course be higher the closer the scintillation is to a particular photomultiplier. The information from all the photomultipliers is collated into an image showing the radionuclide distribution in the organ.

A gamma camera can have one, two or three detector heads. By rotating the entire camera assembly around the patient, the radionuclide distribution in three dimensions can be reconstructed with the aid of a computer, thus producing multiple tomographic sections of the body, SPECT (single photon emission tomography).

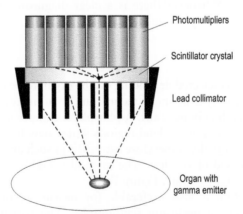

Photomultipliers

Scintillator crystal

Lead collimator

Organ with gamma emitter

Figure 7:14 Lead collimator for gamma camera

Techniques • Box 7:4—Continued

In PET (positron emission tomography) radioactive isotopes are utilized that emit photons in directly opposite directions when decaying. These are then captured with paired detectors on each side of the patient.

SPECT is highly suited for imaging organs located deep inside the body, such as the liver and kidneys. PET was initially used primarily for investigation of brain function, but other clinical applications are now common. The method can give detailed information about metabolism by mapping the blood flow to different cerebral regions, as well as the cerebral glucose and oxygen consumption. This can be achieved by engaging the patient in various forms of thought processes, see Box 7:6 on purpose of colour. The neurotransmitter distribution both in the normal brain and in different disorders can be mapped.

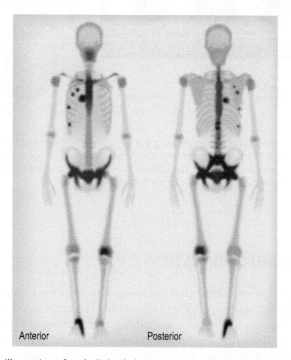

Anterior   Posterior

Figure 7:15 Illustration of a whole-body bone scan of patient with skeletal metastases from lung cancer. The skeleton as a whole has taken up a moderate amount of technetium. The tumour and metastases display a much higher uptake and are clearly defined by black areas against the surrounding normal tissues (only a small fraction of the capillaries are obstructed and the total circulation is not affected). Images are obtained immediately after the injection, and an absence of activity in a lung region indicates obstruction of the blood flow to that region. For comparison with lung ventilation, the inert gaseous isotope xenon 133 is used in **ventilation scintigraphy**. The two methods are often performed during the same examination session in cases of suspected pulmonary embolism. Then the ventilation scintigraphy shows ventilation, whereas the perfusion scintigraphy shows uptake defects in the regions affected by the obstructed blood flow.

Myocardial scintigraphy with thallium 201 or technetium 99m assesses the myocardial perfusion and evaluates the extent of myocardial infarction, Figure 7:16. These radionuclides are taken up by the normal myocardium, but not by the infarction areas.

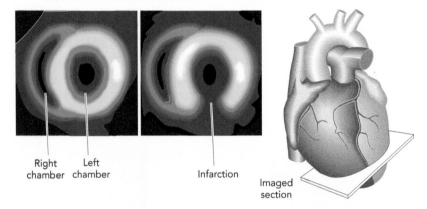

Right chamber   Left chamber   Infarction   Imaged section

Figure 7:16 Tomographic image showing a cross-section through the heart with and without infarction. The bright and yellow areas represent high isotope uptake, and the blue and black ones show areas of low uptake. The area with no uptake in the anterior part of the left chamber corresponds to the infarction area

ULTRASOUND DIAGNOSTICS

The application of ultrasound imaging has increased during recent decades and this tendency is likely to prevail. The reason is that there are few if any known side-effects associated with exposure to ultrasound with the intensities that are common during imaging. Furthermore, soft tissues that are difficult to examine with other methods can be visualized. But the images obtained have relatively low resolution, and can be obscured by interfering noise and artefacts (image details that do not correspond to any real tissue structure).

Techniques • Box 7:5

Functional imaging

A new group of diagnostic methods are summarized under the heading "functional imaging techniques". The method makes it possible to visualize and quantify physiological processes, which generally are local. These methods are denoted by an "f" before the common name, for example **fMRI**, for **functional magnetic resonance imaging**. Other examples of methods suitable for functional imaging are computer tomography (CT), single photon emission tomography (SPECT) and positron emission tomography (PET). Usually functional imaging results in inferior anatomical information, but makes it possible to follow physiological processes.

Functional imaging is of particular value for studying brain processes. Neurophysiologists and psychiatrists have applied functional imaging to many diverse purposes such as visualization of alcohol dependence and autism. A well-known application is for following processes in the brain during various forms of mental activity, Figure 7:20. Functional imaging demands broad competence of the users comprising medicine, physiology and physics.

Principle

All ultrasound machines measure the time it takes for a short ultrasound pulse to travel to the object and be echoed back again. This time is a measure of the distance between the ultrasound transducer and the tissue interface that reflected the pulse. The principle is the same as when using sonar to determine the ocean depth under a ship.

Acoustic impedance

Sound is reflected at the interface between two media of different **acoustic impedance,** such as two adjacent tissue types with different densities and speeds of sound. If the interface is between gas (air, intestinal gas) and soft tissue, the reflection is total. This is because of the very large differences in density and speed of sound between a gas and soft tissues. No sound gets through the interface – it acts like a mirror – nothing can be seen behind it. The lungs cannot be imaged because of their air content. Similarly, the reflection at the interface between bone and soft tissues is also very strong, and it is therefore very difficult to image any structure behind bone, as within the skull. Only when the differences between the two tissues at the interface are very slight, is it possible to observe structures with ultrasound. It is then possible to penetrate the soft tissues to a certain depth.

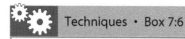

Techniques · Box 7:6

Purpose of colour

With colour the amount of information presented in a picture can be increased. An early application of colour was in thermography, where the skin temperature was represented by colours, Figure 7:17.

The laser Doppler technique produces similar images, but here colour shows the capillary blood flow, Figure 7:18. The method has among other things been applied for measuring the local blood flow after tissue transplantation.

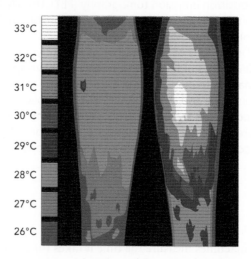

33°C

32°C

31°C

30°C

29°C

28°C

27°C

26°C

Figure 7:17 Illustration of thermographic image of the lower leg showing the skin temperatures. To the right, deep venous thrombosis, which forces the blood flow to the superficial vessels causing an increase in skin temperature

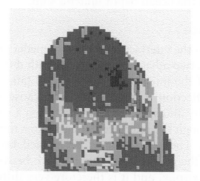

Figure 7:18 Illustration of the laser Doppler image principle showing the fingertip with inflammation of the cuticle. The dark red colour shows where the capillary blood flow has the highest velocity and the blue colour shows where it is normal. The coldest blue area visualizes the nail

Techniques • Box 7:6—Continued

Isodose lines can be coloured in the same fashion to show the dose distribution in radiation therapy (Chapter 11). This makes it easier to avoid irradiating radiation-sensitive organs, such as the spine.

Physiological processes are studied with imaging techniques, and the colour visualizes varying degrees of activity. Blood flow is coded so that red colour represents blood flow towards the ultrasound probe, and blue represents flow going away from the probe, Figure 7:19.

Cerebral metabolism can be measured with positron emission tomography (PET), Figure 7:20. Here, colour, for example, demonstrates oxygen or glucose consumption, or the absorption of labelled substances, such as drugs and neurotransmitters.

Colour is only real in ordinary photographs; otherwise colours are arbitrary. When fine details are depicted, blue and red should be avoided, since the human eye cannot focus sharply on these colours simultaneously with other colours.

Sometimes colour is added to an image without any functional meaning. An example is Figure 7:24 where the three-dimensional image of the fetus has been depicted with a skin-like colour, which has nothing to do with the real colour of the fetus. Presumably this is done to render parents a more life-like image instead a mere black-and-white ultrasound scan.

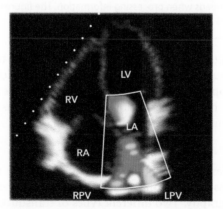

Figure 7:19 Illustration of a cardiac ultrasound image with colour Doppler showing the four heart chambers during systole. The red/yellow area represents the inflow of blood from two of the four lung veins into the left atrium (LA), and the blue area represents the outflow from the left ventricle (LV)

Techniques • Box 7:6—Continued

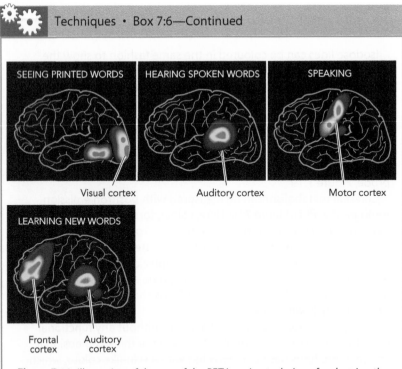

Figure 7:20 Illustration of the use of the PET imaging technique for showing the cerebral centres activated when seeing, hearing and speaking words (top) and when learning a new word when higher intellectual centres are involved in the frontal cortex (bottom). Blood flow changes were registered during these activities. Red, yellow, green and blue colours represent the uptake of glucose, which the brain needs when processing information. The figures are simplified and other centres engaged to a minor degree are not shown

Sectional images can be achieved by **ultrasound tomography** and information about the direction and speed of the blood flow can be obtained with **Doppler ultrasound.** Information about the flow is presented in colour, where red represents flow towards the ultrasound transducer and blue represents flow away from it.

Methodology

Various principles can be applied to demonstrate the reflection of the sound in the tissues. The most common imaging method in clinical practice is tomography. Two different types of transducers are described, **sector transducers** and **linear transducers.**

A sector transducer operates like a radar antenna that rotates to capture the echoes of aircraft. The probe can comprise three ultrasound crystals rotating at the transducer tip, Figure 7:21. The crystals are activated one at a time, and each crystal both sends out signals and receives echoes during the part of the rotation where it is directed

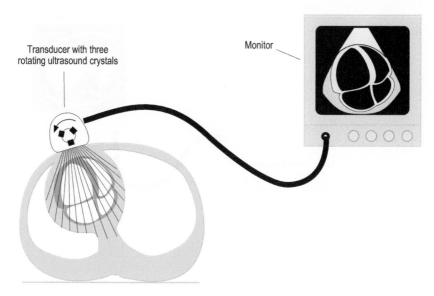

Transducer with three rotating ultrasound crystals

Monitor

Figure 7:21 Sector scanner

towards the body sector being examined. Hence the image obtained is pie-shaped, Figure 7:22.

Sector transducers can be made very small, about 1 mm in diameter, and can be used to examine blood vessels from the inside, such as a coronary artery.

Linear transducers have a large number of small ultrasound crystals arranged in a line, Figure 7:23. The crystals both send out a series of pulses in a complicated sequence and receive reflected echoes that are processed in a computer. The image obtained shows a rectangular section of the body and looks like a slice of paté. Three-dimensional images with

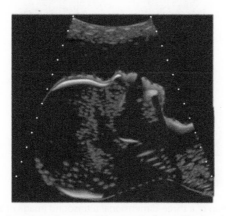

Figure 7.22 Illustration of an ultrasound image of a fetus. The head can be seen better if the book is rotated clockwise

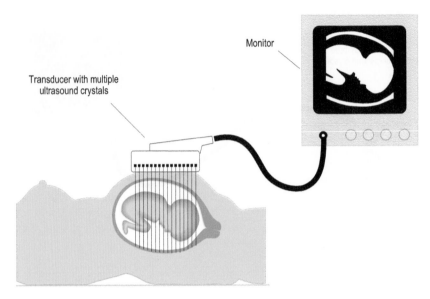

Monitor

Transducer with multiple
ultrasound crystals

Figure 7:23 Linear scanner

volume rendering can be achieved with advanced equipment. A computer can reconstruct a "statue" of the imaged structure, such as a fetus inside the uterus, Figure 7:24.

During the examination, a special gel is applied on the skin to ensure optimal skin–transducer contact and to eliminate any air bubbles that could block the ultrasound transfer.

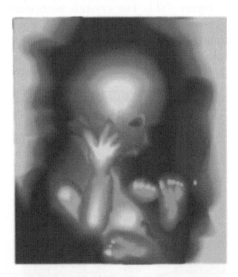

Figure 7.24 Illustration of a three-dimensional ultrasound image of a fetus at term. The skin colour is produced in the image computer to make it more natural, but does not represent the colour of the fetus

Specialized transducers that can be inserted into the body have been developed, for **endoscopic ultrasound**. A tube-shaped transducer is, for example, used to examine the prostate via the rectum. For **intravascular ultrasound** the transducers are miniaturized and placed at the tip of a catheter for insertion into blood vessels. With **biplane imaging** two perpendicular cross-sections can be imaged with longitudinal and transverse axes of the heart from a transducer placed inside the oesophagus.

Use

Ultrasound tomography is performed routinely in **cardiovascular ultrasound**, Figure 7:19. In **cardiac ultrasound** or **echocardiography**, cross-sectional images are used to determine the size and shape of the ventricles, and to observe the movements of the heart valves. The blood flow can be evaluated with the help of Doppler technology. It is of particular interest to investigate the direction of the flow to detect any regurgitation due to a valvular insufficiency, as well as measuring the flow rates for evaluating the degree of a stenosis. The heart can also be imaged from the oesophagus, in **transoesophageal echocardiography**.

Arteriosclerotic plaque can be diagnosed with intravascular transducers that can examine the vessels from the inside. Femoral vein thrombosis can be demonstrated by performing ultrasonography with colour Doppler while simultaneously trying to compress the vein by pressing down from the outside. A vein that collapses is most often normal; if this does not happen the vein most likely has a thrombus.

Obstetric ultrasound is used for determining gestational age, diagnosing multiple pregnancies, evaluating the location of the placenta and diagnosing certain serious malformations such as hydrocephalus, myelocele, abdominal defects and diaphragmatic hernias. Ultrasound imaging also makes it possible to observe the position of the needle when taking a foetal blood sample from an umbilical blood vessel for diagnosing hereditary diseases, such as haemophilia. The procedure is not entirely without risk, as it can occasionally lead to a miscarriage.

In **gastroenterology** ultrasound is used to examine the liver, kidneys, pancreas and spleen, primarily to identify tumours and cysts. Ultrasound is an excellent method for examination of gallstones since it requires no patient preparation, as opposed to a radiological examination for gallstones.

In **urology** ultrasound is employed, for example, to examine the prostate for tumours. A special ultrasound transducer is inserted into the rectum. As many false positives are obtained, the prostate is often biopsied for collection of samples for histocytological investigation. Also ultrasound is regularly utilized to determine the amount of residual urine after the patient has tried to empty their bladder.

Ultrasound is also used in **ophthalmology**, to diagnose retinal detachment when the vitreous body is too cloudy to allow examination of the retina with an ophthalmoscope.

Techniques • Box 7:7

Ultrasound

The ultrasound frequency is selected based on the organ to be investigated. The choice is a compromise between resolution capabilities and penetration depth. The resolution capability is usually limited to about half a wavelength, and at 1 MHz, for example, it is in the range of 1 mm. The tissue attenuation increases with increasing frequency. At 1 MHz, the ultrasound penetration depth is about 30 to 40 cm; after that the signal becomes fainter and no echoes are detected from deeper structures. At 10 MHz, which is common in ophthalmology, the attenuation prevents the ultrasound from penetrating more than a few centimetres, but the resolution is very good – down to a tenth of a millimetre.

For most abdominal investigations, frequencies between 3 and 5 MHz are used, which give a penetration depth of about 10 cm, with acceptable resolution capability.

One disadvantage with ultrasound tomography is in fact the limited resolution, which is linked to the very principle of ultrasound imaging.

The echoes are caused by the varying speeds of sound and densities in tissues of different composition. But because of these differences, the time it takes for the echo to return to the crystal also varies somewhat depending upon which path the sound has taken through the tissue. These differences cannot be distinguished, and echoes from the same tissue structure will be placed in slightly differing locations on the monitor, resulting in a fuzzy picture and a somewhat incorrect rendering of the shape of the imaged structure.

Where there are parallel tissue layers in the body, multiple echoes may be created as the sound bounces back and forth between the layers before returning. These echo structures are repeated periodically deeper down in the imaged organ, although no real corresponding tissue structures exist – an artefact is created.

In addition, the echo signal from a small tissue structure will broaden as the tissue depth of the structure increases. This is due to the fact that the sideways scattering of the ultrasound increases the longer it has to travel – the deeper the object, the fuzzier the image. Because of these flaws, images by **reflected** ultrasound will never be as clear as those by computer tomography or magnetic resonance.

Recent developments with **transmitted** ultrasound with many ultrasound emitting and receiving detectors on opposite sides of the body have yielded very high resolution images. The technique involves a reconstruction of the image resembling that in computer tomography.

8

Ventilation

Few machines in a modern hospital can seem as intimidating as ventilators. The great number of controls apparently has frightened people, resulting in an inordinate respect for these devices. But this is unwarranted, as ventilators are in principle not complicated. It is not necessary to know how the machine is constructed to operate it. The major difficulty that doctors and nurses actually face is to decide the individual patient's need for ventilator treatment. This requires medical education, physiological insight and extensive practical experience. But the functions of the devices are simple.

This chapter therefore explains how **ventilators** may be used to provide respiratory support and how ventilation may be controlled by means of various types of **anaesthetic machines.** Everyone should know the basics of **oxygen treatment,** as it is given both in hospitals and in the patient's home. A special kind of oxygen treatment is given in **incubators.** Finally, this chapter describes methods for **monitoring** ventilation – it is primarily by such monitoring that the risks of anaesthesia can be reduced.

VENTILATORS

The technical devices that are used depend entirely upon the patient's need for **ventilator treatment.** In an emergency situation a **manual breathing bag** may suffice, whereas long-term care requires ventilators. In order to demonstrate how simple in principle these technical devices really are, we will here describe the **fundamental parts** of a ventilator. Then we will describe their **use.**

Ventilator treatment

A healthy person does not have to exert his muscles very much in order to breathe. But in many types of disorders, the body cannot sustain adequate ventilation. As a result the carbon dioxide level in the blood increases and oxygenation becomes inadequate, and a state of **respiratory insufficiency** has developed.

The disease process may be localized in the lungs, the chest cage or the respiratory muscles, the nerves controlling these muscles or in the respiratory centre in the brain stem.

The most common reason for ventilator treatment is that the breathing centre of the brain is unable to control respiration, for example, in sedative-hypnotic poisoning resulting from a **suicide attempt**, or during surgery when patients are given general **anaesthesia**. Many **neuromuscular diseases** can lead to respiratory paralysis, such as various forms of muscle atrophies, or Guillain–Barre syndrome (polyradiculoneuropathy), as well as toxins that affect the nervous system (diphtheria, botulism, tetanus). Myasthenia gravis may also require ventilator treatment. Ventilator support can be essential for survival in severe **trauma cases**. Babies with underdeveloped lungs may need ventilator support during the **neonatal period**. All these conditions require either temporary or life-long ventilator treatment.

Ventilators are not only needed in intensive care and surgical departments, but also at home in the care of chronically ill patients. A special kind of ventilator employed for home treatment of sleep apnoea is called a **CPAP (continuous positive airway pressure) machine**.

Manual breathing bags

A breathing bag can be used to ventilate a patient when a technically more sophisticated ventilator is unnecessary or unavailable, for example, during transportation and in emergency situations. Various systems are available – a common type, Figure 8:1, consists of a mask connected to a breathing bag and a reservoir balloon.

The breathing bag is designed with inner springs that expand it, so that it fills automatically after compression. It is also equipped with one-way valves, which direct the gas flow to the patient during compression. Oxygen is obtained from a reservoir balloon that is continuously filled with a steady flow of gas from an oxygen tube. The reservoir balloon reduces the oxygen drain from the gas cylinder. If the oxygen was supplied directly from the oxygen tube for each breath, a much higher flow would be required, which would go to waste when the patient exhales. The reservoir balloon instead acts as a buffer, evening out the intermittent oxygen consumption. If the oxygen flow becomes greater than that required, the reservoir balloon releases the surplus, thus preventing the patient from being subjected to excess pressure from the oxygen tube, which could potentially lead to a pneumothorax through a puncture of the pulmonary pleura, resulting in collapse of the lung.

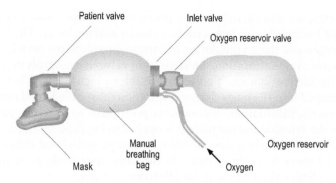

Figure 8:1 Manual breathing bag used for ventilation in case of failing spontaneous breathing

A manual breathing bag can also be used without an oxygen supply – it then automatically fills with air. Oxygen is given only as a supplement after surgery or in accidents.

Fundamental components of a ventilator

A pump that can take over the patient's respiratory work is an essential part of the ventilator system. The simplest system conceivable is an electric motor driving a piston up and down in a cylinder, Figure 8:2. The cylinder is connected to the patient via a tracheal tube. As a result, the air in the cylinder is alternately pumped into and sucked out of the patient's lungs. By varying the motor revolution rate, the respiration rate can be adjusted. This simple arrangement provides a **power source** that can take over the patient's respiratory work.

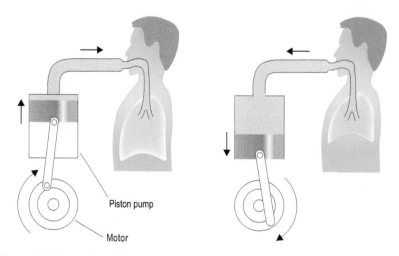

Figure 8:2 When the piston travels upwards, air is forced into the patient's lungs; when the piston travels downwards, air is sucked out

However, we immediately have a problem. The same volume of air is travelling back and forth between the cylinder and the lungs. The lack of fresh oxygen and the accumulation of carbon dioxide in the breathing air would soon cause suffocation. An **expiration valve** that controls the direction of the airflow can easily solve this problem, Figure 8:3. When fresh air is pumped into the lungs during **inspiration** (also called **inhalation,** or more exactly, **insufflation**) the valve is positioned so that the passage between the cylinder and the patient is open. During expiration, the valve closes so that the carbon dioxide-filled and oxygen-depleted exhaled air is directed away from the system. At the same time fresh air is sucked into the cylinder via a one-way (unidirectional) valve.

In principle, it would be possible to sustain ventilation in a patient indefinitely with this simple arrangement. But since the volume of every inspiration is determined by the size of the cylinder, it would not be possible to treat a larger patient who needs more air, or a child who requires only a fraction of this volume. To do this, the **tidal volume** (the volume of each breath) needs to be adjusted. This could be achieved by placing a suitably sized balloon inside the cylinder, a large one for adults and small one for children, Figure 8:4. The maximum volume of the balloon would then limit the volume of each inspiration. If the piston continued its upward travel after the balloon was emptied, the air in the cylinder would simply be compressed, and no air would pass from the cylinder into the patient tube.

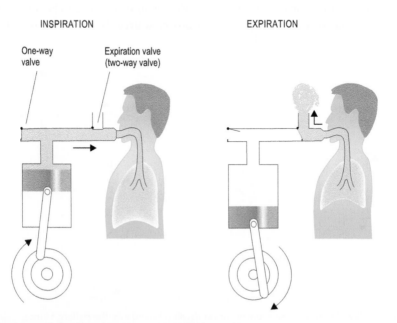

INSPIRATION   EXPIRATION

One-way   Expiration valve
valve   (two-way valve)

Figure 8:3 The airflow direction is controlled by two valves

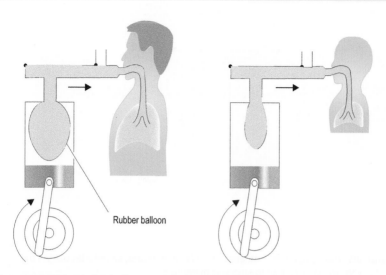

Rubber balloon

Figure 8:4 With suitable balloon size, the inspiratory volume can be adjusted to the patient so that the appropriate tidal volume is achieved

To be able to use this ventilator in real life without risk, one further detail is required. The powerful electric motor could produce such high pressure that the patient's lungs could puncture (if too large a balloon were used) leading to a pneumothorax and immediate collapse of the lungs. Therefore a **pressure release** is needed, which is accomplished by connecting a **safety valve**. This can be achieved by connecting the pump to a pipe that is inserted into an open cylinder filled with water, Figure 8:5. This assembly works like a water seal. If the pressure becomes too high, the air bubbles out of the system, and the patient is protected.

The ventilator described is no imaginary construction. It is similar to the **Engström ventilator**, named after a physician who invented it in the 1950s. This ventilator design was still being used in the 1990s – a long lifetime for a medical device.

The real Engström ventilator differed somewhat from the one we have just described. The tidal volume was adjusted by changing the degree to which the balloon was filled and not as described here by choosing a suitably sized balloon. Further, the design had been adapted for use during surgery, so that oxygen and anaesthetic agents could be mixed into the inhaled air.

Various methods for **humidifying** the air have also been developed. The reason for doing this is that the patient's airways dry out unless the inhaled gas mixture is saturated with water vapour, as happens in the nose in normal breathing, Box 8:1. Nowadays, this is best achieved with a single-use **humidity exchanger**, which is also called an **artificial nose** and consists of a plastic tube filled with a porous substance that has a great capacity to absorb and release water vapour. During expiration,

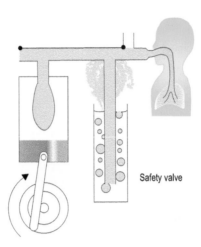

Figure 8:5 The completed ventilator. At positive pressures, air bubbles out via the safety valve and puncture of the lungs is prevented

the moisture in the exhaled air is absorbed by the substance and again released into the fresh dry air at inspiration.

Using disposable materials in a life-support system does carry the risk of manufacturing defects with serious consequences:

CASE 8:1 Manufacturing defect in artificial nose

A patient with respiratory problems after contracting a virus infection involving the neuromuscular system was placed on a ventilator for respiratory support. The ventilator was connected to the patient via a disposable humidity exchanger. But the patient did not receive sufficient ventilation, which was quickly discovered and no damage resulted.

When investigating the cause, a plastic membrane was found in the humidity exchanger connecting tube, which was 1.5 cm wide. The plastic membrane, however, had a hole only 2 mm wide, which of course did not allow enough air to flow through. Similar defects have been reported on other occasions. Cases like these emphasize the importance of carefully testing the function of a ventilator patient circuit before it is connected to a patient.

Various types of ventilators are needed. For short transport of patients, a simple ventilator without advanced functions will suffice. Similarly, a ventilator for home use should be simple to operate, small, lightweight and silent. But for surgery and in intensive care units several special functions are required. Some facts about different types of ventilators are given in Box 8:2.

Fundamentals • Box 8:1

Relative humidity

The capacity of the air to hold water vapour varies greatly with temperature. For example, when we breathe out on a cold winter day, our breath looks like a white cloud. The water vapour in the exhaled air is cooled and condenses, and is transformed from an invisible gas to a cloud of tiny water droplets.

At 25°C, the air can contain only half as much water vapour as at 37°C. A quantity of air that at 25°C is **saturated** and unable to absorb more water has a **relative humidity** of 50% at 37°C. At this temperature, the air can again absorb the same quantity of water if it comes into contact with a moist surface, such as the mucus membranes in the airways. Inhaled air is normally humidified in the nose and the pharynx so that the relative humidity of the air is 100%, i.e., it is saturated by the time it fills the alveoli.

The relative humidity of indoor air normally varies between 30 and 70%. The humidity indoors is usually lower in winter than in summer, as the incoming external fresh air, even if saturated with water vapour at external temperatures, cannot hold as large a quantity of water as is possible during the summer season. When the cold air is heated the relative humidity decreases, despite the fact that the absolute humidity, i.e., the water content per volume unit, for example, expressed in milligrams per litre, is constant.

All medical gases are dry at delivery, i.e., their relative humidity is 0%. This means that the ventilator treatment would dry out the patient's mucus membranes unless water vapour was somehow added. This is not a great problem for short procedures, but for procedures of long duration the gases must be humidified.

The ventilator described above is tidal-volume controlled, which means that at every inspiration, it delivers the volume of the breathing bag, which has been set to correspond to the desired tidal volume. One practical advantage with this ventilator type is that the respiration can be monitored by observing the rhythmic and ventilation-synchronous movements of the breathing bag.

Ventilator use

The rule that staff must always read the **instructions for use** before operating a machine for the first time is particularly applicable to ventilators, as these provide life-support treatment. The general information given here must always be supplemented with the special instructions that accompany

Techniques • Box 8:2

Ventilator types

Ventilators are categorized according to the principle used to interrupt inspiration and start expiration. There are **time-controlled, flow-controlled, pressure-controlled** and **volume-controlled** ventilators. In more advanced designs, the different principles are often combined.

In **time-controlled systems**, the patient is connected via a timing circuit to a propellant gas at appropriate pressure. The timing circuit opens the system to allow momentary gas flow, thereby portioning out the gas in cycles. Since the reduced pressure is constant, it is the timing that primarily determines the tidal volume obtained. Time-controlled ventilators have the disadvantage of being sensitive to pressure changes in the propellant gas. These ventilators are, however, small, light and simple to use, and are often suitable during patient transport.

In **flow-controlled** systems, inspiration is interrupted when a certain preset minimum flow has been achieved – the lower the set minimum flow, the larger the tidal volume. The flow normally decreases as the lungs fill with gas. Purely flow-controlled ventilators were previously used in inhalation therapy, but today this principle is incorporated as a partial feature in more advanced ventilators. The advantage with flow-controlled ventilators is that lung pressures are kept low.

In **pressure-controlled** systems, it is the patient airway resistance that determines when inspiration stops. Pressure-controlled ventilators are technically uncomplicated. The disadvantage, however, is obvious, as the tidal volume will be dependent on the airway resistance of the patient. This ventilator type has been used for inhalation therapy (such as administering bronchial dilators in asthma) and in the treatment of sleep disorders.

Volume-controlled ventilators are functionally superior and are used for more demanding applications. Here, the ventilation may be controlled by tidal volume or minute volume.

The ventilator described above is controlled by tidal volume, which means that at every inspiration, it delivers the breathing bag volume which has been set to correspond to the desired tidal volume. One practical advantage with this ventilator type is that the respiration can be monitored by observing the rhythmic and ventilation-synchronous movements of the breathing bag.

Since the minute volume is the most important physiological factor, **minute-volume-controlled ventilators** have become increasingly more common. This type of ventilator can be given a more compact design than the tidal volume-controlled ventilators, and is easy to use and clean.

Techniques • Box 8:2—Continued

In modern **intensive-care ventilators**, the above principles are combined. These ventilators are used primarily as minute-volume-controlled ventilators, but when required can momentarily be switched to flow- and pressure-controlled ventilation. A control unit calculates the required flow from the minute volume, tidal volume and respiration rate settings.

In the servo ventilator the flows and pressures to and from the patient are continuously monitored by sensors on both the inspiratory and expiratory side. The sensor signals are compared with the ventilator settings. The ventilator instantly corrects any differences between the measured and the preset values, so that the correct flows, pressures and time intervals are maintained at all times. This is done by mechanically reducing the cross-sectional areas of the gas tubes going to and from the patient.

each specific type of ventilator. Before the actual **ventilator treatment** is initiated, all necessary **preparations** must first be carried out.

Preparations

The preparations consist of **assembly, connection** of gas and electricity, **functional testing** and **setting of initial values** for the treatment. The functional test includes, but is not restricted to, ensuring that the displays and gauges for minute volume, tidal volume and airway pressure are at the zero level prior to any connection of gas tubes. The functional test also includes ensuring that the system is **airtight** and that the pressure, volume and flow **alarms** are operational. It is important to detect any leaks. Many accidents have occurred due to leaky systems and because of **accidental disconnections of gas tubes** during treatment that were not discovered in time.

CASE 8:2   Disconnected gas tube leads to irreversible brain damage

A 16-year-old girl fell off a horse and broke her shoulder. During surgery she was connected to an anaesthetic machine with a ventilator. In order to obtain X-ray images of the fracture and for other reasons as well, the ventilator was moved several times during the procedure.

The anaesthetic nurse finished her shift during the course of the operation and was relieved by a colleague. Soon thereafter, the patient's blood pressure dropped and her pulse rate increased. The anaesthetic nurse then tried to increase the oxygen delivery to 100%, but the breathing bag failed to inflate, as a tube between the anaesthetic machine and the ventilator had become disconnected. The patient had in fact received no ventilation at all following the disconnection of the tube.

The patient was treated using the ventilator for 6 hours, but upon recovery from the anaesthesia she could not see properly. Computer tomography demonstrated brain damage in the occipital lobe where the visual centre is located. The patient's condition deteriorated and she became totally paralysed (spastic tetraplegia) and unable to communicate with her surroundings (pharyngeal and bulbar paralysis). All this occurred because of one disconnected tube.

Ventilator treatment

In order to determine the initial ventilator settings, various estimations can be made. One method is to calculate the tidal volume needed from the patient's body weight – approximately 10 ml is needed per kg. For an adult patient, a respiratory rate of approximately 12 breaths per minute is selected. For a patient weighing 60 kg, this results in a minute volume of $10 \times 60 \times 12 = 7200$ ml or 7.2 litres per minute. In practice the ventilation is continuously checked by measuring the exhaled carbon dioxide level by capnography (see below). The anaesthesia might be started giving the 60 kg patient 7 litres per minute. Thereafter, the **respiratory rate** or **tidal volume**, which among other factors is dependent on the patient's age, is set according to

Respiratory rate = (minute volume)/(tidal volume)

Other parameters are initially set at the normal values, often indicated by special markings on the respective scales: **inspiration flow, inspiration/expiration ratio** (usually 1:2) and **upper pressure limit** (the maximum pressure allowed in the airways). Several **alarm limits** are also set to facilitate monitoring.

The patient should be neither over- nor underventilated. To achieve this balance, experience and physiological insight are both required. Underventilation carries the greatest risk, while a certain degree of overventilation is less dangerous. The accidents that happen are most often caused by simple handling errors, which may, however, be disastrous.

CASE 8:3 Anaesthetist forgot to check settings

A patient who had recently undergone heart surgery had to undergo a second procedure because of haemorrhage. The patient was connected to the same ventilator as was used in the intensive care unit. The anaesthetist heard the ventilator running and connected the patient, thinking that the breathing volume settings were the same as before.

During transportation, however, the gas volumes had been reduced to zero. This would normally have been discovered by the alarm going off, had the minimum acceptable expiration volume alarm limit been set. In the hurry triggered by the haemorrhaging, when many other devices, such as ECG, were also being connected, no one remembered to check the alarm limit setting.

The patient developed arrhythmias and sinking blood pressure, which was erroneously diagnosed as being caused by cardiac tamponade, for which he was treated. Only later was it discovered that the ventilator was not ventilating the patient. When the ventilator was reset, the patient quickly regained normal circulation. However, due to the lack of oxygen the patient suffered permanent brain damage.

Treatment with increased airway pressure is, however, also disadvantageous in that it affects the circulation negatively – the increased intrathoracic pressure reduces the venous return to the heart, which in turn reduces the cardiac output.

Types of ventilation support

Modern ventilators can be set to accommodate various breathing patterns. For example, the tidal volume can be set to occasionally generate inspirations of higher than the standard tidal volume. This way a "sigh" is generated, which helps to prevent pulmonary atelectasis from developing.

Pulmonary atelectasis can also be prevented from forming by ensuring that a positive pressure is maintained at the end of the expiration – this method is called **PEEP** (positive end-expiratory pressure). The PEEP level is normally set at a value between 5 and 10 cmH_2O.

During ventilator treatment, the ventilator should not take over more of the respiratory workload than necessary. This is especially important in long-term treatment, where the patient can quickly become dependent on ventilator support to the point where he can no longer do without it. Before a patient can be completely taken off the ventilator support, he must be gradually **weaned** by receiving **pressure support ventilation** only. Here, the ventilator provides increased inspiration pressure only after the patient tries to inhale – the patient "triggers" the pressure support. The added pressure relieves the patient of some of the respiratory workload. During weaning, the pressure setting is successively reduced from about 20 to about 5 cmH_2O.

A special form for ventilatory support is **CPAP** (continuous positive airway pressure). A positive pressure is maintained during both inspiration and expiration with spontaneous breathing. CPAP is used in the treatment of pulmonary oedema and RDS (respiratory distress syndrome), in both children and adults. It is also used to treat sleep apnoea, brief interruptions of breathing during sleep due to excessive snoring. Overweight men are often afflicted by this condition. During sleep, the patient wears a nose mask connected to the CPAP machine, which can be used at home.

When a patient is recovering from general anaesthesia, it is important to use the appropriate amount of ventilatory support, so that the ventilator does not disrupt the patient's spontaneous breathing. Modern ventilators are therefore equipped with a number of functional settings that allow the user to adjust the ventilator support to the needs of the individual patient, Figure 8:6.

The ventilator support ranges from completely controlled ventilation, where the ventilator handles all gas exchange, to spontaneous breathing, where the ventilator for all practical purposes is functionally disconnected, despite being physically connected to the patient. Various settings are thus used depending upon the patient's level of consciousness and general condition.

Compression losses

The volume delivered by the ventilator at each inspiration does not correspond to the actual tidal volume received by the patient. This is due to the gas compression that occurs when the pressure is increased, known as **compression losses**. Another reason for the tidal volume being smaller than the set value is the expansion of the somewhat elastic tubes connecting the patient to the ventilator. These losses must be compensated for. The smaller the patient lung volume and the larger the gas

		Type of ventilation	Abbreviation
PATIENT COMPLETELY AWAKE, BREATHING SPONTANEOUSLY			
	1	Spontaneous breathing	SPONT
	2	Spontaneous breathing with pressure support ventilation	SPONT PRESS SUPPORT CPAP
	3	Spontaneous breathing with synchronised intermittent mandatory ventilation	SIMV SIMV + PRESS SUPPORT
	4a	Assisted controlled mechanical ventilation	ASSISTED CMV
	4b	Controlled mechanical ventilation with sigh	CMV + SIGH
	4c	Controlled mechanical ventilation	CMV VOLUME CONTROL
PATIENT IN DEEP ANAESTHESIA			

Figure 8:6 The level of ventilator support needed depends upon the patient's condition. On the right, examples are given of abbreviations used on two common types of ventilators

volumes in the ventilator and tubes, the greater the relative losses – these factors all need to be taken into consideration when compensating for the losses.

ANAESTHETIC MACHINES

The purpose of an anaesthetic machine is to administer volatile anaesthetics (nitrous oxide or volatile liquid anaesthetics) and oxygen. The anaesthetic machine must also be equipped with a suction system for the removal of excess mucus from the airways.

During anaesthesia, the patient can often carry out the respiratory work himself by **spontaneous ventilation,** and in these cases the anaesthetic machine is employed only to deliver a suitable gas mixture to the patient. But if the patient has received muscle relaxants, which have paralysed the respiratory muscles, or if the patient's spontaneous ventilation has ceased, then **controlled ventilation** must be administered. Ventilators that are equipped to administer various anaesthetic agents are often used. Special anaesthetic machines are also available without the many features of the ventilator.

Anaesthetic systems

An anaesthetic machine consists of a **fresh gas system** that generates an appropriate mixture of nitrous oxide and oxygen. The fresh gases are ordinarily supplied via the hospital central pipeline system and occasionally via gas cylinders. Liquid **anaesthetics** are vaporized in a **vaporizer** and added to the fresh gas. The patient circuit includes a gas reservoir in the form of one or two rubber balloons. These serve two purposes. They ensure a continuous delivery of an appropriate gas mixture and can also be used for controlled ventilation when compressed by the anaesthetist, that is, manual ventilation. The balloon is connected to an **inspiratory tube** that delivers the gas mixture to the patient, either via a mask or more commonly through an endotracheal tube. An **expiratory tube** directs the exhaled gas away from the patient. Depending on the type of anaesthetic system, the exhaled gas can either be eliminated by a scavenging system in the operating room or returned to the gas reservoir.

The gas flow is controlled by valves, so that fresh gas is delivered to the patient and the exhaled gas is eliminated in the correct direction.

Anaesthetic systems can be divided into **non-rebreathing** and **circle-breathing systems.** The latter can be classified as either **partial rebreathing** or **total rebreathing systems.** In the non-rebreathing type, new fresh gas mixture is supplied continuously and the excess gas is eliminated by a scavenging system connected to the operating-room ventilation system, Figure 8:7. The unused gas is directed to a **reservoir tube.** During expiration, the tube becomes partly filled with gas; during inspiration, when no further used gas mixture is added, the tube is emptied by the scavenging

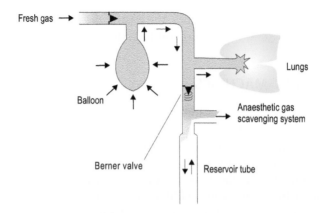

Fresh gas

Lungs

Balloon

Anaesthetic gas
scavenging system

Berner valve

Reservoir tube

Figure 8:7 Gas flow in a non-rebreathing type anaesthetic system. Several essential components, such as the vaporizer, have been left out

system. Since the tube thus acts as a buffer, the required flow in the scavenging system is limited. The reservoir tube must always be open at the free end, so that the scavenging system is prevented from generating a vacuum, which could otherwise affect the anaesthetic machine valve functions.

One disadvantage of non-rebreathing systems is the high gas consumption. The advantage is the ease of use. Non-rebreathing systems are often advantageous when anaesthetizing children.

In **partial rebreathing** systems, the exhaled gas mixture is partially reused, Figure 8:8. A **carbon dioxide absorber** eliminates the carbon dioxide from the exhaled air. The absorber consists of a container with calcium hydroxide, which is converted into calcium carbonate when the carbon dioxide is added. During anaesthesia induction, nitrous oxide and volatile anaesthetics (if they are used) are administered until the required anaesthesia level is reached. When this has been achieved, the primary function of the system is to deliver enough gases for the patient's needs while simultaneously eliminating the exhaled carbon dioxide. The gases are supplied at a slight surplus, to compensate for any leaks. The technique is also called **circle breathing**.

The carbon dioxide absorber function can easily be checked during the anaesthesia, as the absorber generates heat when the carbon dioxide is absorbed.

One advantage with partial rebreathing systems is that the gas consumption remains low. But the savings are only moderate because of the added cost of the carbon dioxide absorber. Another advantage is the fact that the humidity from the respired air is maintained in the circuit, which prevents the airways from drying out. A disadvantage is the more complicated handling.

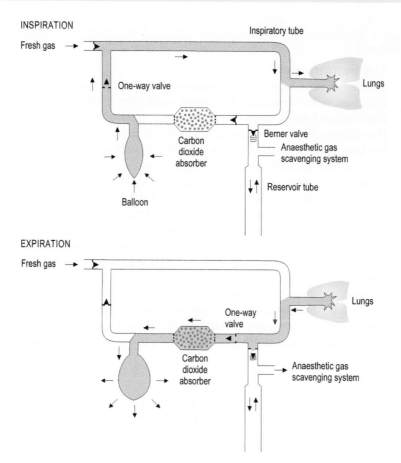

Figure 8:8 Simplified diagram of the gas flow in a circle-breathing anaesthetic system

Total rebreathing anaesthetic systems are being used to an increasing extent. These are similar to the type of system described in Figure 8:8, for partial rebreathing, with the only difference being that they are completely closed. Careful monitoring is essential to ensure that the exact oxygen quantity required is being delivered, once equilibrium has been reached.

To prevent too high a pressure from developing in the anaesthetic machine, the expiratory tube is equipped with a special pressure relief valve, for example, a Berner valve, Box 8:3.

If the patient is not connected to the system via an endotracheal tube, an effective local evacuation system must be used, such as a double mask (Chapter 4).

Risks during anaesthesia

Staff must constantly be aware of the fact that mistakes can occur during anaesthesia (a few cases have already been described above, and more

Techniques • Box 8:3

The Berner valve

The Berner valve is part of the expiration circuit. It serves two purposes: while controlling the patient ventilation, it also handles the elimination of waste gas. A reservoir tube is attached to the outlet of the valve, and acts as a buffer to momentarily store waste anaesthetic gas before it is sucked out by the anaesthetic gas scavenging system.

The Berner valve can be used for both pressure-controlled and volume-controlled ventilation. The valve is shown in Figure 8.9, and a simple schematic describing its function in Figure 8.10. The valve has two valve seats, enabling the valve plate to close in both the lowermost and uppermost positions. It contains two springs, the upper of which is in use during only pressure-controlled ventilation when the pressure on the valve plate can be adjusted by turning the control knob.

The valve has four positions. In the closed position, when the knob is in its lowest position, no waste gas can leave the system, and the valve is closed. This position is used for the tightness check performed prior to anaesthesia initiation. By turning the setting knob,

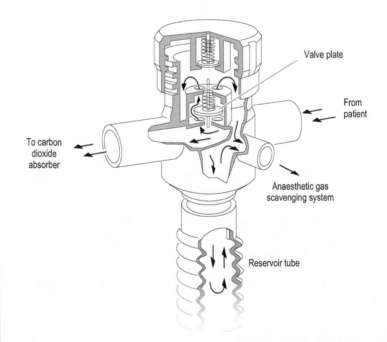

Figure 8:9 The Berner valve. It is set to volume-controlled mechanical ventilation position and illustrates patient expiration

Techniques • Box 8:3—Continued

which is graduated in cmH$_2$O, the desired value at which the valve opens during pressure-controlled ventilation can be set. When the valve knob is opened further the upper spring is disengaged, and the lower spring with the smaller spring tension allows the valve to open with the small pressures caused during spontaneous breathing.

With the valve knob in its fully open position there is no obstruction to the valve plate moving fully with a small pressure rise, which then closes the valve with the valve plate in its upper position. This is used for volume-controlled ventilation so that whenever the pressure rises during ventilation the valve closes and none of the volume to be used for ventilation is lost in the expiration circuit.

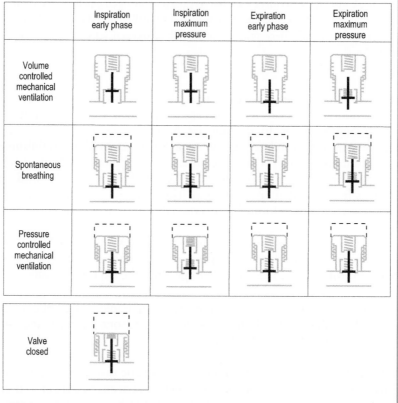

Figure 8.10 The four settings of the Berner valve

instructive cases follow below). **Technical problems** are unfortunately not uncommon. **Mix-up of pipes** in the central gas line systems in hospitals have led to several serious accidents. The most serious situation is of course when no oxygen is supplied from the oxygen outlets. Pipes have in the past repeatedly been mixed up after repairs, resulting in air or nitrous oxide being delivered instead of oxygen:

CASE 8:4 Fatal birthmark cosmetic surgery

A 14-month-old girl was undergoing a laser procedure to lighten a birthmark. It was the first surgery requiring general anaesthesia in a new building.

After the procedure the girl was found to have brain damage. The girl was immediately transported to an adjacent hospital but never recovered and was pronounced dead two days later.

The cause of the accident was that oxygen and nitrogen pipelines had been interchanged. The gas piping system was not labelled and did not follow a common hospital safety practice of installing oxygen sensors in relevant gas lines.

Rigorous administrative routines have therefore been implemented for all installation and repair work on central pipeline systems. The routines vary among countries. In all countries, hospitals need to decide on who holds which responsibilities, and in some this is achieved by establishing a gas committee which is held accountable at that hospital. In the USA, National Fire Protection Association (NFPA) standards require that medical gas lines be checked after installation. The check requires that a "cross-connection test" be performed to ascertain that gas carried in lines matches the labels on the outlets.

However, because of the human factor, mix-ups still happen. Staff must therefore always be ready to supply gas from gas cylinders, in case the desired treatment for obscure reasons fails to produce the expected results.

> **Tip** Never forget that air consists of 21% oxygen (old anaesthetic safety rule). If the gas distribution does not work for one reason or another, then ventilate the patient with air.

As the patient's life may depend on the anaesthetic machine being operational, certain checks must be performed before each anaesthesia induction. The US Food and Drug Administration (FDA) has issued recommendations for checking apparatus, including detailed procedures for the following major steps:

1. Verify that backup ventilation equipment is available and functioning.

2. Check oxygen cylinder supply.

3. Check central pipeline supplies.

4. Check initial status of low-pressure system.

5. Perform leak check of machine low-pressure system.

6. Turn on master machine switch.

7. Test flow meters.

8. Adjust and check scavenging system.

9. Calibrate O_2 monitor.

10. Check initial status of breathing system.

11. Perform leak check of the breathing system.

12. Test ventilation systems and one-way valves.

13. Check, calibrate and/or set alarm limits of all monitors.

14. Check final status of machine.

Most accidents and incidents are caused by **simple handling errors**. Many of these could have been avoided if the above rules had been followed.

CASE 8:5 Six mistakes cause patient's lungs to puncture

A new ventilator design was being tried. The device was connected to the patient, who, however, did not receive any ventilation.

The anaesthetist then opened the oxygen supply to the maximum but there was still no gas flow. A helpful person rushed to the oxygen wall outlet and checked the tube connection. The tube had been incorrectly inserted and after correction, full gas flow was obtained.

The patient's lungs instantly punctured, filling not only the pleural cavity with gas but penetrating the parietal pleura, forcing the gas far into the tissues, reportedly all the way to the rectum. The patient died instantly on the operating table. The new ventilator design included an electrically controlled pressure-limiting valve that could be switched off, rendering this safety feature inoperational. Further, the oxygen valve allowed an unnecessarily high gas flow.

Six mistakes had been perpetrated, and they all contributed and led to the accident. (1) The newly designed ventilator had not been inspected by an independent clinical engineer before it was used for the first time. If such an inspection had been performed, it would have been discovered that both (2) the pressure limiting valve and (3) the oxygen valve were wrongly constructed. Neither (4) the oxygen supply, nor (5) the ventilator function had been tested before patient connection. (6) The medical leadership during the anaesthesia was flawed and probably constituted the main reason for the accident.

Anaesthetic machines have also been influenced by electrical interference (Chapter 3). On one occasion, interference from an electrosurgical unit caused changes in the set volume and pressure. Fortunately, such errors are very rare.

Other serious accidents have occurred when the gas supply for some reason has been disconnected. Dirt in narrow channels of the anaesthetic machine have on occasion caused operational disturbances. Gas leakage or completely disconnected tubes are much more common causes.

An interrupted oxygen supply can be difficult to detect in certain anaesthetic systems equipped with one-way valves in the oxygen tubing. In this design, a tube can actually get disconnected and the user may still continue the manual ventilation, thinking that the oxygen supply is functional. The reason for this is that the patient circuit may appear tight, since the one-way valve prevents the anaesthetic gases from leaving the system via the open oxygen connection. The patient is then ventilated with no oxygen supply whatsoever.

CASE 8:6 Fresh gas connection disconnected

A partial rebreathing system with a carbon dioxide absorber was used during a shoulder operation. A function and tightness check of the anaesthetic system had been performed immediately before the procedure. After a while the nurse discovered that the colour of the patient's face had changed, so she switched to manual ventilation. She attempted to temporarily increase the oxygen supply by "flushing", but since the fresh gas connection had become disconnected, the manual ventilation bag did not expand. Despite this the patient had been ventilated but with continuously decreasing oxygen levels. The patient suffered serious and permanent brain damage.

CASE 8:7 Nurse forgot to plug in the ventilator

A patient, who was to undergo hip surgery, was anaesthetized in the preparation room and moved into the operating room unconscious. At this time, an alarm indicating interrupted central gas supply was activated. In this stressful situation, the anaesthetic nurse responsible for the patient forgot to plug the ventilator into the wall power. The patient, who was without ventilation for 5 to 10 min, died from the resulting brain damage.

Mistakes can also lead to **insufficient anaesthesia**. As the following case shows, this can be hard to detect.

CASE 8:8 Several patients received inadequate anaesthesia

During a major abdominal operation, a patient was ventilated with a ventilator that received its fresh gas supply via a gas mixer. After a while, the pulse rate and blood pressure increased, and the patient displayed signs of inadequate anaesthesia. An arterial blood gas sample was obtained, which indicated that the patient had only received pure oxygen despite the mixer being set to supply a mixture of oxygen and nitrous oxide. The ventilator was replaced and the patient was properly anaesthetized.

During a subsequent study of anaesthesia reports, it was discovered that several patients had "slept badly" during surgery and required unusually large doses of analgesics. In all these cases, the ventilator in question had been used.

The gas mixer was examined at the hospital clinical engineering department (one of the largest departments in the country, connected to a medical school). Black particles were found in the gas mixer. The particles had most probably come from the pipelines from the central gas supply and they had obstructed the nitrous oxide flow.

CASE 8:9 Weeping patient had her eyes taped shut

A 33-year-old woman was to undergo abdominal laparoscopy. After intravenous anaesthetic induction, she was intubated and connected to the anaesthetic machine, which was equipped with a gas analyser for monitoring the anaesthetic concentration.

The attending anaesthetist, who was actually a gynaecology resident and worked at the surgical department only in order to receive supplementary training in anaesthetics, set the anaesthetic vaporizer for delivery of 2% volatile anaesthetics. During the operation, the anaesthetist found that the patient's eyes were open and that she had tears in her eyes. But nobody remembered to examine the pupils (the anaesthesia depth is normally checked by assessing the pupil size). Instead, the eyelids were taped shut. The operation was completed as planned.

Towards the end of the operation, the anaesthetist noticed that the patient was moving her head. He then discovered that the gas analyser indicated 0% anaesthetics, despite the vaporizer being set for delivery of 2%. A new gas analyser was fetched and warmed. When the new gas analyser was to be exchanged for the one presumed defective, the doctor noticed that the vaporizer had never even been connected. The patient had not received any anaesthetic at all, and had been awake the entire time since waking up when the surgeon started carrying out the laparoscopic operation. She had experienced excruciating pain and had heard everything that was being said during the operation.

A similar situation has been described in Case 1:12. Many reports from many countries show that the risk of patients not receiving the intended anaesthetic is substantial. Since muscle-relaxing drugs are administered, the patients are unable to draw attention to the situation. Patients who have experienced such situations often suffer from severe and longstanding anxiety after the operation. Not only are they subjected to unbearable pain, but the fact that the surgeon and other staff chat about matters unrelated to the operation makes the patient worry that proper attention might not be being paid to the surgical procedure.

Hazard communication

Most countries have hazard communication standards or incident reporting, which stipulate that employers in health care facilities must develop, implement and maintain at the workplace a written hazard communication programme. The programme must, among other things, include any operations and equipment in the work area where anaesthetic agents and hazardous chemicals are present.

Also an employee training and information programme must be included involving the physical and health hazards of the chemicals in the work area. Furthermore, the programme must include measures employees can take to protect themselves from hazards, and methods and observations that may be used to detect the presence or release of anaesthetic gases and other hazardous chemicals in the workplace.

OXYGEN TREATMENT

Although oxygen is indeed often administered via a ventilator, the primary objective of ventilator treatment is to relieve the patient of the respiratory workload. But in other situations the patient may be able to breathe spontaneously, but is still suffering from a lack of oxygen.

Need for oxygen treatment

Oxygen treatment is indicated primarily for various lung diseases. We have to distinguish between two patient categories – those with and those without carbon dioxide retention, that is, increased partial pressure of carbon dioxide in arterial blood.

Patients with a long history of respiratory insufficiency develop a tolerance for increased carbon dioxide levels, as the brain's respiratory centre can adapt to increased levels. Respiration in these patients is stimulated by a reduction in the oxygen partial pressure (the hypoxic drive) as opposed to being stimulated by increased carbon dioxide partial pressures (hypercapnic drive), as is the case in normal people. If such patients receive unlimited amounts of oxygen, their respiratory drive will fail, since their respiratory centre will not react to the increased carbon dioxide level in the blood. These patients will instead suffer steadily increasing carbon dioxide retention and may die as a result. In such cases, which are most often caused by chronic obstructive lung disease, oxygen must be administered with great caution. The effect of the treatment must be closely monitored by blood gas analyses, a procedure called **controlled oxygen treatment.**

Examples of conditions with no carbon dioxide retention are pulmonary diffusion defects, pulmonary fibrosis and pulmonary embolism. In such patients, the brain's respiratory centre functions normally and oxygen can be administered without restrictions.

Risks

Pure (100%) oxygen should not be administered indiscriminately, even if the patient's respiratory centre permits it. Because of **free oxygen radicals,** oxygen has damaging effects on the organism. At high concentrations, these may induce various types of cell damage, partly by causing contraction of the arterioles – this might possibly be the body's way of protecting itself against large amounts of free radicals. The arteriole contraction instead paradoxically results in localized oxygen deficiency in the tissues, which can result in permanent damage. Local high concentrations of oxygen can also irritate the mucus membranes in the airways.

CASE 8:10   Bed linen explodes killing patient

A 42-year-old cardiac patient was receiving ventilator treatment, as he also suffered from respiratory failure. The patient suddenly went into cardiac arrest, and resuscitation was initiated. During the resuscitation efforts, the ventilator tube became disconnected and oxygen flowed out and into the bed linen. During defibrillation, the bed linen ignited and an explosive fire erupted that spread to the mattress and completely destroyed the ventilator as well as other items.

The patient died instantly, most probably as a result of the cardiac arrest, which could not be reversed. However, even if the resuscitation efforts had been successful, he would probably still have perished due to extensive burns.

The smoke forced the evacuation of 11 other patients in the same intensive care unit.

The direct cause of the fire was the use of an electrode gel with poor electrical conductivity, resulting in a spark being generated during defibrillation.

Treatment at home

In certain lung diseases, oxygen treatment can contribute to increased life span and enhanced quality of life, provided that it is correctly administered over a long period of time, months or even years. Thus there is good reason to carry out the oxygen treatment in the patient's home. A prerequisite is, however, that the patient is able to accept and understand the treatment, and that the patient or relatives can handle the equipment. Due to the fire hazards, another prerequisite is that smoking is very strongly discouraged and in some countries is not allowed. Treatment at home requires preparations which will vary between countries, but will generally include:

1. The patient and the relatives must be properly informed and instructed.

2. The primary health care provider must be involved.

3. The fire service must be informed.

4. The provider who will be responsible for the gas quality, and who normally handles the delivery of gas cylinders or oxygen concentrators, will be involved at an early stage.

The best alternative is to supply the patient with an oxygen concentrator (Chapter 4). Another alternative is to supply liquid oxygen, which is precooled and stored in an installed thermally insulated storage vessel. Supplying oxygen in gas cylinders is the most expensive alternative. Never underestimate the risks involved in keeping oxygen cylinders at home.

CASE 8:11 Explosive house fire

The fire service was called to an explosive house fire that started when the husband changed oxygen cylinders for his sick wife. Both husband and wife suffered burn injuries – the husband was so severely burned that he died one week later.

The fire service had approved the use of the equipment, which had been installed by the hospital clinical engineering department, and both the patient and the husband had been instructed on equipment handling. They had signed a copy of the handling instruction including the safety rules. The consumption of oxygen was such that the husband had to change cylinders at least once a week for several months – thus he was quite used to handling the cylinders.

Despite all this, on this particular occasion, oxygen had leaked out and ignited flammable materials, seemingly without there being any open flame nearby.

Significant preparatory work is required to carry out long-term treatment at home. It can also be a heavy responsibility for those who are to handle the equipment.

TREATMENT WITH NITRIC OXIDE

An effective measure for improving blood circulation locally is to administer **nitric oxide (NO)**. This is a gas with surprising biological qualities given its simple chemical structure. It is of importance in a large number of processes that involve among other things the body's immune response, learning mechanisms, memory and penile erection.

The circulatory effect of nitric oxide works by dilating the blood vessels, and is used for various lung disorders. The patient inhales the gas, which has immediate effects that can be monitored with a pulse oximeter (see below). The treatment can be life saving and is especially useful for new-borns. Careful dosage and monitoring is important since the gas is also very toxic.

PRESSURE CHAMBER TREATMENT

Oxygen is transported in the blood mainly bound to the haemoglobin in the red blood cells and partly physically dissolved in the plasma. At normal atmospheric pressures, the physically dissolved part is of less importance. But at increased pressures, tissue oxygenation can largely, or even completely, occur via the dissolved oxygen.

The latter phenomenon is utilized in **hyperbaric oxygen (HBO) therapy**. This type of treatment is given in cases of carbon monoxide poisoning (which occurs in fires and in suicide attempts with car exhausts) where the haemoglobin is blocked in such a way that the normal oxygen transport is disrupted. HBO therapy is also used in the treatment of certain infections with anaerobic bacteria (gas gangrene) and for severe crushing injuries with tissue oxygen deficiencies. Another use is for treatment of the bends, or decompression sickness in scuba divers. Then nitrogen gas bubbles form in the tissues and blood vessels when the diver ascends too rapidly to the surface from a great depth (at the increased ambient pressure, large quantities of nitrogen are dissolved in the tissues and are later released in the form of gas bubbles during the ascent).

In all such emergency situations, it is important that the HBO treatment is administered without delay. The patient is placed in a pressure chamber, which is often of the one-person type that can accommodate only one patient in the supine position. In other cases larger chambers may be required, where nursing staff can be present and where there is space for additional equipment, such as a ventilator.

Due to the toxicity of oxygen, the treatment cannot be given for a very long period. Burn patients might be treated three times the first day and thereafter twice daily. Each treatment usually lasts about 90 min. To avoid accidents it is essential that all textiles and other materials do not retain static charge:

A patient with inadequate cerebral blood flow was treated in a hyperbaric chamber. Suddenly the chamber exploded instantly killing the wife. The patient also died later. Three hospital workers were also slightly injured.

Static electricity in a synthetic blanket placed in the chamber was assumed to be the cause of the accident.

Wool and man-made fibres are capable of producing static electricity, whereas pure cotton or linen materials are safe. Conventional dressing materials may be used. But all plastic-based materials must be avoided. Also Vaseline (petroleum jelly) or alcohol-based ointments or lotions are forbidden. Organic dust, lint and fluff are fire hazards, so the chamber interior must be kept exceptionally clean.

INCUBATORS

The use of incubators for the creation of the correct temperature environment has been described above (Chapter 6). Incubators are also used to treat newborn babies with respiratory problems. The fluid balance in such newborns may also be disrupted, which contributes to the drying out of the airways.

Regardless of whether extra oxygen is administered, the incubator must of course be ventilated so that consumed oxygen is replaced and carbon dioxide vented out. A moderate amount of air circulation accomplishes this.

The baby often requires extra oxygen. Oxygen has in the past been given directly into the incubator, but now it is usually supplied with special means such as catheters in the nostrils, a mask for CPAP treatment or an endotracheal tube for respirator treatment.

Oxygen must be administered with caution due to the risk of eye injuries, **retinopathy of prematurity**. High oxygen levels can cause constriction of the immature blood vessels in the retina. This results in an inadequate oxygen supply, which stimulates growth of new vessels as well as fibrous tissue, which protrudes into the vitreous body. Eventually, the baby may go blind. In the 1940s, before these risks were known, more than 10,000 children all over the world went blind due to the treatment of premature babies with oxygen; at the same time, many of course were saved and escaped other injuries. A large number of incorrect treatments using pure oxygen have inadvertently occurred due to gas mixers that were hard to read (see Case 1:13).

The oxygen level has to be carefully balanced. It must be low enough to avoid eye injuries, but high enough for adequate ventilation.

MONITORING

Without the aid of measuring devices, it would be impossible to determine a patient's ventilatory needs. The **blood gas levels** are either measured directly, or indirect readings are obtained of the haemoglobin oxygenation using **pulse oximetry**, and of the exhaled carbon dioxide levels using **capnometry**. Anaesthetic gas analysers provide additional safety during anaesthesia.

Blood gas analysis

The best method is to analyse a sample directly in a **blood gas analyser**. This gives quantitative measurements of the carbon dioxide and oxygen levels as well as the blood pH value. This type of instrument is invaluable in intensive care. The most reliable values are obtained from arterial blood samples, often from the radial artery.

In children, capillary samples may also be used, and can be obtained from the earlobe, fingertip or heel (should be avoided as it is painful) and from the scalp during delivery after rupture of the fetal membrane.

Pulse oximetry

In less critical situations, it suffices to monitor the blood oxygenation by measuring the **oxygen saturation**. This is easily done with a **pulse oximeter**, Figure 8:11. The sensor of the oximeter is simply clipped onto a finger or earlobe. It detects the changing blood volume below the sensor with each heartbeat. Because it can determine blood colour, it is possible to estimate how red or blue the blood is, and hence how much oxygen it contains.

In smokers, this method can, however, give falsely high values. Smokers inhale carbon monoxide, which is then chemically bound to the haemoglobin, but the pulse oximeter cannot differentiate between oxyhaemoglobin and carboxyhaemoglobin. Readings obtained from heavy

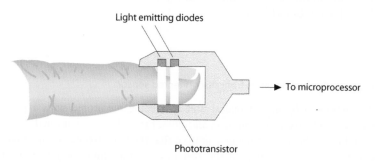

Figure 8:11 Pulse oximeter sensor

smokers may therefore erroneously be interpreted as normal. In cases of carbon monoxide poisoning (smoke inhalation accidents) the method cannot be used at all. Nail polish can eliminate the signal if of a colour that absorbs the light. A low haematocrit can also contribute to inaccurate readings.

Similarly, if the peripheral circulation is severely impaired and the sensor has been placed on the finger, the method will not work. In such a situation placing the sensor on the earlobe or the nose may be attempted.

The pulse oximeter may also malfunction due to entirely **technical reasons**. Some devices have actually indicated a seemingly normal oxygen saturation value as well as pulse rate even after the sensor has been disconnected from the patient, Box 8:4.

 Techniques • Box 8:4

Pulse oximeter

The pulse oximeter sensor consists of a measuring clip, Figure 8:11. The patient's earlobe or fingertip is placed between the two clip jaws. One jaw contains two LEDs, which emit light at two wavelengths (often 660 and 940 nm). The other jaw contains a phototransistor that measures the intensity of the two transmitted wavelengths. As the haemoglobin colour varies with the oxygen saturation, the phototransistor signals will vary with the saturation level. With the help of a microprocessor and by utilizing empirical relationships, the oxygen saturation percentage can be calculated.

The pulse rate is obtained simultaneously, since the light transmission for the two wavelengths varies with the amount of blood present in the tissues.

Certain pulse oximeters may show "normal" values even when the sensors are not placed on a patient. The reason for this phenomenon might be that sensor and room light interfere with each other, resulting in the device misinterpreting the signal as one generated by pulsating blood flow.

CASE 8:13 Normal readings from disconnected sensor

A newborn baby in a neonatal unit was being monitored with a pulse oximeter. The oxygen saturation and pulse rate values were normal.

Suddenly, the paediatric nurse noticed that the pulse oximeter sensor had come off and was lying on the bed next to the child. Despite this, it continued to give normal readings.

In this case luckily no accident happened, but falsely normal values could of course have delayed the initiation of appropriate treatment had the child's condition deteriorated.

 Protect the pulse oximeter sensor from fluorescent tube light. Check that it is correctly applied to the patient.

The convenience of pulse oximetry makes it an extremely valuable tool in routine monitoring, for example, during and after surgery and for continuous monitoring in intensive care. The method is also used as a supplement to transcutaneous blood gas monitoring in children.

Transcutaneous blood gas monitoring

In some cases, blood gases can be analysed by sensors placed on the skin. The method is based on the fact that the corneal layer of the epidermis is permeable to oxygen and carbon dioxide, and that the skin's top layer consists of dead tissue and thus gas levels do not change during diffusion through the skin.

A round sensor unit about a centimetre in size, with an integrated electrical heating element, is placed on the skin. The skin is warmed to 43–44°C, which results in hyperaemia in the underlying tissues, thus facilitating the diffusion of oxygen and carbon dioxide from the capillary blood through the corneal layer of the epidermis to the sensor. In the sensor, the oxygen partial pressure is measured using a Clark electrode. For analysing the carbon dioxide partial pressure, a Severinghaus electrode is normally used (here, the carbon dioxide pressure changes the pH value of a buffer, which is measured with a glass electrode). The method is useful for monitoring relative blood gas changes in children, who have thin skin; the method can be unreliable in adults.

Capnography

By continuously monitoring the exhaled carbon dioxide levels, the patient's respiratory status can be assessed. Gas is suctioned, **sampled** and the concentration measured during the respiratory cycle. During inspiration the concentration is low, and thereafter it increases, reaching its maximum value at the end of expiration, the **end tidal concentration**. For patients with healthy lungs, this value gives a good indication of the blood carbon dioxide level.

The method is of great practical value, as it very quickly indicates whether or not the ventilation is sufficient. Very importantly, the method also provides an immediate indication of whether the tracheal tube in intubated patients is positioned in the trachea or in the oesophagus. Every year patients die due to incorrect intubation, and these deaths could be prevented by routine capnography.

Capnometers have alarms that are triggered when the carbon dioxide level is too high or too low.

Monitoring during anaesthesia

Many guidelines for the monitoring of patients have been suggested. The one below comprises the basics. During anaesthesia, monitoring must be carried out using devices including, but not limited to:

1. Oxygen monitor, the sensor of which is, for example, placed in the patient inspiratory tube.

2. Anaesthetic gas analyser.

3. Volumeter for checking exhaled gas volume.

4. Capnometer.

5. Pulse oximeter.

6. Continuous ECG monitor.

7. Body thermometer for long procedures.

8. Alarms for high pressure in the ventilatory system, low oxygen levels, low expiration volumes, and for low blood oxygen saturation levels.

The value of monitoring

The accidents described above are typical cases that have unfortunately been repeated on several occasions in many countries. Thanks to the increasing use of technical monitoring devices, such as analysers for oxygen, carbon dioxide and anaesthetic agents in anaesthetic machines, safety has gradually improved. Capnography is one of the most important monitoring methods, since it provides a direct measure of how efficiently the ventilation is able to eliminate carbon dioxide.

Pulse oximetry, which provides information about oxygen saturation and pulse rate, is widely used for continuous monitoring of the patient's respiratory status. And the ECG is still of fundamental value for monitoring the function of the heart. Together the two methods complement each other, and among other things enable staff to check that the pulse oximeter is operating correctly – the pulse rate should of course correspond between the two methods; if this is not the case, this is an indication that there could be a problem with the pulse oximeter.

Fatalities because of anaesthetic accidents have gradually decreased to less than one death in 100,000 operations. By careful use of modern technology and the lessons learned from previously common accidents, this number could be reduced even further.

9

Parenteral administration of drugs

It is often necessary to give fluids and drugs **parenterally**, in ways other than via the gastrointestinal tract. The most common method is to give an **intravenous infusion**, but solutions consisting of low-molecular-weight substances may also be injected subcutaneously. Occasionally, the infusion is given **intra-arterially** in order to deliver chemotherapeutic drugs to a certain organ with a tumour. **Intraperitoneal administration** may be of value, as the substances are ultimately delivered to the portal vein, thereby reaching the liver, which is the normal route for substances absorbed by the intestines. In cases of chronic pain in the lower parts of the body, morphine can be delivered through an **epidural** catheter, which is placed outside the dura mater – the dense membrane that protects the spinal cord, adjacent to the spinal nerves that conduct the pain impulses to the brain. Such analgesics may also be injected **intrathecally**, via a catheter inserted through the dura.

Various methods will be described that are needed to meet different requirements. First, common infusion methods are covered when **infusion sets**, various types of **infusion rate regulators** and **infusion pumps** are used. Then more specialized **implantable devices** will be explained, which have been developed to facilitate repeated intravenous injections and also to enable long-term treatment of patients.

Parenteral administration of drugs always involves certain **risks** mainly for the patients, but to some extent also for the nurses when handling certain drugs and treating infected patients.

Risk for hospital staff

Some modern drugs require particular caution when used. Thus most cytotoxic drugs are particularly dangerous and necessitate special equipment and procedures. Closed systems have been developed that effectively prevent anyone from coming in contact with the drugs when brought from the pharmacy to the patient. Yet during the infusion of such drugs protective clothing and goggles are needed, since connections might leak and tubes might burst because of wrong handling, as will be described.

A major health issue is to avoid catching an **infection** from the patients. This is particularly important for potentially fatal diseases such as AIDS and hepatitis. Several such lethal infections have been caused by accidental puncture of the skin by syringe needle. Special designs have therefore been developed to minimize this risk. Unfortunately, some such "safe" designs have proved not to be safe when standard syringes have been combined with an attachment that folds around the needle after the injection. A better design is where the needle, when the injection has been completed, withdraws into a specially designed syringe. The use of such advanced syringes is preferable, and likely reduces total expenses even though initially somewhat costlier – each prevention of an infection is a considerable financial saving and, more importantly, may save a life.

Medical requirements

Infusion therapy is especially important in **intensive care,** where it is most commonly used to maintain an appropriate fluid balance after major surgery, in severe burn cases and for treating dehydrated children who cannot be made to take fluids by mouth.

An infusion system must be able to handle various solutions, such as those containing electrolytes and glucose, lipid emulsions and blood. It must also be possible to set the amount of solution to be infused, as well as the infusion rate. Moreover, it is of fundamental importance that air is prevented from entering the solutions, as this could otherwise cause air embolism. Of course, the solutions must be clean, sterile and free of foreign particles, as well as prevented from being mixed up with other types of liquids.

CASE 9:1 Gastroenteral feeding formula given intravenously

Patients who have become debilitated, for example, by a major surgical procedure, are often too weak to eat normally, and therefore receive nutrition by means of a tube that is inserted through the nose and reaches down to the stomach (nasogastric tube). Nutritive solutions can also be administered by intravenous infusions, often by drip infusions. The compounds supplied by these two different routes naturally differ greatly from one another – those given intravenously must consist of substances that are already broken down in the way they would have been had they been absorbed via the gastrointestinal tract. The feeding formulas given via the nasogastric tube may consist of ordinary liquid foods.

A nurse assistant accidentally mixed up the tubes in such a way that the tube intended for the nasogastric feeding instead was connected to the intravenous cannula. The patient went into shock and respiratory distress, but recovered after ventilator treatment. Because of this accident, feeding tubes are now fitted with connectors that cannot be connected to intravenous cannulae (compare Case 1:5).

Unfortunately, however, there are no technical solutions that can prevent the mix-up of several infusion catheters in the same patient:

CASE 9:2 Fatal mix-up of three-way stopcocks

A 62-year-old woman, being treated for pain because of breast cancer metastases, suffered a complication in the form of bacterial meningitis. She had two catheters inserted, one that was connected to a subcutaneous infusion port (see below) for administration of fluids and medications, and one that was placed in the spinal canal for intraspinal administration of morphine with an infusion pump. Both catheters were fitted with three-way stopcocks.

A nurse, who was going to give a penicillin infusion to the patient, placed a clamp on the glucose infusion tubing and turned the three-way stopcock to stop the glucose infusion. She then connected the penicillin infusion set.

Half an hour later, the nurse discovered that the infusion pump was no longer working, and realized that she had inadvertently also turned the infusion pump three-way stopcock in addition to the glucose infusion stopcock. She also realized that she had injected the penicillin into the wrong catheter. The nurse had cared for this patient before, and had not understood that the infusion pump had also been fitted with a three-way stopcock, which explained the mix-up. The patient had been lying in the supine position with her gown buttoned only half-way, thereby hiding the catheter going to the subcutaneous infusion port from the nurse's view.

The patient suffered generalized seizures and was transferred to the intensive care unit where she was treated with general anaesthesia and artificial ventilation. She died four days later, never having regained consciousness. Penicillin is extremely toxic to the central nervous system.

There are no types of catheter or tubing connections that have never been mixed up with catastrophic results.

Whenever you are going to give an infusion to a patient equipped with more than one catheter, always ensure that you are using the correct route by tracing the catheter to its port of entry to the patient.

Patients can sometimes do the most unimaginable things:

CASE 9:3 Elderly patient connects oxygen to infusion tubing

An 83-year-old man had received an intravenous infusion in connection with a surgical procedure, and had been returned to the surgical ward.

The patient was later found dead in his bed, with the nasal oxygen tubing connected to a Y-connector attached to the infusion set. The infusion fluid had drained into the bed. It appeared that the infusion tubing had become disconnected from the Y-connector, and the elderly patient had himself inadvertently connected the oxygen tubing instead of the infusion tubing, which both unfortunately were of the same diameter.

At autopsy, death was shown to have been caused by emboli, gas bubbles in the blood vessels, which had blocked the blood circulation.

The requirement for **infusion rate accuracy** varies considerably, depending on the type of infusion. During a blood transfusion, the rate is not crucial unless the patient is in shock. But in many situations greater accuracy is required than can be achieved with an ordinary infusion set. Then some form for active control of the amount of substance given per time unit is needed. This is, for example, necessary when supplying heparin for anticoagulation, or vasopressors and inotropes in cardiac failure to maintain blood pressure, or oxytocin for stimulation of uterine contractions during labour. In underdeveloped infants, extremely small volumes are given each hour, and here exceptional accuracy is required, especially at low flow rates.

As emphasized in Chapter 5, it is necessary to be cautious when assessing the accuracy ratings provided by the manufacturers. This is especially true for infusion pumps delivering low infusion rates. In one investigation of devices from five different manufacturers, it was shown that the stated measurement uncertainty of ±5% was correct as long as the flow rates remained between 5 and 10 ml/hour. But at a setting of 1 ml/hour, flows of only 0.65 to 0.90 ml/hour were obtained, thus rates for the five pumps were between 35% and 10% lower than the rate set.

It is also well known that the infusion rate can differ greatly during an ongoing infusion and thus cause fluctuations in the patient's condition, such as varying blood pressure during vasopressor or inotrope infusions.

INFUSION SETS

A simple **infusion set** consists of an **fluid container**, most often in the form of a pliable plastic bag, a **drip chamber** where the drip rate can be observed, a **roller clamp (tubing clamp)** that is used to adjust the drip rate, and an **infusion cannula**, most often inserted into a vein, Figure 9:1. The container is hung 0.5 to 1 metre above the patient, and the fluid flows through gravity infusion into the patient.

There are many advantages with this simple type of set. It is easy to handle and also inexpensive. It carries little risk for the patient, especially when the fluid container consists of a pliable plastic bag and the roller clamp is placed at a low level, close to the IV cannula.

The risks that do exist are due to the possibility of air entering the vascular system, thereby causing air emboli. This risk exists in particular when using rigid containers made of glass or plastic, for example, for infusion of certain drugs, Figure 9:2. When the fluid is emptied from such a rigid container, it is replaced by air, which enters the bottle via a special tube running through the bottle rubber stopper. The tube diameter must be large enough to prevent a vacuum from forming when the fluid is emptied from the bottle. If there is negative pressure, air may be sucked into the tubing via a set connection that is not tight. This does not

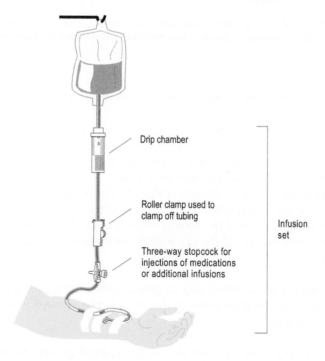

Drip chamber

Roller clamp used to
clamp off tubing

Three-way stopcock for
injections of medications
or additional infusions

Infusion
set

Figure 9:1 Gravity infusion of fluids

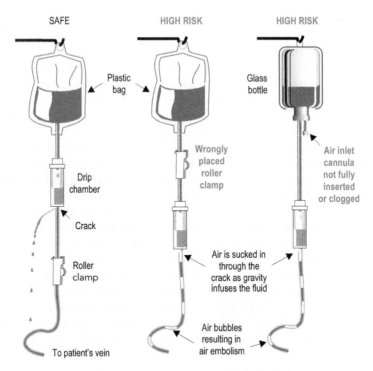

SAFE   **HIGH RISK**   **HIGH RISK**

Plastic bag

Glass bottle

Drip chamber

Wrongly placed roller clamp

Air inlet cannula not fully inserted or clogged

Crack

Roller clamp

Air is sucked in through the crack as gravity infuses the fluid

To patient's vein

Air bubbles resulting in air embolism

Figure 9:2 Manufacturing errors or improper handling of infusion sets may result in cracks. It is of fundamental importance that the risks involved are fully understood

happen when using soft plastic containers, as these containers collapse as they empty.

All types of container, however, carry a certain risk of air embolism if the tubing clamp is placed high up on the tubing and the drip rate is low. In this situation, a vacuum may be created in the tubing segment below the clamp, thus allowing air to be sucked in.

The first sign of air embolism is that the patient gets dyspnoea. The air bubbles are transported to the lungs where they will block the passage of blood around the alveoli because of the high surface tension between blood and air. If the cause of the embolism is not discovered it is lethal.

Tip Gravity is an excellent way to give patients liquids, since normally there is no risk of air entering the veins. But be aware, if you err even gravity kills.

Drip chambers are often equipped with filters, which prevent any particulate matter from entering the patient along with the fluid, Figure 9:3. Blood transfusion filters are larger.

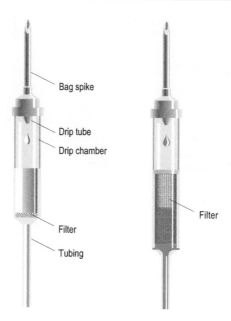

Figure 9:3 Drip chamber for gravity infusion of solutions (left) and blood (right)

For treatment of shock or serious haemorrhaging, a **high-pressure infusion** may be given. This can be achieved by placing the plastic infusion fluid container in a high-pressure cuff, which is similar to a blood pressure cuff. The cuff is connected to a pressure regulator that maintains a certain preset pressure during the entire infusion.

For blood transfusions, it is often desirable to prewarm the blood. A **blood warmer (haemowarmer)** can be used. This device may consist of two thermostat-controlled metal plates between which the blood bag is placed, so that the blood is warmed before it leaves the bag. Another design consists of a cylindrical, thermostat-controlled housing with a spiral-shaped groove into which the infusion plastic tubing is threaded so that it describes three to six turns, Figure 9:4. The blood is warmed as it passes through the tubing in contact with the warmer. There are many other types as well, such as those where a coil of the tubing is immersed in a temperature-controlled water bath, and another where the blood is led through a pre-sterilized stainless-steel tube inserted in a battery-driven thermostat-controlled device suitable for transport of critically ill patients.

There have been many accidents with blood warmers of faulty design, which have caused excessive warming of the blood, above 40°C, causing haemolysis of the red cells. For this reason, all blood warmers must now be furnished with an independent safety circuit in addition to the main thermostat circuit, which is activated if high temperatures are reached. The user must, however, always remain vigilant and keep in mind that errors do occur in safety circuits. It is a good idea to check the tempera-

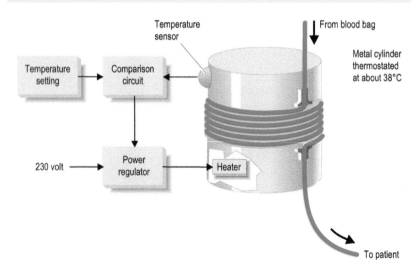

Figure 9:4 One type of blood warmer

ture by simply touching the bag or the tubing with the outer surface of the fingers (where the temperature sensitivity is better than on the inner surface).

Blood warmers do not provide entirely ideal warming of the blood, as the blood cools off in the tubing on its passage from the warmer to the intravenous cannula.

There are rigorous regulations aimed at avoiding transfusion with an incorrect blood group. In spite of this, mistakes still happen:

CASE 9:4 Nurse gives wrong blood group

A 66-year-old woman with advanced cancer was to receive a blood trans-fusion. A nurse went to the hospital blood bank to bring the blood bag. A colleague had asked her to also bring another blood bag that was intended for another patient.

When she returned to the ward, she placed the bags along with the blood group reports in the nurse's office. Half an hour later, she took one of the bags and one of the reports and went in to the patient. She checked that the name on the report matched the name of the patient and the name in the patient medical record. Thereafter she connected the transfusion set to an existing catheter and started the transfusion.

Ten minutes later, the patient complained that she was feeling cold, and the nurse covered her with two blankets. Five minutes later, the patient rang the bell, and told the nurse that she had pain in the lower back. The nurse then gave the patient a morphine injection and a morphine tablet and went back to her office. There she met her colleague, who told her that she could not find the blood bag that she had asked the nurse to fetch for the other patient. At that point, the nurse realized that she had given the patient the wrong blood. She went to the patient and stopped the transfusion. A total of 100 ml blood had been transfused. Thereafter she gave the correct blood to the patient.

The patient was transferred to an intensive care unit and was released after five days. She died one month later from her cancer.

The nurse had committed a number of errors. (1) She had not checked that the blood group printed on the blood bag matched the blood group listed in the patient's medical records. (2) She had not reacted when she pasted the check label from the blood bag, which was red, into the patient's medical record, where other check labels of green colour had already been pasted from previous transfusions. (3) She should have stopped the transfusion immediately when the patient displayed the symptoms of shivering and lower back pain, which are the classic symptoms of transfusion with the wrong blood group. (4) It was a mistake to give the patient morphine, without first checking whether the symptoms might be caused by something other than the underlying disease. (5) It was a mistake to start administering the correct transfusion without first having notified the physician in charge.

Following the second transfusion, the nurse tried to cover the erroneous red label from the wrong blood bag in the patient medical record with the green label from the correct blood bag, in order to cover up her mistake. This action was considered especially serious.

DROP COUNTERS

The original type of drop counter is rarely used today because of its poor accuracy. But its principle is still described here, as it is sometimes combined with infusion pumps for added safety. The drip rate in an infusion set is controlled by a regulator, as shown in Figure 9:5. Each drop is detected optically when it passes the drip chamber, and an electronic control circuit activates a valve mechanism that pinches the tubing so that the set drip rate is achieved.

The low accuracy of the drop counters is due to several factors. Even if these work perfectly and deliver the exact set drip rate, the amount delivered per unit of time may still vary by more than ±20%. This is due to the fact that the droplet size is affected by several factors. Of importance is the surface tension, which may vary greatly with minute amounts of certain substances, temperature, viscosity and drip rate – the higher the drip rate the larger the droplet. Therefore, drop counters cannot be used if accurate infusion rates are needed.

Another problem with drop counters is that the fluid level in the drip chamber may become too high, resulting in the detector being occluded and unable to detect each droplet. The drip chamber may also be hanging at an angle, thus enabling droplets to pass through without being

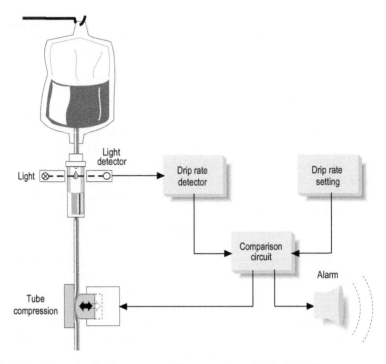

Figure 9:5 Principle of a drop counter. The comparison circuit checks for any difference between the preset and the detected drip rate. If there is a difference, the pressure exerted on the tubing is immediately and automatically adjusted, so that the intended drip rate is restored

counted. Splattered fluid can also obstruct the light pathway through the chamber and thus prevent the counter from functioning correctly.

CASE 9:5 Patient received four times the prescribed dose

A patient was being treated for a suspected pulmonary embolism with an infusion containing 10,000 IU heparin in 500 ml fluid, with a drip rate of 14 drops/minute. It was calculated that this infusion would last about 12 hours. After three hours, however, the entire infusion had been delivered. The counter alarm had not gone off, which should have happened whenever the drip rate was incorrect.

No fault could be found with the drop counter. Most likely the drip chamber had been hung up at an angle or the drip detector had been positioned wrongly.

Although drop counters have several advantages, one of them being the small risk of air embolism (infusion stops when the fluid cannot flow with gravity), the disadvantages dominate. Therefore, these devices are nowadays being replaced by various types of infusion pump.

INFUSION PUMPS

Peristaltic pumps

A common way to regulate the infusion rate accurately is by means of a peristaltic pump. These can be of the **linear peristaltic** or **rotating peristaltic** type. The maximum infusion rate error with these pumps is often as low as ±5%.

For linear peristaltic pumps, the infusion tubing is inserted into a channel where a number of peristaltic fingers compress the tubing in a wave-like motion, Figure 9:6. In rotating peristaltic pumps, the tubing is instead compressed by two or more rotating rollers. The desired infusion rate and total volume can be preset. A disadvantage of older pumps of the linear type is that the fluid flows freely into the patient if the tube is not clamped, such as when the door is opened. Pumps of newer design prevent this by blocking the flow. Other pumps use tubing sets where the flow is stopped as soon as the set is removed from the pump. To further increase safety, modern pumps issue audible alarms for:

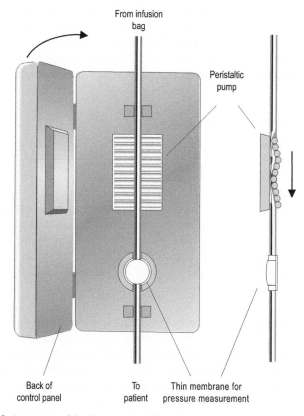

Figure 9:6 Infusion pump of the linear peristaltic type

- low battery voltage
- open door
- air bubbles in tubing
- closed clamp
- stopped infusion
- completed infusion
- empty bottle/bag
- internal error

When the preset infusion volume has been delivered, modern peristaltic pumps continue to infuse the solution at a very low flow rate, 1 to 3 ml/hour for adults and 0.1 to 0.3 ml/hour for children. This is to prevent the formation of blood clots that would otherwise cause obstruction in the infusion cannula or the vein, a procedure often referred to as KVO – keep veins open.

Some designs use an extremely sensitive transducer that continuously monitors the infusion tubing pressure. This provides two advantages: alarms may be triggered early if infusion stops, and the central venous pressure can be measured provided that the infusion tubing is connected to a catheter placed in the vena cava. Peristaltic pumps without pressure guards can cause unexpected complications if used incorrectly:

CASE 9:6 Burst infusion tubing

Two infusion pumps were connected to the same patient, with the two tubing sets connected to the same three-way stopcock. Both pumps were running. After a short while, one of the tubes burst.

A three-way stopcock can only admit fluid from one of two possible directions, and therefore the flow in one of the two tubes was completely blocked. In this case, the pump was connected to the tube that was connected to the closed stopcock port. As the infusion set was not equipped with any pressure guard, the pump kept on running in spite of the fact that no flow was possible. The tube simply kept on expanding until it finally burst.

The most common method to detect air bubbles in the infusion tubing is by an optical device; the disadvantage is that such designs work poorly with opaque fluids such as blood and lipid emulsions. A better method has detectors that are based on ultrasound detection of bubbles, with air reflecting the ultrasound. These detectors are, however, more complex in design.

CASE 9:7   Infant dies from air embolism

An infant was receiving an intravenous feeding solution. When the solution had been used up, the device did not trigger the alarm, but it continued to pump air into a catheter that had been placed in the vena cava. The baby died.

During the subsequent investigation at the clinical engineering department, no technical fault with the device could be found. But it was discovered that this device, as well as others of the same type, did not work correctly with the particular kind of solution used. The solution was too opaque, and it also formed a foam when the solution was used up. This was the reason why the air detector had not worked.

In the instructions for use for the device, it was stated that at least 5 ml solution must remain in it when the treatment is completed. This accident was thus caused by two major errors – unsatisfactory treatment monitoring and the wrong device having been selected for this kind of treatment.

Infusion sets of the wrong type are sometimes used. They are not keyed like pin-indexed gas connections. It is the user's responsibility to choose the correct infusion set:

CASE 9:8   Premature baby receives overdose

A premature baby was being treated with an intravenous infusion. The dose required was 120 ml/24 hours, and the infusion pump was set at a rate of 5 ml/hour. After a couple of hours the paediatric nurse discovered that the 200 ml infusion bag was almost empty. The infusion pump had seemed to function normally during the treatment.

The reason for the incorrect dose was that an infusion set of the wrong brand had been used. This brand had been stored alongside those of the specialized sets intended for this particular pump. The staff had been aware of the risk of confusion as the sets looked deceptively alike, but in spite of this the accident still happened. Luckily, the baby was not seriously affected by the accident.

Staff must always be aware of the risk of faults due to wear and tear. A common fault with linear peristaltic pumps is that the pressure plate mechanism that presses the tubing against the rollers is worn out, causing fluid in the tubing to leak past the fingers. Leakage can also occur when the door on which the pressure plate is mounted is not properly closed, and in such situations gravity may cause large volumes of infusion fluids to flow rapidly into the patient.

CASE 9:9 Incorrectly mounted infusion tubing

An infusion was started with the rate of 16 ml/hour, and the maximum infusion volume set at 235 ml.

During a check more than 7 hours later, everything was functioning normally and it was noted that 130 ml solution remained. Half an hour later, however, the bottle was found to be empty. The total volume listed on the infusion pump was 140 ml, which is less than what the bottle had contained originally. Thus 95 ml had been delivered without being recorded.

The clinical engineer found that the infusion tubing was placed in a loop towards the hinge side. When mounted this way, no resistance to the flow was provided although the door had been closed. The fluid had thus been able to flow freely into the patient.

A contributing factor to the incident was that for unknown reasons, the tubing was abnormally pliable to the extent that it easily ended up in a bent position. There was also some play in the hinge of the pressure plate that provides counter-pressure for the peristaltic rollers, and therefore the plate did not provide enough pressure on the tubing at the hinge side.

Peristaltic pumps have the advantage of being easy to handle and relatively inexpensive to run. But they do carry a risk of air embolism when the safety systems are malfunctioning.

Syringe pumps

Sometimes the requirement for accuracy in drug administration is exceptionally high. For example, the amount of vasopressors or inotropes used to normalize the blood pressure in shock treatment must be very carefully adjusted. In such cases, a syringe pump ("power pump") is used, Figure 9:7. The flow rate may be varied within a very broad range, such as 0.1 to 150 ml/hour. The maximum error is often less than ±3%.

Syringe pumps are accurate, compact and carry little risk of air embolism. They must, however, be used with prudence:

CASE 9:10 Girl receives multiple dose

A young girl suffering from asthma was to receive a theophylline infusion delivered by a syringe pump. As there were air bubbles in the tubing, the nurse increased the pump infusion rate to the maximum in order to get rid of the air bubbles. She then connected the infusion tubing to the IV cannula and started the pump.

The nurse had, however, forgotten to reset the pump infusion rate, and 27 ml were delivered to the patient before she realized her mistake. The patient had received a dose of 800 mg, which should normally have been

distributed over at least two hours. The girl displayed symptoms of intoxi-
cation, but her condition stabilized after treatment in the intensive care unit.
Wrong handling of the pump caused the incident.

The syringe in this type of pump must be properly secured, Figure 9:8. If
there is play between the syringe barrel and/or plunger and the pump
mechanical parts, this can lead to a sudden infusion of an unintended
bolus dose, as well as overlong periods where no medication is delivered
at all.

If the pump is positioned at a level higher than the patient when the
stopcock is opened, gravity will suck the plunger into the syringe barrel
if not properly secured. Some of the fluid in the tubing will then be
delivered suddenly to the patient as a bolus dose, with the accompanying
risk of an overdose, especially in children.

If the pump is instead positioned at a level lower than the patient,
gravity will act in the opposite direction. This results in a positive
pressure build-up in the syringe, which pushes the plunger away from the
main body of the syringe barrel. In this situation, the patient will not
receive any medication at all until the pump has moved far enough to
compensate for the play. With low flow rates, this delay may last an hour
or more.

SAFETY ASPECTS

Risk of interference

In all types of infusion systems where microprocessors are used, there
is a risk of operational interference caused by devices such as surgical
diathermy units and mobile telephones (Chapter 3), which may, for

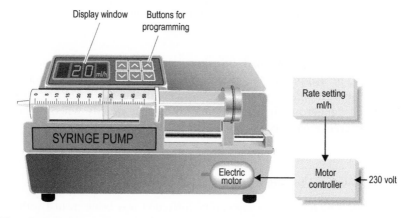

Figure 9:7 Syringe pump

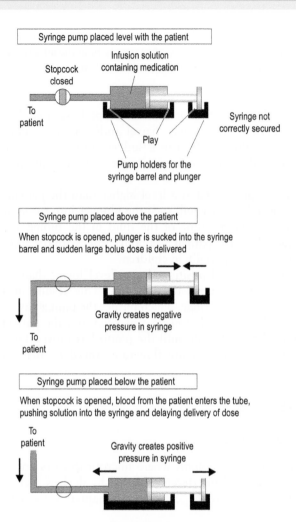

Figure 9:8 If there is play between the syringe pump and the syringe the delivered dose can be lower or higher than intended depending on level of pump

example, cause unexplained infusion interruptions or infusion rate increases. The distance to the interfering device has often been just a few meters, but with older-type telephones much greater distances have been considered dangerous. It is impossible to predict exactly when or how such interference will occur.

CASE 9:11 Infusion to cardiac patient suddenly interrupted

A patient suffering from a myocardial infarction was being treated with vasopressors delivered by a cassette pump in the intensive care unit. On several occasions, the pump suddenly stopped running without triggering the alarm. The pump was replaced with another pump of the same make and type, but despite this, the problem persisted. Clinical engineers immediately suspected that electrical interference was causing the malfunction.

When investigating the activities in nearby rooms, it was found that a patient on the floor above had started using a cellular phone of the older analogue type, which emits much stronger electromagnetic fields than modern types. No technical faults were found in the two cassette pumps.

Electrical interference of different types can also cause problems:

CASE 9:12 Infusion pump runs amok

While a patient's bed was being made, a static discharge occurred between the bed and the assistant nurse, who was wearing clothes made of synthetic fabric. Immediately, the battery-operated infusion pump connected to the patient exhibited several malfunctions. It triggered a continuous alarm consisting of short signal bursts, the valve motor ran uninterruptedly and the pump roller stopped. The pump could not be turned off.

The alarm ceased only after the pump had been disassembled and the battery removed. When the battery was again inserted, the pump operated normally again. This demonstrates the weakness with modern electronic devices, which may react completely unpredictably when subjected to electrical interference.

CASE 9:13 Batteries must be charged

An infusion pump, which could be powered either by the power lines or by an internal battery, suddenly stopped working without warning while running on the battery. The pump was immediately connected to the power lines, but still refused to resume operation. A functions check revealed that the battery was discharged, even though the battery charging functioned as expected. But when switching from battery to power lines, the pump needed to be restarted, and during the course of the incident, this had been overlooked.

Someone had probably put the device into storage without first recharging the battery. The pump then functioned only as long as the remaining charge lasted.

Tip Depleted batteries held in store can appear to function correctly for a short time. If a device with batteries has been held in store for some time, check the device again after it has been in use for a short time. Always be prepared to switch to power lines.

Delays

One disadvantage with infusion pumps is that it may take a relatively long time for the drug to pass through the tubing or catheter and into the patient's bloodstream. This may be true both when using an ordinary intravenous cannula and to an even greater extent when using a central venous catheter; in the latter case, at an infusion rate of 2 ml/hour, it can take about 10 minutes for the solution to get through. If a three-way stopcock is connected to the tubing system (for example, in order to be able to measure the central venous pressure with a catheter, Chapter 6) the increased total system volume may increase the time required to 15 minutes.

In emergency situations such as cardiac failure, this delay constitutes a major drawback, as it is necessary to rapidly inject an initial vasopressor bolus dose, immediately followed by a maintenance dose. As the peripheral circulation fails, it is preferable to give the medications centrally, via a catheter placed in the vena cava. At the same time, infusions of large volumes of fluids are undesirable, and for this reason it is not a good idea to dilute the solution to be able to increase the infusion rate. There has to be a compromise between, on the one hand, delivering the minimal amount of fluid, and on the other hand, supplying the medication as fast as possible.

Note that other medications must never be administered in the form of a bolus dose via the same tubing used for treating, for example, cardiac failure with vasopressor drugs. If this were done, the patient would immediately receive the entire amount of this medication present in the tubing (the amount intended for delivery over a period of perhaps 10 to 15 minutes). And after this delivery, the patient would not receive any maintenance dose during the following 10 to 15 minutes because the remaining bolus dose will have replaced the vasopressor drug. Unintentional delivery of such undesirable and large doses of vasopressor drugs to the patient must be avoided, as this can cause a dangerous increase in blood pressure with accompanying elevated myocardial oxygen demands, since the heart then has to deliver a higher work output. This increases the risk of myocardial ischaemia and possibly life-threatening cardiac arrhythmias.

In the care of critically ill patients, it is not uncommon to have the patient hooked up to three or four infusion pumps simultaneously. If more than one infusion pump is to be connected to an infusion port, the consequences must be considered, Figure 9:9. For simplicity's sake, suppose that two pumps, A and B, are connected to a common tube, and that both pumps are set at the same infusion rate. If both pumps are running, the intended volumes will be infused at the desired rates. However, if one pump is turned off, B for example, the flow rate in the tube is now only half what it was. Since the fluid column between the Y-connector and the blood vessel consists of an equal mixture of the drugs

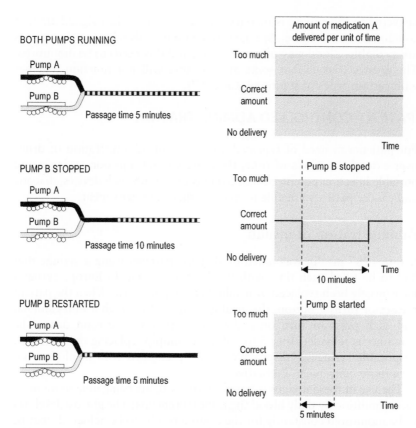

Figure 9:9 When two or more pumps are interconnected and one of them stopped or restarted, the infused volume per unit of time from the running pump is affected. The figure demonstrates what happens to the medication from infusion pump A when pump B is stopped and then restarted

from the two pumps, the column will contain only half the concentration of the drug that is supposed to be delivered from pump A. The patient will receive only half the dose until the fluid column has been replaced by solution from pump A.

If B is then restarted, the infusion rate is doubled, and the patient receives a double dose of the drug from pump A until the fluid column in the tube has been replaced by a mixture of the two solutions.

Effects of various types of infusion solutions

The most common infusion solutions, such as those with electrolytes or glucose, do not pose any particular hazards, as long as spills onto the pumps are avoided. But some solutions can create problems. Insulin and nitroglycerine are adsorbed to glass and plastic, and the drug amount delivered to the patient is therefore not the same as the original amount contained in the solution. Special tubes with nonadsorbing inner surfaces are available. Blood may obstruct filters, and this needs to be monitored. The greatest risk is that some air detectors will not function together with certain types of solutions (Case 9:7).

PATIENT-CONTROLLED ADMINISTRATION

For patients in need of repeated and frequent administration of drugs over extended periods of time, there are **special injection syringes** and **portable injection pumps,** also called **injectors.** With such devices, diabetic and cancer patients are able to manage their own treatment.

Administration of insulin

Before 1987 insulin was taken by diabetic patients using a syringe that had to be filled each time with insulin from a vial. In Europe syringes have largely been replaced by insulin pens, Figure 9:10. When the patient presses or turns a button, the insulin is injected through a thin cannula, and each press or turn on a dose dial provides a certain dose. The container is reloaded after 3 to 7 days by simply replacing the cartridge. **Disposable syringes** ("disposable pens") preloaded with insulin are an even more convenient alternative.

The use of these designs is based on the patients being able to monitor their condition by daily blood sugar measurements. The glucose level has to be monitored constantly for the desired results to be achieved, that is, an even and normal blood sugar level.

Treatment with short-acting insulin can be simplified by using a **portable infusion pump** controlled by an automatic mechanism, Figure 9:11. The mechanism nowadays consists of a small microprocessor unit programmed so that appropriate doses are injected according to a dose schedule.

The pump delivers a basic dose, which constitutes about half of the daily requirement. In addition, the patient can inject **bolus doses** 15 to 30 minutes before a meal, which provides for greater mealtime flexibility than does conventional treatment. Just like the nonautomatic methods

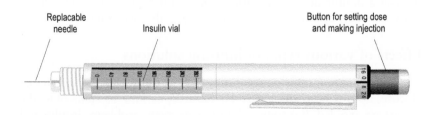

Figure 9:10 Insulin pen

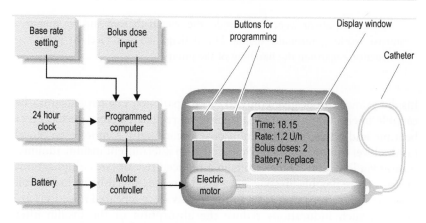

Figure 9:11 Example of insulin pump

for delivery of short-acting insulin, the insulin is delivered to the patient via a tube and a cannula that are kept in the same place for about 3 days. The patient can adjust the insulin amount for both the basic and the bolus dose.

An insulin pump must be capable of triggering an alarm in an error situation (low battery voltage, empty insulin cartridge or flow blockage). In addition to any such safety functions, the pumps must of course also be programmed correctly and must not be subjected to abnormal external conditions, such as excessive cold.

CASE 9:14 Insulin patient received double dose

During a check-up at the hospital, a diabetic patient had his old type of insulin of concentration 40 IU/ml, changed to a new, stronger type, with a concentration of 100 IU/ml. At the same time, the pump was reprogrammed.

For 2 days thereafter, the patient had constant symptoms of an insulin overdose and returned to the hospital. After disconnection, the pump was checked and at first seemed to function normally, but when measuring the amount of insulin pumped out on an analytic balance, it was discovered that the pump delivered almost twice as much insulin as intended.

The patient was in good condition at the examination and was given a new pump of the same model. The first pump had been programmed incorrectly.

CASE 9:15 Patient's insulin became frozen

A patient used to carry his insulin pump in a bag on top of his clothes. After being outdoors during a winter day when the temperature was down to −12°C, the insulin had become frozen, and as a result the pump stopped.

When the patient went back inside, the insulin thawed and the pump started working normally again. The patient had not received proper instruction regarding the handling of the pump.

Insulin pumps can be given only to certain patients. The patients must be capable of checking their blood sugar level regularly before meals and at bedtime and adjusting the insulin dose accordingly. A more even blood insulin level can be achieved compared with intermittent insulin administration via injections. This results in a reduced risk of late complications in life, a more flexible lifestyle and a greater sense of well-being in general. Also the indurations that form in the tissues after repeated injections are avoided; such indurations reduce the absorption of the insulin after subsequent injections.

The portable pumps are equipped with replaceable cassettes that contain between 10 and 100 ml. They remain stable for at least 5 days.

The pump is connected via a catheter inserted into the abdomen, chest or back. The catheter is normally placed subcutaneously. The catheter skin insertion site is protected by a small transparent self-adhesive cover. This allows for inspection of the skin and early detection of any infection. The pump is usually carried in front and attached by a belt around the waist. During showering, bathing or swimming the pump is generally removed, even if pumps are advertised as waterproof.

CASE 9:16 Eight-day insulin dose delivered within an hour

A patient with an insulin pump had been snorkelling when she suddenly became ill with severe hypoglycaemia and was taken to a hospital. After treatment with, among other things, glucose infusions the glucose level in the blood stabilized after 13 hours.

The patient examined the pump after the accident and discovered a minute crack in the case and condensation of water on the inside of the display window. The pump had been advertised as being safe to wear during water sports.

Portable pumps for analgesia

Pumps for administration of morphine and other types of analgesic drugs (as well as for antibiotics and chemotherapy) are similar to the portable insulin pumps, Figure 9:12. There are several advantages to using a pump as opposed to giving ordinary injections. Thanks to the continuous administration, a more even plasma level can be achieved. When applied for **patient-controlled analgesia (PCA)**, the patient can control the amount of painkiller delivered by pressing a particular button that gives an extra dose. The pump is equipped with a thin tube connected to a catheter, which can be placed subcutaneously, intra-venously or in the epidural or intrathecal spaces.

CASE 9:17   Respiratory arrest and cramps

A patient who had received a pump for delivery of analgesics was found cramping and in respiratory arrest.

It was discovered that the medication cassette was sitting loose as it had been mounted incorrectly. It had therefore delivered too much medication. According to the accompanying instructions for use, the pump must be placed on a firm surface when loading the cassette, so that the cassette can be locked in place.

The nurse had not received any training in the handling of the pump.

The patient recovered and did not seem to suffer any lasting effects of the incident.

IMPLANTABLE DEVICES

For medications that need to be given by frequent injections over extended periods of time, an implantable device can be very useful. These can, for example, consist of **injection ports** and **catheters. Implantable medication pumps** are available but not commonly used.

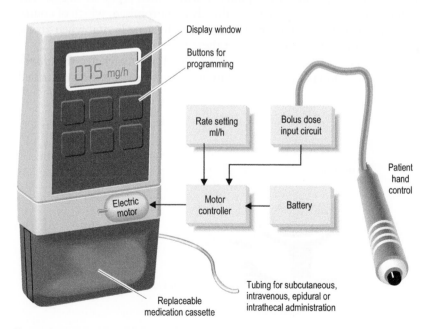

Figure 9:12 Portable analgesic pump

Injection ports

An injection port consists of a chamber that is placed subcutaneously, and is connected via a catheter to a vein, artery, the epidural space or the abdominal cavity, Figures 9:13 and 9:14. The chamber is made of tissue-friendly materials such as stainless steel or titanium. It has a thick membrane that is punctured when drugs are delivered to the device. A special injection cannula is used, which penetrates both the skin and the membrane. Ordinary injection cannulae must not be used, as these may damage the membrane. The membrane is capable of withstanding around 1000 to 2000 penetrations.

The chamber is implanted under local anaesthesia. The catheter is often inserted in a neck vein that has been exposed by surgical cut-down. In such cases the chamber is placed in the chest wall about 5 to 10 cm below the clavicle, and sutured to the underlying tissue. One advantage with injection ports is that medications can be administrated with the same ease as a subcutaneous injection. In addition, the patient's super-ficial veins are not damaged by repeated injections. The pain during the injection is negligible, and anaesthetics are not needed for adults; for children, a surface anaesthetic sticking plaster can be applied prior to the injection, see below.

A disadvantage with injection ports is that they may carry an increased risk of septicaemia in patients with certain diseases. Several such cases have been reported in treatment of childhood leukaemia with chemo-therapeutic drugs and AIDS patients with other types of drugs. The immune system in such patients is already compromised, which of course increases the risk of septicaemia. Meticulous hygiene is vital when giving infusions and in the general care of these patients.

On occasion, catheters have fragmented and been carried in the blood-stream to the lungs. The implantation procedure must not be trifled with:

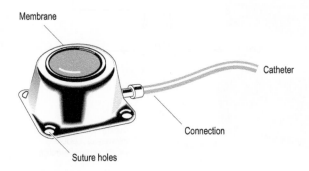

Figure 9:13 Infusion port

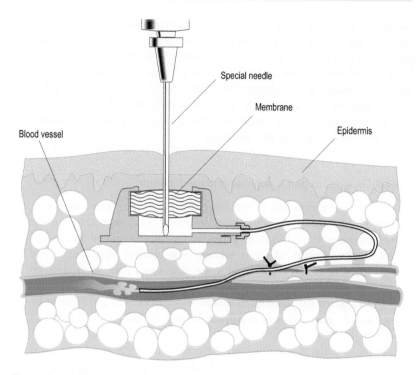

Special needle

Membrane

Blood vessel

Epidermis

Figure 9:14 Infusion port with catheter inserted into a blood vessel

---

CASE 9:18 Catheter came loose

A patient was to receive an injection port. The accompanying catheter was not used, as it did not fit the introducer used by the anaesthetist. Instead a thin catheter made of silicone rubber, which was normally used for other purposes and supplied on a roll, was cut to length. The catheter was pushed onto the infusion port outlet tube, and attached by two ligatures.

Five years later, the patient had recovered from his illness, and no longer needed the injection port. As the patient was uncomfortable with the port, it was surgically removed. Upon removal, one ligature remaining on the port outlet tube was found, and another one was found lying separately in the soft tissues. The catheter, however, could not be found. It must have been carried off in the bloodstream and became stuck somewhere. The catheter could not be localized, as silicone is not visible with X-ray.

At the time of removal, the patient had not had any symptoms from this complication.

A technical problem with injection ports is that they sometimes can be obstructed by blood clots, for example, when drawing blood samples via the port. The port must therefore be flushed with saline immediately after taking the sample. If several samples are taken at one session, the port must be flushed after each sample. After taking the sample, a heparin solution is injected to prevent clotting. If clots have already formed, attempts at dissolving them can be made with a special solution that is allowed to remain in the port for a short period.

It is very important to ensure that the cannula is positioned correctly in the port before giving the injection:

CASE 9:19 Injection port leakage leads to painful death

A 50-year-old man suffering from myeloma was to receive treatment with chemotherapeutic drugs. During the insertion of an injection port, the surgeon encountered difficulties in placing the catheter around the clavicle, and bleeding ensued. The port function was checked with X-rays after completion of the procedure, and it was discovered that the catheter tip had been placed in the right atrium.

The following day the surgical wound area was swollen and "ugly look-ing" and the port was hard to palpate. In spite of this, chemotherapy was started.

In the evening, it was discovered that the patient's hospital gown was wet, and that a swelling had emerged behind the armpit. The patient was sent to the regional hospital, where a radiograph with contrast media demonstrated a leakage between the injection port outlet tube and the catheter. Large areas of the chest cage became necrotic, and in spite of three plastic surgery operations, the patient died after 17 days.

An infusion port can remain implanted in the body for up to 2 years if there are no complications. On average, they remain operational for about 250 days.

Catheters

Sometimes it is necessary to administer medications locally, such as around the spinal nerves that carry the pain signals (for example, caused by cancer metastases) from a part of the body to the central nervous system. A catheter is inserted and then brought out through the skin, so that it may be connected to an infusion pump. It is often tunnelled, or advanced under the skin, over the shoulder and made to exit at the upper front chest, or to the abdominal side, Figure 9:15. This procedure facilitates the infusion of analgesics and also allows for attachment of an infusion pump for administration of analgesics.

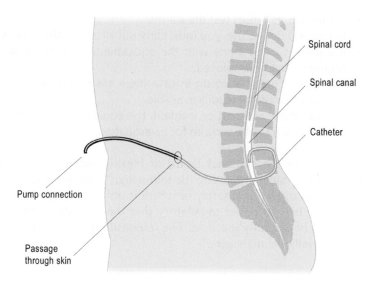

Spinal cord

Spinal canal

Catheter

Pump connection

Passage
through skin

Figure 9:15 Tunnelling of catheter to the spinal canal

Skin absorption

Before injections are given to children, the skin is preferably anaesthetized with the help of a sticking plaster containing an anaesthetic agent that can penetrate the skin. The same principle has been used for other drugs, for example, insulin and nicotine to adults. By conducting an electric current from the medication to the skin, the absorption of certain drugs can increase several times. Ultrasound can also be used to agitate the tissues, resulting in an increased absorption of certain drugs.

SAFETY HAZARDS

Because of the high number of accidents in connection with the use of infusion pumps, a number of countries have issued special notices. The content of the notice below is still highly topical. The document summarizes the duties of the person responsible for the treatment. Some of the responsibilities that need to be given special emphasis can be reworded to apply to any personnel handling infusion devices. Some of these statements reiterate what has already been stated in Chapter 1:

 Whenever handling infusion devices remember the following:
- Read the instructions for use.
- Make sure that you have received appropriate training and document the training.
- Your knowledge of the equipment must be checked by a superior.

- Before use, you must test the alarms.
- Before and during use, you must carry out all other safety checks.
- If a patient is left alone with the equipment, established safety routines must be employed.
- Instructions on what to do in case there are problems with the equipment must be readily available.
- In case of any accident or incident, the equipment, including all accessories, must be secured for investigation.

A notice issued by the National Board of Health and Welfare in one European country ended by stating the following: "Equipment is an aid, the function and operational safety of which is ultimately dependent on human factors. It is therefore mandatory that the local distribution of responsibilities be carefully specified. The responsibility for ensuring that this is done befalls the managers."

10

Artificial organs and stimulators

A prosthesis is an artificial substitute for a body part or function that has been lost. Prostheses implanted in the body are called **implants,** and must be manufactured with **biocompatible materials** that will not harm the body tissues or cause inflammatory reactions.

For several decades it has been possible to reconstruct joints and other parts of the skeleton with **endoprostheses,** and to replace the valves in the heart and sections of vessels with **cardiovascular prostheses.** Semi-permeable membranes in **oxygenators** (also called **artificial lungs**) and **dialysis machines** have enabled the addition and elimination of gases and soluble substances to and from the body. **Hearing aids** have long been used to compensate for hearing loss. With a simple electromechanical device, a so-called **electrolarynx,** the function of the larynx can at least partly be replaced.

Stimulators are electric devices that affect nerves and muscles. Some types of stimulators, such as **pacemakers,** are implanted. **Defibrillators** are of vital importance for rapid treatment of ventricular fibrillation in cardiac arrest. Electric pulse generators are also used as **muscle** and **nerve stimulators** to compensate for loss of nerve function, for pain relief and for improved peripheral blood circulation.

Biomaterials

Biomaterials, also called **biocompatible materials,** are needed to replace a part or a function in the body. A large number of different types of materials have been developed for many varying needs. Examples of common application areas are given in Table 10:1 and the repaired organs in Table 10:2.

Table 10:1   Various application areas of biomaterials

Usage	Example
Replacement of diseased tissue	Hip prosthesis, dialysis machine
Healing aids	Sutures, bone plates, screws
Improved function	Pacemaker, implantable lenses
Cosmetic	Breast implants
Diagnostic tools	Catheters, probes
Therapeutic tools	Drainage, dialysis filters, dressings

Table 10:2   Examples of organs and some available artificial functions

Organ	Examples
Heart	Pacemaker, artificial valves, cardiac pumps
Eye	Contact lenses, intraocular lenses
Ear	External ear, cochlear implants
Kidney	Dialysis machine

Implants can be divided into two main groups: those that are not in direct contact with the circulating blood and those that are constantly immersed in the bloodstream. Whereas many different biomaterials may be used for the first group, it has proved considerably harder to develop materials for implantation in the vascular system that will not cause the blood to coagulate. Many artificial heart designs have failed mainly because of formation of blood clots at the blood–prosthesis interface. The clots have become dislodged and the emboli carried in the bloodstream to the brain and other organs, causing infarctions.

Most foreign materials, if implanted, would trigger tissue reactions such as rejection or formation of scar tissue. At the same time, the materials themselves would be adversely affected, resulting in weakening or deterioration of the prostheses. Therefore, all components in direct contact with body tissues must therefore be subjected to rigorous requirements. Besides being tissue-friendly, a biocompatible material must also be **biostable,** meaning that its chemical and physical properties must remain unaltered.

To prevent the prostheses from becoming fibrin-coated and causing blood clotting, materials have been covered with a layer of heparin. The long-term effects of such **heparinized prosthetic** biocompatible materials in contact with blood have been positive. Another possibility is to coat the prostheses with **pyrolytic carbon,** that is carbon that has been heated to above 1200°C to acquire a very dense and hard structure. Following implantation, prostheses coated with pyrolytic carbon become covered with a thin, non-degrading and thus tissue-friendly protein layer.

New methods have been developed, where prosthetic materials are coated with **organic polymers** (such as polyethylene oxide) by means of vacuum vaporization. It has been shown that such materials remain essentially free of fibrin coatings, which indicates that they are highly tissue-friendly.

Implants are made of many different materials – **metals, ceramics** and **polymers** – which are used either separately or in various combinations.

Metals and alloys

Due to its excellent manufacturing properties, stainless steel was originally the main material for joint endoprostheses, but its importance has decreased as it elicits tissue reactions, including nickel allergies. Today, most orthopaedic prostheses are made of chrome–cobalt or titanium–aluminum alloys. The element **titanium** possesses a great advantage, in that a peroxide layer with anti-inflammatory and bactericidal properties forms on its surface, rendering it highly biocompatible. The titanium grows on to the bone tissue.

Because of the excellent properties of titanium, this metal can be utilized for fixation of various external prostheses. The prosthesis is then attached by a screw to a titanium implant that has already grown on to the bone – an osseo-integrated implantation. Thus artificial external ears and eyes as well as larger constructions, for example, facial prostheses required after surgical removal of facial tumours, can be attached using titanium implants. Some types of hearing aids, which operate on the principle of bone sound conduction (the sound is conducted to the inner ear through the skull bone), are also attached to a titanium implant that is screwed into the bone behind the ear. The implant penetrates the skin, allowing it to connect to the sound transmitter of the hearing aid.

More commonly, single tooth implants are fixed with the help of a titanium implant, or several implants are utilized to fix an entire dental bridge. Each implant consists of a cannulated screw, which has an outer thread that is screwed into the jawbone, and an inner thread into which a smaller screw fits. The smaller screw is used to attach the artificial tooth or dental bridge, which, if necessary, can be removed at a later time.

Ceramics

In ceramic materials, china-like substances, silicon is substituted by calcium phosphate, resulting in a material with a surface structure so similar to bone that tissue can grow into it. These materials do not trigger any tissue reactions or change once implanted in the body. Previously these materials were brittle, but modern development has overcome this disadvantage and ceramics can today replace articulating surfaces and cover metallic prostheses in thin layers, enabling these to merge with the bone.

Polymer biomaterials

Synthetic polymer materials are common for a large number of medical applications, Table 10:3. The main advantage of polymers in comparison with metals is that they are much more easily formed to fit different applications. They are also much less expensive and are available with highly varying mechanical properties.

Applications of medical polymers

Special **silica materials**, substances where the organic carbon has been replaced by silicon, have been used extensively for plastic surgery, such as reconstructive breast surgery. This type of prosthesis consists of an outer, solid silicone sheath, filled with either a softer silicone mass or saline. The silicone-filled prostheses unfortunately age after implantation, and can rupture and leak. The silicone released may then trigger neo-formation of fibrous tissue and scarring. The mechanical durability of silicone materials is low.

Several **polyurethane compounds** offer considerably superior mechanical properties with regard to both durability and flexibility. These compounds have, for example, been used as pump membranes in artificial hearts, where the requirements are quite exceptional – such membranes must be able to withstand some 40 million reshapings per year.

For a long time, it has been possible to replace blood vessels with **grafts** made of knitted or woven **PET** (**polyethylene tetraphtalate**). Today, knitted **polyurethane** and other types of porous materials with excellent biocompatibility, such as expanded **PTFE** (**polytetrafluoroethylene**) are used.

Table 10:3   Examples of use of different synthetic polymers

Synthetic polymers	Use
Polyvinyl chloride (PVC)	Packaging materials, blood bags, infusion sets, syringes
Polyethylene (PE)	Catheters, orthopaedic implants, pliable containers
Polypropylene (PP)	Disposable syringes, membranes, suture materials, vascular grafts
Polyurethane (PU)	Films, tubing and tubing components
Polymethyl methacrylate (PMMA)	Blood pumps, dialysis membranes, intraocular lenses, bone cement
Polytetrafluoroethylene (PFTE)	Catheters, vascular grafts

The purpose of these porous materials is to enable tissue ingrowth to anchor the graft, as described below.

The fact that a damaged eye lens may be replaced by an implant was discovered by accident. During World War II, a British ophthalmologist noticed that splinters originating from the plastic shield in fighter planes did not appear to damage the eye. He then had artificial lens implants made of the same material, **polymethylmethacrylate**. It worked, and was used for decades. One disadvantage with these lenses, however, is that they are rigid, forcing the surgeon to make an incision of at least 6 mm in the eye during the implantation. Therefore, the lenses mostly used today are made of a soft sheath, filled with a **hydrogel**. Such lenses are small prior to implantation, but once implanted in the eye, they absorb water and swell to the correct size.

ORTHOPAEDIC PROSTHESES

Joints should be painless, mobile and stable. This normal state can be affected by any of several chronic diseases. **Rheumatoid arthritis** and **osteoarthritis** often cause such severe changes that entire joints need to be replaced by endoprostheses. The hip and knee joints are most often reconstructed, but other joints such as the shoulder and the carpometacarpal joint of the thumb may also be treated by arthroplasty.

Types of prostheses

An orthopaedic endoprosthesis may either consist of a device that completely replaces the surgically removed bony parts, a **total implant,** or it may replace only a part of the joint, a **partial prosthesis,** Figure 10:1. A prosthesis may also merely replace the articulating surfaces, an **articulating prosthesis,** Figure 10:2. The latter type may suffice in cases where the ligaments of the joint are intact. Such simpler implants carry the advantage of requiring a less extensive surgical procedure.

In a total implant, the two articulating surfaces are made of different materials, which results in less friction and wear than would be the case if both surfaces were made of the same material. In a hip implant, for example, the femur head might be manufactured of metal and the acetabular cup of polyethylene. To reduce friction, the head is made considerably smaller than a normal femur head, which has a diameter of about 50 mm; common implant diameters are 32 and 22 mm. Nowadays, ceramics are also used for articulating surfaces.

Fixation of prostheses

Orthopaedic prostheses are most often attached with **bone cement,** consisting of fast-curing polymethylmethacrylate, which fixes the prosthesis in place during the implantation procedure. The disadvantage is that over time

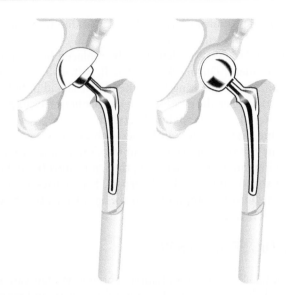

Figure 10:1 Left: A total hip implant, where both the acetabulum and the femur head are replaced by implanted materials. Right: A partial implant, where only the femur head has been replaced

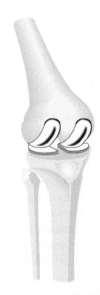

Figure 10:2 Articular surface prosthesis of the knee joint

this material becomes brittle and rigid, and broken-off cement fragments may cause pain. It is also not completely biocompatible, as a fibrous membrane may form at the bone–cement interface. At the same time, bone tissue is resorbed, resulting in compromised fixation and decreased stability.

For this reason cementless fixation methods, **biological fixation**, have been developed, where the implant is given a porous texture, enabling fibrous tissue ingrowth into the surface. The result is a longer lasting fixation. The disadvantage is that the fixation process requires a certain amount of time; less pain relief is sometimes obtained immediately after surgery.

Complications

The most serious complication for all types of implants is infection. The risk is relatively small, less than 1%, but when it does occur, the implant must most often be replaced.

Sometimes the implant does not stay in situ because of mechanical problems with the fixation, called **aseptic loosening**. Good surgical technique is essential for minimizing this risk. When cementing hip prostheses, it is thus important that the femoral medullary cavity is properly prepared and flushed, that the intramedullary canal is plugged, that it is properly filled with cement, and that appropriate proximal pressure is maintained until the cement is sufficiently cured.

CARDIOVASCULAR PROSTHESES

Several diseases of the circulatory system can now efficiently be treated with surgically implanted cardiovascular prostheses. For vascular abnormalities such as birth defects, aneurysms and arteriosclerotic changes, **vascular grafts** can replace diseased vessel segments. Stenotic (obstructed) or leaking cardiac valves can be replaced with **artificial heart valves**. **Cardiac pumps** can be used to temporarily relieve the heart muscle. Even **artificial blood** is being developed.

Vascular grafts

A common application for vascular grafts is in the treatment of aortic aneurysms. This can be done using two principally different methods. First, the aorta may be surgically freed, transected and then both ends sutured to the graft. Second, the procedure may also be performed using a **transluminal technique**, where the graft is inserted through a small incision in the vessel wall and then advanced to its proper position. During such procedures, the graft is inserted via the femoral artery in the groin on one side, the so-called **transfemoral** approach, and an abdominal incision is thus not needed. During the insertion, the graft is kept compressed to a small diameter inside the tube-shaped introducer that is inserted into the artery. When the graft is deployed from the introducer, it expands and attaches to the non-diseased parts of the arterial inner wall, where endothelial ingrowth will anchor the graft.

A common type of vessel graft consists of knitted or woven PET. Following implantation, blood leaks through the loops, where it coagulates and seals the graft. The coagulated blood is subsequently transformed to fibrous tissue, and endothelial ingrowth from the adjoining vessel will eventually completely cover the inside of the graft. Modern vascular grafts made of **expanded PET** are tighter and somewhat easier to implant. The long-term results of such reconstructions of the aorta and the greater arteries have been very good; for smaller vessels the outcome has not been as favourable, as these can become occluded after some time.

Vascular grafts can be furnished with a metal mesh, a **stent**, Figure 10:3. Such stent grafts may be fitted with tiny hooks at the ends, which anchor the graft in the correct position inside the artery. Stents can be either self-expanding or be expanded with a balloon. Stents are also used separately, without a graft, for supporting and expanding arteriosclerotic blood vessels, often following balloon dilatation (Chapter 11).

Valvular prostheses

Stenotic as well as incompetent cardiac valves may be treated surgically by implantation of valvular prostheses. A disc valve prosthesis can consist of a metal orifice ring with an outer layer of synthetic woven fabric, a round disc with struts on the ring to hold the disc in such a way that it is free to move, Figure 10:4a. The disc opens and closes in the same way as a hinged lid. Another design utilizes two crescent-shaped discs which open and close against each other like butterfly wings, Figure 10:4b. Replacement valves can also be obtained from pigs, **xenografts**.

During the implant procedure, the patient's damaged valve is first removed, and the prosthesis then sutured into place in the annulus. The outer fibrous layer around the prosthetic ring then fills with blood, which then coagulates and transforms into fibrous tissue, thus anchoring the prosthesis to the tissue.

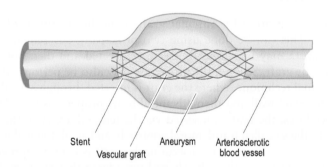

Stent   Aneurysm   Arteriosclerotic
        Vascular graft   blood vessel

Figure 10:3 Aneurysm with a vascular stent graft

CASE 10:1 Many perish due to inadequate reporting

A patient with a mitral prosthesis with a single disc suddenly developed severe heart failure and died shortly thereafter.

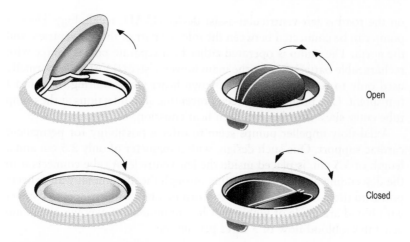

Figure 10:4 (a) Valvular prosthesis of the type described in Case 10:1. (b) Modern valvular prosthesis where the discs move like butterfly wings

Autopsy demonstrated that the strut that had held the mobile disc in position had fractured, resulting in the disc breaking free from the valve. This was caused by a manufacturing design defect.

In one European country alone 43 patients died because of the same manufacturing defect. The reason for such a large number was the initial failure to report the cases to the authorities with subsequent follow-up, resulting in many new patients still being fitted with the same type of valve. It was without comparison the largest medical-technical accident ever to occur in that country. It could have been avoided at least in part had reporting and follow-up, known as post-market surveillance, been effective.

Tip No medical device is perfect. You must always look out for problems and failures and immediately report any incident. Never assume that the failure you have observed is an isolated event. Reporting saves lives.

Cardiac pumps

For temporary cardiac support during surgery, **intra-aortic balloon pumps (IABP)** are generally used. These consist of a long, thin balloon that is inserted into the descending aorta and inflated during diastole when the aortic valve is closed, thereby facilitating the blood flow to the tissues, and deflated during systole to aid the blood flow into the aorta.

The dream of being able to design an artificial heart has been difficult to realize but now seems to be approaching a solution. An important step on the road is **left-ventricular-assist device (LVAD)** technology. Here, a pump can be connected between the inferior part of the left ventricle and the aorta. The pump is operated either by a separate power source with rechargeable batteries or by the main power system. LVADs are normally used only to support the patient's own heart while waiting for a heart transplant. One problem has been preventing skin infections at the pump tube entry sites. Another has been heat emission.

Axial-flow impeller pumps seem to offer a possibility for permanent cardiac support. One such design, with a diameter of only 2.5 cm and a length of 5.5 cm, is placed inside the left ventricle. A tube connects it to the descending aorta. A small cable through the abdominal wall delivers power to the pump from a battery worn in a belt. All surfaces in contact with blood are made of highly polished titanium. On average, the pump generates a blood flow of 5 litres per minute.

Artificial blood

The lack of donor blood of the appropriate blood group is a constantly recurring problem. Different techniques are tried to replace the need for donor blood in acute situations. One method involves the use of human or bovine haemoglobin in various preparations. **Polymerized** or **cross-linked haemoglobin** can still retain its oxygen- and carbon dioxide-carrying capabilities. A similar approach is to envelop haemoglobin with a thin lipid membrane to obtain artificial blood corpuscles.

Another method is to replace the haemoglobin completely by a "breathing liquid" consisting of an **emulsion of perfluorocarbons**. Potential uses for such emulsions include surgery, trauma, open heart surgery, and oxygenation of tumours during radiation or chemotherapy. The emulsion is eliminated from the blood by phagocyte cells.

OXYGENATORS

In blood oxygenators, oxygen is transferred through a membrane. In one type the membrane consists of a large number of heparin-coated tubes, with a diameter of approximately 0.2 mm. The tubes are arranged just like beverage straws packed into a glass. Oxygen passes through the tubes, while the blood flows in the opposite direction outside the tubes. During this process, gas exchange takes place, resulting in oxygenation of the blood and elimination of carbon dioxide from the blood.

Oxygenators are an important part of **heart–lung machines**, which are used during open heart surgery. Here, the blood is pumped from the vena cava to the oxygenator and then back to the aorta.

Oxygenators are also used for temporary care of pulmonary patients, using **ECLA (extracorporeal lung assist)** and **ECMO (extracorporeal membrane oxygenation)**. Here, the oxygenated blood can be retransfused into either an artery or a vein. When reintroduced through a vein, which is the common procedure in adults, the blood can be led out of the body through the femoral vein and routed back to the body via the subclavian vein.

This way, oxygenated blood is supplied to the right side of the heart and thus also into the pulmonary circulation, thereby facilitating the healing process in the lung. The disadvantage compared with arteriovenous ECMO is that some admixture of blood does take place in the vena cava, resulting in reduced blood oxygen saturation.

This treatment may be given for several weeks in cases of temporarily impaired pulmonary function, such as in newborn babies. In hiatus hernia the intestines slip upwards into the thoracic cavity, thereby preventing the baby's lungs from developing normally. Here, ECMO may be of vital importance in providing a few days preparation before a planned operation. Children with foreign objects occluding a main bronchus, leading to an entire lung, may receive ECMO treatment during the bronchoscopy that is performed to retrieve the foreign object. ECMO has also been employed in the treatment of patients with chronic lung diseases to give the lung tissue a greater chance to heal.

Extracorporeal oxygenation in respiratory insufficiency is advantageous as it not only takes care of the immediate gas exchange, but also avoids administration of pure oxygen to the patient, which may otherwise have a harmful effect on the lungs because of formation of free oxygen radicals.

DIALYSIS MACHINES

Completely ceased or severely impaired kidney function results in uraemia. Chronic kidney failure may, for example, be caused by previous **nephritis** or by **circulatory disturbances** in the kidneys. **Acute kidney failure** may be due to various temporary causes, such as poisoning (suicide attempts with sleeping pills) and extensive tissue degradation in severe trauma cases. Both chronic and acute kidney failure may be treated with dialysis. The physical procedures are described in Box 10:1.

The dialysis may be **extracorporeal** or **intracorporeal.** In extracorporeal dialysis, blood is led from the patient to an artificial "kidney", where waste products are eliminated, whereupon the blood is routed back into the body. Such treatment can be given by means of **haemodialysis,** where waste products are transferred to the dialysis solution, or by **haemofiltration,** where all compounds of low molecular weight are filtered from the plasma in a fashion that simulates the function of the glomerulus. For intracorporeal dialysis, the abdominal cavity is used as a "kidney"; this is known as **peritoneal dialysis.**

These methods complement each other. Extracorporeal dialysis is superior where quick elimination of waste products is concerned, and carries little risk of infection, but it requires expensive equipment. Intracorporeal dialysis is technically simpler to carry out, and can often be administered by the patient. But this method does carry a slight risk of peritonitis, as the dialysis solution is infused directly into the abdominal cavity.

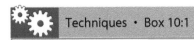

Techniques • Box 10:1

Physical processes in dialysis

Dialysis can in principle be achieved by **diffusion**, **osmosis** and **ultrafiltration**. In all three processes, the blood is purged with the aid of a semi-permeable membrane with a total area of about 1 to 2 m². Such a membrane permits only substances of low molecular weight to pass through, while all high-molecular-weight molecules, such as albumen and gammaglobulins, are retained.

Diffusion of substances through the membrane is directed toward the side with the lowest concentration. Accumulated waste products in the blood are transferred to the dialysis solution until equilibrium is reached. In the same fashion, whenever the dialysis solution levels are higher, low-molecular-weight substances diffuse from the dialysis solution (which has a composition similar to the body's extracellular fluids) to the patient. Equilibrium is reached and the body's internal environment is restored.

The process of **osmosis** may draw water out of the patient. If the **osmotic pressure** of the dialysis solution is high, for example, due to a high glucose level (7%), water is drawn from the patient to the dialysis solution. If less dehydration of the patient is desired, a lower glucose level is chosen.

In **ultrafiltration**, the hydrostatic pressure of the blood is increased to the point where low-molecular-weight substances are forced through the semi-permeable membrane and eliminated from the blood.

Haemodialysis

In haemodialysis, the blood is directed to an extracorporeal dialysis machine, Figure 10:5. For temporary treatment, a double lumen catheter may be inserted into the femoral vein. For long-term treatment, an arterio-venous fistula is created surgically, most commonly in the left arm. The fistula is a permanent connection between an artery and a vein. The fistula dilates due to the arterial pressure, facilitating the constantly recurring puncture that needs to be carried out to connect the patient to the dialysis machine. Efficient dialysis treatment requires a well-functioning fistula. The blood flow is usually 200 to 300 ml per minute.

Before the patient is connected to the dialysis machine, the dialysis side of the machine is filled with dialysis solution, and the blood side with normal saline. After a check that no air bubbles are trapped in the system, the blood tubes are connected to cannulae inserted into the fistula or to the double lumen catheter. Heparin is continuously administered to prevent any blood clotting in the machine. After completing dialysis, the blood in

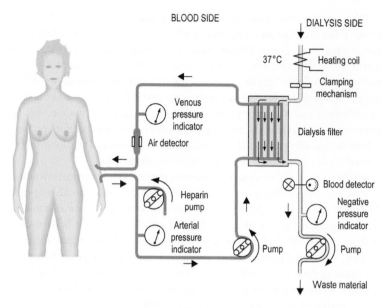

Figure 10:5 Haemodialysis

the machine and the tubes is reinfused into the patient. A haemodialysis session usually lasts 3 to 5 hours and is carried out three times per week, normally in the hospital, but it may also be performed at home. In intensive care units, continuous slow blood flow dialysis is also sometimes used.

Haemodialysis machines must be equipped with certain control circuits. To avoid a massive loss of blood, should a membrane rupture, a blood detector is connected to an automatic mechanism that shuts off the blood pump in case of a leak. The pressures in the tubes coming from and leading to the dialysis equipment are measured, and the composition of the dialysis solution is monitored, for example, by measuring its electric conductivity. A thermostat circuit ensures that the temperature of the dialysis solution is kept at 37°C.

CASE 10:2 Elderly woman dies of pulmonary embolism

An 82-year-old woman was receiving care for advanced uraemia, and had just undergone surgery. She was receiving heparin-free dialysis treatment – no anticoagulant had been added so as to avoid the risk of postoperative haemorrhaging. (To avoid clotting in the tubing when administering heparin-free dialysis, the dialysis should be continuous, with no interruption of the blood flow.) A physician prescribed albumen to be given via arterial infusion. A verbal "rule" for this type of infusion dictated that the patient not be left alone due to the risk of complications.

When only a small amount of albumen remained in the vial, the nurse lowered the drip rate and went to attend to another patient. She then went for a coffee break. About 10 minutes after lowering the drip rate, the system alarm went off, indicating air in the system. The nurse went back to the patient, noticed that "the air guard was filled with blood", and assumed that the alarm was due to "turbulence in the air chamber". She did not notice that the albumen vial was empty. She carried out a couple of manoeuvres to lower the blood level in the air chamber, which failed. She therefore pressed a button that allowed blood to bypass the air chamber. The blood pump started again, whereupon she reactivated the air guard.

At this time, an alarm went off at another patient. While she was attending to this, another air alarm came from the dialysis circuit of the 82-year-old. The nurse assumed that the new alarm was due to the same cause she thought had triggered it the last time. As she was afraid to stop the heparin-free dialysis for fear of clotting, she panicked and pressed the air guard bypass button. The blood pump started again, and this time she noticed that air was passing through the tube to the patient. Another nurse, who had been assigned to this particular patient, came in and shut off the dialysis.

The patient died a week later from air embolism.

Several mistakes had been made. The nurse who had originally been assigned to the patient should never have left the patient during the arterial albumen infusion. The clinical management had erred with regard to the delegation of responsibilities in the ward, the transfer of information between nurses and the organization of the entire unit. Written instructions regarding arterial infusions and other routine procedures were not available.

 If you do not feel fully able to handle a certain situation, or if you feel you are about to panic, never disconnect an alarm without first consulting a more experienced colleague.

Haemofiltration

This method is similar to haemodialysis, but here a dialysis solution is not always used. The blood flows alongside a **semi-permeable** membrane, that is highly permeable to water and small solutes, but impermeable to plasma proteins and blood cells. When negative pressure is applied to the external side of the membrane, ultrafiltration takes place in a fashion analogous to that in the glomerulus. All substances of low molecular weight are carried with the blood fluid and a kind of primary urine is obtained. Typically 20 litres are filtered per treatment session. The loss of water and other substances of low molecular weight are usually replaced through intravenous electrolyte infusion.

During haemodialysis, the patient often suffers from headaches, muscle cramps and falling blood pressure; these problems are not as pronounced during haemofiltration.

Peritoneal dialysis

In peritoneal dialysis, the peritoneum functions as the dialysis membrane. A catheter is inserted through the patient's abdominal wall via a small incision just below the navel. Sterile dialysis solution is introduced into the peritoneal cavity, diffusion takes place, and the solution is again drained out of the abdomen, Figure 10:6. There are two types: **continuous ambulatory peritoneal dialysis (CAPD)** and **intermittent peritoneal dialysis (IPD)**.

In CAPD, the patient has about 2 litres of dialysis solution in the peritoneal cavity at all times, and the solution is exchanged four times per 24 hours; this procedure does not have to be done in the hospital. The treatment does not require any machines, and the patient can carry out the exchange. Sterile sets, consisting of a collection bag, a bag with dialysis solution and special couplings are available, enabling easy and sterile connection of the peritoneal catheter to the set, Figure 10:6.

CAPD has a particular advantage for diabetic patients, who often suffer from kidney failure as a complication of their disease, as insulin can be added to the dialysis solution. This provides for a more even blood glucose level and better blood glucose control.

In IPD, which is normally carried out in hospital, the peritoneal cavity is rinsed using a special device over a period of 8 to 15 hours, two to three times per week. A volumetric pump injects the dialysis solution, which

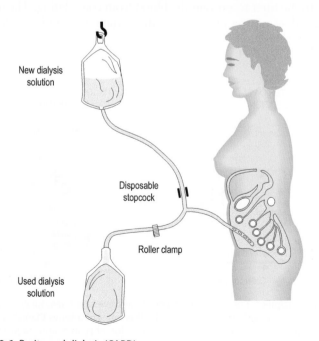

New dialysis solution

Disposable stopcock

Roller clamp

Used dialysis solution

Figure 10:6 Peritoneal dialysis (CAPD)

has been pre-warmed to body temperature, into the peritoneal cavity. As the pump drains the peritoneal cavity about 30 minutes later, the volume is again carefully recorded, as it is important to make sure that the solution is not left behind after each exchange. Leftover fluid can otherwise collect over a couple of cycles and cause breathing difficulties as the accumulated fluid pushes up on the diaphragm.

Renal replacement therapy in intensive care

In intensive care, a modified form of haemofiltration is used. As the patient is bedridden, it is possible to filtrate the blood on a continuous basis, **CRRT (continuous renal replacement therapy** – if not continuous shortened to **RRT**). This has several advantages, among other things it places less stress on the circulatory system than intermittent techniques. Several methods are available, for example, the original technique, **CAVH (continuous arterio-venous haemofiltration)**, Figure 10:7. Usually the femoral artery is punctured and blood passes through a filter that cleans the blood in much the same manner as in the kidneys. The patient's own blood pressure is thus used to drive the filtering. The pressure difference between the blood and the filtrate is regulated by elevating and lowering the collection bag 10 to 50 cm relative to the filter. The arterial pressure forces water and low-molecular-weight molecules through the filter membrane. The fluid loss is replaced and the blood is then returned to the patient through the femoral vein. Heparin is usually infused continuously proximal to the filter to prevent the blood from coagulating. The method is simple, it does not require complicated equipment, and is of low risk

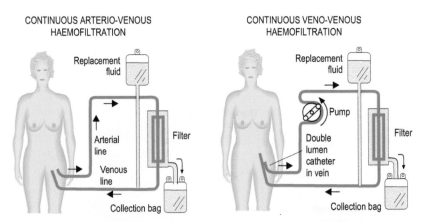

Figure 10:7 Principles for two common types of intensive care haemodialysis devices. The connection to the patient may go through other veins or arteries than shown in the figures. Not shown are common items such as those for infusion of anticoagulant (heparin). The replacement fluid may be added before the filter rather than after it

to the patient, apart from the risks connected with the arterial puncture. An obvious disadvantage is that the method has limited capacity to purify the blood when the blood pressure is low, which is often the case in a critically ill patient.

CVVH (**continuous veno-venous haemofiltration**) is then to be preferred, Figure 10:7. A large vein, such as the femoral or internal jugular vein is punctured, and a double lumen catheter is inserted. Blood is sucked out by means of a peristaltic pump from a hole on the side of the catheter. After having passed the filter it is returned to the patient through the other opening at the tip of the catheter. The method has the advantage that it eliminates the need to puncture an artery. If no replacement fluid is supplied, the method is called **SCUF** (**slow continuous ultrafiltration**).

A further improvement is to apply also a haemofiltration technique, **CVVHDF** (**continuous veno-venous haemodiafiltration**), Figure 10:8. The dialysate passes the filter in a direction opposite to that of the blood flow. By controlling the flow of the dialysate in or out of the filter, a negative pressure is obtained relative to the blood on the other side of the membrane.

Continuous renal replacement therapy is increasingly used in critically ill patients to treat, besides renal failure, conditions such as trauma, shock, sepsis, poisoning (suicide attempts), and correction of electrolyte and acid–base abnormalities. Severely ill patients often have to be given large amounts of infusions resulting in an overload that results in increased interstitial water and pulmonary oedema, which can be handled effectively. CRRT also offers a simple means to control a patient's body temperature.

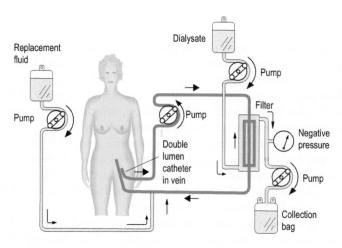

Figure 10:8 Continuous veno-venous haemodiafiltration

EXTRACORPOREAL IMMUNOADSORPTION

Extracorporeal adsorption can be used to eliminate certain harmful antibodies from the blood. This method resembles haemodialysis, but here the dialysis membrane is replaced by adsorption columns coated with a protein that binds the antibodies to be eliminated from the patient's blood. This method has been used for removal of circulating immune complexes associated with a number of diseases such as idiopathic thrombocytopenic purpura (ITP), haemolytic uraemic syndrome, red cell aplasia, and treatment of haemophilia by removing antibodies against vital coagulation factors.

HEARING AIDS

It is estimated that 10–12% of the population have a hearing loss of practical importance, and that a half of these have a need for and could use an aid. But at present only about half of those needing an aid have access to one. Mostly elderly people need hearing aids, and about half of these patients are over about 70 years old.

Assessing patients for hearing aids is achieved using a standard hearing test. This is a very safe procedure, but like any clinical test, users need to be aware of complications:

CASE 10:3 Patient deafer than ever

A patient was undergoing a hearing test. The sound level was increased to a level that worsened the loss of hearing.

After similar occurrences with other patients, protocols have been changed.

A hearing aid consists of a **microphone**, which captures the sound, an **amplifier** with **volume controls** for adjustment of the sound level, and a **receiver**. The volume control could be manual, but it is often automatic in modern aids relieving the patient from adjusting the volume. A hearing aid should also be equipped with a **telecoil**, which picks up magnetic signals from special teleloops. Such listening systems can be installed for wireless transfer to the hearing aid of, for example, radio/TV programmes, sermons and lectures. The hearing aid often has a switch, marked **M** for microphone and **T** for telecoil, so that the user may choose the appropriate function. The hearing aid is powered by a replaceable cell or **battery**, which normally lasts about a hundred hours.

A hearing aid must be adjusted to the particular needs of the individual user. These depend on the type of hearing loss and in what surroundings the hearing aid will be used.

Types of hearing aids

There are four major types of hearing aids, depending on the external shape. In the **body aid**, the microphone, amplifier and setting controls are held in a case, connected by a wire to the receiver, which is placed in a customized ear mould. The case is carried in a pocket or holder. The advantage of the body aid is that the case allows for large, long-life batteries, and easier-to-handle volume and tone controls. The large case is the reason why this type of aid may be beneficial for patients with impaired fine motor skills. However, because of the unnatural placement of the microphone and the long wire, this type of aid is not used to any great extent.

One of the dominating types is the **behind-the-ear** (**BTE**) aid where all electronic components including the receiver are placed inside a small, crescent-shaped case, which hangs behind the outer ear, Figure 10:9. The sound is conducted from the integrated receiver via a transparent plastic tube to a customized ear mould inside the ear canal. As the aid is placed on the side of the head, the patient's impression of the sound becomes more natural. The controls are located on the back of the device and are therefore easily accessible.

Advanced types have a separate control unit to be placed in the user's pocket or in a handbag. The control unit allows the user to adjust the settings by remote control.

Hearing glasses are a variation of the behind-the-ear aid, where the circuits are integrated into the frame of the patient's glasses. This design has, however, proved to be rather impractical, as the glasses and the hearing aid are not necessarily needed at the same time.

A growing number of patients prefer the **in-the-canal** (**ITC**) hearing aid, where the entire device is placed inside a customized, moulded shell in the ear canal, Figure 10:10. Depending on the volume of the components and the size of the patient's ear canal, the entire aid may reside in the canal, a **completely-in-canal** (**CIC**) hearing aid. This design, however, cannot accommodate the telecoil. Since the microphone is placed just

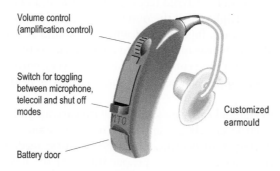

Volume control
(amplification control)

Switch for toggling
between microphone,
telecoil and shut off
modes

Customized
earmould

Battery door

Figure 10:9 Behind-the-ear hearing aid

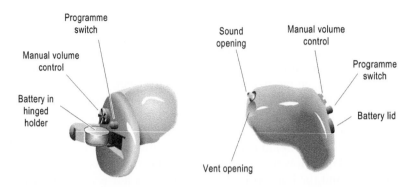

Figure 10:10 In-the-canal hearing aids, shown actual size. The aids are depicted in a position as if they were to be inserted into the reader's ears with the head slightly turned to the left. Many ITC aids have automatic volume control and no manual control. The programme switch allows selection of normal mode, noise reduction mode and telecoil reception

inside the ear canal entrance, the effects of the skull bone and the outer ear on the sound field may be utilized, enabling the patient to determine the direction of the sound.

> **Tip** It is not immediately obvious how to help a patient to insert an in-the-canal device if you have not done it before. Look at Figure 10:10 to discover how to distinguish right from left and up from down. First note that the part that goes into the ear canal is above the outer part protruding down into the cavity of the outer ear. Next note that the part that goes into the ear canal is somewhat bent with the convex side towards the forehead and the concave side towards the neck.

Normally, the ear mould has a **vent channel** or **bore** for equalization of the pressure in the ear canal with the atmospheric pressure. Without a vent channel, the pressure would build up and cause the ears to feel blocked.

One major problem is to avoid feedback from the sound output in the ear canal to the microphone on the outer side of the aid. If such **acoustic feedback** occurs, a loud, high-pitched whistling sound is generated. To avoid such feedback the ear mould of old devices had to fit closely to the patient's ear canal and the vent channel had to be very narrow. Acoustic feedback can also happen when a telephone receiver is held against the hearing aid.

As the sound channel easily gets clogged with earwax and dirt, it must be cleaned regularly; elderly patients may need assistance with this, as well as with battery replacement. To avoid acoustic feedback, elderly patients also often need help with proper fitting of the hearing aid, as well as the volume settings.

> **Tip** First lower the volume control until the noise stops, then adjust the ear mould so that it fits properly, and finally increase the volume again, to a level where the patient can hear ordinary speech.

Modern advanced hearing aids avoid acoustic feedback with special electronic circuits, using **acoustic feedback cancellation**. Such designs allow wide vent openings in the ear canal, and this has the advantage that the patient can use their own hearing ability in the low-frequency sounds as described below.

Sound level

The normal human hearing sense has a great capacity to adapt to the sound situation at hand. We are able to discern a spoken voice while in the midst of noisy traffic, and we can also recognize a distant bird far away in the forest. But people with hearing loss lack this adaptive capacity.

Setting the volume control at the appropriate sound level is a constantly recurring practical problem for users of simple types of hearing aids. Various technical solutions are utilized to facilitate this procedure, or, as in the most advanced designs, entirely eliminate the need for a volume control. The simpler aid types have a **sound level limiter**, which prevents sound pressures above a certain level from being produced. The disadvantage of this simple solution is the pronounced distortion of the sound – when the sound increases to the limiter activation level, it sounds "cracked". Modern aids are therefore equipped with an **automatic gain control** (**AGC**), which allows the sound level to determine the degree of amplification.

Frequency characteristics

Human speech consists of consonants, with sounds of mainly high frequencies, and vowels, which are dominated by sounds of low frequencies. As the consonants convey most of the speech information, they must be amplified to a greater extent than the vowels, for discrimination of the spoken words. The vowels, on the other hand, contain more energy and must instead be attenuated.

The degree of hearing loss at different frequencies almost always varies. The treble range, with high-frequency sounds, is affected more often and more extensively than the bass range, the low frequencies. For this reason, the amplification of different frequencies, the **frequency response**, of each hearing aid should be individually adjusted. Some advanced hearing aids can be programmed for different sound reproduction in various sound environments, enabling the user to choose the reproduction type that is best suited for specific listening situations. Switching between these modes is easily done by wireless transmission from the control box.

One further modern development is **noise reduction**, Box 10:2. As most people afflicted with hearing loss are elderly, they may have less need for highly sophisticated functions, and may be better served with aids that are simpler to use.

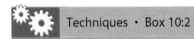

Techniques • Box 10:2

Noise reduction in hearing aids

The single most difficult technical problem with hearing aids is to improve the performance in noisy surroundings. People with hearing impairment have a lower tolerance for noise than those with normal hearing. Most patients are disappointed with their hearing aids in noisy surroundings.

In industrial workplaces and in airplane cabins, it is easy to suppress noise to a large extent. The pure noise signal is then picked up, phase shifted 180° and mixed with the sound channel, whereby the noise is reduced or cannot be heard, for example, in a headset. This is possible if the noise signal can be obtained completely separated from the signal carrying the desired information, be it spoken words or music.

This option is not available in hearing aids since the microphone usually is placed in the aid inside or behind the outer ear. Then the information and the noise sounds are indistinguishable. One option left with digital techniques is, however, to reduce the amplifier gain when no speech is detected by the aid and increase it to full volume when speech is present. This relieves the patient from hearing amplified noise during periods when no information signal is present. One method to achieve such an automatic detection of speech is to analyse the spectral components in the recorded signal. Each vowel in speech, as distinguished from noise, has a characteristic overtone pattern. Thus, if the vowel "a" has a fundamental frequency of 100 Hz, overtones occur at 200, 300, 400, 600 up to perhaps 8000 Hz. For each vowel the overtones usually have a certain amplitude relative to other harmonics. An example of one approach is the detection of typical overtone patterns, followed by the adjustment of the amplification. When no typical overtone patterns are present, the amplification drops to a low value within some 5 to 10 seconds.

Thus, so far, the acceptability of hearing aids in noisy surroundings can only be improved by decreasing the gain when the microphone does not pick up any speech signal.

Hearing implants

People with severe to profound hearing loss may be helped by an electric stimulator with electrodes, which can be implanted into the cochlea of the deaf ear. It is known as a **cochlear implant**. This device stimulates any remaining functioning nerve fibres in the auditory nerve, and a sound perception can thus be achieved. Usually, 22 or more electrodes are arranged on a very thin silicone tube, which is inserted into the spiral cavity of the cochlea. The electrodes are connected to a tiny receiver unit implanted under the skin behind the ear. An external microphone and transmitter in the specialized hearing aid, which looks like the ordinary body aid, sends information to the receiver.

The sound perception thus generated is completely different from that of normal hearing. But the user regains a certain degree of contact with the sound world. Sounds in the nearby environment may be perceived and the patients also gain the ability to control the volume of their speech – it is very difficult for profoundly deaf individuals to learn to speak, as they cannot hear their own voice. Most patients obtain a greatly enhanced ability to understand speech, in particular when this technology is combined with lip-reading. A few are helped to such an extent that they are even able to talk on the phone. Children benefit from early implantation, typically at about 2 years, so that they are able to hear when they learn to speak.

Another somewhat similar type of hearing aid, but not yet common, is the **auditory brainstem implant (ABI)**. It uses electrodes to stimulate a part of the brain surface close to the brain's hearing centre. This device is designed to help patients who have no functioning auditory nerves.

VOICE AIDS

Patients who have had their larynx surgically removed can usually learn to speak again by using the oesophagus, so-called oesophageal speech. The patient swallows air, releases it or "burps" in the form of a sound, and modulates the sound by shaping the resonance cavities in the pharynx and oral cavity just as in normal speech. However, the sound becomes coarse as well as hoarse, which can be hard to accept, especially for female patients. The speech is also faint, and difficult to hear over the telephone.

For this reason, electric larynx prostheses, such as the **electrolarynx**, have been developed, which replace the voice generation of the larynx. The electrolarynx consists of an electric vibrator held against the neck just below the jawbone. The vibrator generates a basic tone, which the speaker then processes by articulation, or reshaping of the resonance cavities in the pharynx and mouth.

The **voice prosthesis** offers a more advanced solution for patients who have had a tracheostomy (opening into the trachea through the neck). The prosthesis is placed between the trachea and the oesophagus, and it comprises a vibrating sound source called the **oesophageal sphincter** or **neoglottis**. When the patient intends to speak, the tracheostoma is closed forcing air through the neoglottis. This can be obtained by two different designs. Either the patient closes the tracheostoma by hand or by a built-in automatic obstruction of the opening when the patient increases the airflow from the lungs, whereas it remains open during normal breathing. The patient speaks by forming words in the mouth as usual. The neoglottis remains closed during eating thus preventing food from entering the trachea.

PACEMAKERS

Some abnormal heart rhythms can be treated by implanting a pacemaker. The most common indications are disturbances in the propagation of impulses from the atria to the ventricles, that is heart block (Chapter 6). The treatment is very successful in complete heart block, and the survival rate for such patients is the same as that of comparable groups without heart block.

The pacemaker is usually placed subcutaneously below the clavicle on one side, and connected most commonly with one or two leads (containing electrode wires), which are inserted through a peripheral vein and advanced to the right side of the heart via the superior vena cava, Figure 10:11. Correct positioning of the lead electrode tip is then first verified with fluoroscopy. A pacing system analyser is used to check the pacemaker's ability to pick up signals and stimulate the heart to contract. The procedure is done under local anaesthesia and normally takes less than 1 hour.

A typical pacemaker measures about $5 \times 4 \times 0.6$ cm and weighs about 20 g; simpler types are even smaller, Figure 10:12. The hermetically sealed case is usually made of titanium. A pacemaker is driven by a power source with a lithium battery, enabling a service life of 10 to 15 years depending on the power consumption. A lead, which has a diameter of about 2 mm, can have silicone rubber or polyurethane insulation and the electrode tip can be made of platinum, carbon, iridium oxide or titanium nitride.

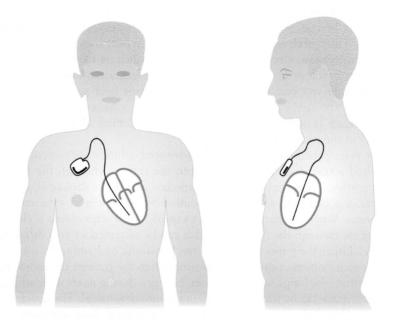

Figure 10:11 Implanted pacemaker

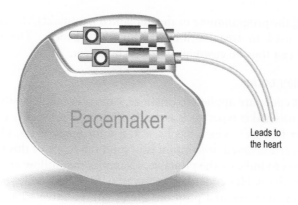

Figure 10:12 Pacemaker, shown actual size

The electrodes are used both to sense the spontaneous heart rhythm for regulation of the pacemaker stimulation activity, and to stimulate the myocardium to initiate the contraction of the heart muscle. There are several reasons why the sensed heart activity is used to control the pacemaker. Rhythm disturbances may occur sporadically, such as when the patient has a normal heart rhythm most of the time, and in these cases energy would be wasted if the pacemaker were to continuously stimulate a heart that beats on its own. Another reason is that pacemaker stimulation during a normal heartbeat would pose a hazard, as ventricular fibrillation might be triggered should the stimulating impulse occur during the vulnerable part of the cardiac cycle.

The threshold for eliciting a contraction of the myocardium is in the range 2 to 3 µJ. The pulse amplitude and duration are set with a certain safety margin, to ensure that a contraction will result. The pulse amplitude is usually set between 2.5 and 10 volts, and the pulse duration between 0.25 and 1 ms.

Pacemaker types

Many different pacemaker types have been developed, and these are categorized in various ways, and include the number of leads. When only one electrode is used in the right atrium or ventricle, we speak of **single-chamber systems**. When electrodes are placed in both the right atrium and the right ventricle, this is called a **dual-chamber system**. There are also three electrode systems used for stimulation of the right atrium and right ventricle, and in the coronary sinus to activate the left ventricle.

Another categorization is based on the type of arrhythmia being treated. **Antibradyarrhythmia pacing** is used to treat various forms of block that cause bradycardia, or too slow a heart rhythm. **Antitachyarrhythmia devices** are used to treat heart rhythms that are too fast, tachycardias. By adjusting the programming of the implanted pacemaker, the same design may be used to treat various rhythm disturbances. The pacemaker function can thus be customized for each patient.

Pacemaker codes

Different codes are applied to organize, categorize and classify the many different pacemaker types, such as the **ICHD code** (Inter-Society Commission for Heart Disease), which has been in use for many years. Other codes are similar; a detailed description is beyond the scope of this text, which only serves to indicate the principle. Examples that follow are essentially based on the ICHD code. It consists of a five-letter code, but in daily usage only the three first positions are listed, see Table 10:4.

T = triggered means that a pacing impulse is triggered by an impulse from the same chamber or chambers.

I = inhibited means that a pacing impulse is prevented whenever there is normal activity in the chamber or chambers.

D = dual in the first position means that both the atrium and ventricle are paced; in the second position that both the atrium and ventricle are sensed; and in the third position that the atrium is triggered and the ventricle output is inhibited.

O = "none" stands for the absence of the function in question.

Some examples:

VOO = pacemaker with ventricular pacing (stimulation) but no sensing function. The rate is asynchronous, that is, not determined by any natural heart impulses.

VVI = pacemaker with ventricular pacing, which is inhibited whenever the sensing electrode placed in the ventricle senses ventricular activity.

DDD = a pacemaker that both paces and senses in both the atrium and the ventricle, and is inhibited by patient-generated normal cardiac activity.

There are more descriptive synonyms that are used in daily language. A VOO pacemaker is said to be a **fixed rate** or **asynchronous** pacemaker, as it cannot adjust to any spontaneously occurring, normal cardiac activity.

Table 10:4   The ICHD code

Position I	Position II	Position III
Paced chamber	Sensed chamber	Response to sensing
A = atrium	A = atrium	T = triggered
V = ventricle	V = ventricle	I = inhibited
D = A + V	D = A + V	D = T + I

A pacemaker with the designation AT in the second and third position respectively, is called an **atrial synchronous** pacemaker. Correspondingly, an AI or VI pacemaker is called a **demand pacemaker**, meaning that it will only generate stimulating, or pacing, impulses when needed. Pacemakers that stimulate both cardiac chambers in sequence, and thus have a D ("dual") in the first letter position, are called **AV sequential** pacemakers.

Pacemaker syndrome is a problem for patients with single-chamber ventricular pacemakers. The patient experiences strong palpitations when the atria beat against already contracted ventricles with closed atrioventricular valves. The syndrome can be caused either by the atrial rhythm being asynchronous with the paced ventricular rhythm, or by retrograde conduction from the ventricles to the atria. Switching to a DVI or DDD pacemaker, for example, can often alleviate the problem.

Physiological rate regulation

There is a great principal difference between the kinds of pacemakers described above, where the rate is regulated by cardiac activity, and where the rate is regulated by other parameters, as in **rate response** or **sensor-controlled pacemakers**, such as the DDDR. The impulse rate generated by such pacemakers is regulated by one or several parameters, which vary with the patient's physiological needs, so that the pacing rate can increase in response to physical activity or metabolic demands. This is useful, for example, when the patient does not have a functioning sinus node, which could otherwise be used to regulate the pacing.

Activity-sensing pacemakers have been utilized for some time. In these pacemakers, a mechanical motion sensor is used to sense the patient's movements or acceleration. Thus when the patient exercises or performs manual labour the heart rate increases. An obvious disadvantage is that the heart rate also will increase when the patient travels in, for example, a car; the design is, however, both simple and reliable.

Minute ventilation pacemakers are controlled by the respiratory volume, which is recorded by a sensor that measures thoracic electric impedance changes (**bioelectric impedance measurement, BIM**) during the respiratory movements.

QT interval pacemakers utilize the fact that the levels of circulating norepinephrine affect the QT interval, and thus an indirect hormonal regulation of the heart rate is achieved.

Pacemakers are fairly insensitive to external electromagnetic fields (EMI, Chapter 3). But close contact with automotive ignition systems can, for example, cause inadvertent pacemaker inhibition. Patients with pacemakers should not be treated with transcutaneous nerve stimulation (TENS, see below).

Pacemaker programming

Pacemakers may be programmed from outside the body so that the function matches the patient's needs. Pulse duration and amplitude are set so that electric energy is conserved. The pacing rate may be set between 30 and 150 impulses per minute. The programmed rate determines the lowest heart rate. Modern types can even automatically set the amplitude just above the stimulation threshold which they can determine themselves.

The choice of pacemaker type and programming depends primarily on the condition of the sinus node in the atrium. If the patient's sinus node is dysfunctional, resulting in bradycardia, the condition may be corrected by an AAI pacemaker, provided that the rest of the heart's conduction system is intact. If the patient has heart block, ventricle-stimulating types are selected, such as VDD or DDD pacemakers. They are chosen when the sinus node function is intact, allowing the pacemakers to be controlled from the atrium.

Reprogramming of the pacing mode (such as VVI, DDD) may be done directly, through the intact skin. Modern pacemakers can also automatically switch from, for example, a DDD mode to another type depending on the impulses picked up from the heart. Telemetry enables remote downloading of data stored in the pacemaker, so that professional staff may review information such as the program used, pacemaker model, serial number, patient ID, the clinic where the pacemaker was implanted, telephone number, implantation date programmed, pacing mode and a very detailed history of the delivered therapy depending on changes in the patient's heart condition. The pacemaker can also store intracardiac ECGs before and after any such change in delivered therapy. This is of particular importance for antitachyarrhythmia devices and implantable defibrillators.

DEFIBRILLATORS

The technique of resuscitating patients by administering an electric shock might have been used for the first time in the 1790s in England. The method was recommended due to the "the admirable powers of the electrical shock" in resuscitation of cases of "suspended animation". However, the world was not ready for the new discovery, and the technique fell into oblivion until the 1950s.

Most physicians and nurses working in hospitals or ambulances may at some point face the need to defibrillate a patient. Few technical methods have gained such importance for saving lives in emergency situations.

The principle is simple. In external defibrillation, electrodes are placed on the chest in such a way that the current will be conducted along the long axis of the heart, Figure 10:13. Upon discharge of a capacitor, which has been charged to a voltage level of about 4000 volts, an electric pulse of about 50 amperes and a duration of 5 to 10 milliseconds is generated, Box 10:3. This causes all cardiac muscle fibres to contract, and following a short refractory period, the heart should resume its normal activity.

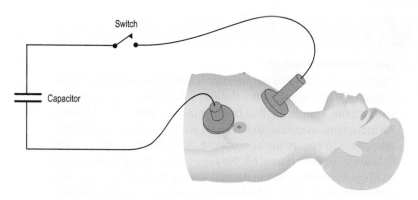

Figure 10:13 Simple design principle of a defibrillator

Indications

The most common indication for defibrillation is **ventricular fibrillation**. This arrhythmia is often a complication to a heart attack, and it can occur even when the infarction area is small. Defibrillation is usually carried out with external electrodes as already described. In open heart surgery, fibrillation is deliberately provoked to facilitate the surgical procedure, as the heart then remains almost motionless, and after completion of the surgery defibrillation is carried out using two internal "spoon"-shaped electrodes that have a concave inner surface to ensure good contact with the heart.

Atrial fibrillation, atrial flutter and **ventricular tachycardia** may also be treated with defibrillation. In these cases, the electric defibrillation shock must be synchronized with the cardiac cycle, so that a shock is avoided during the T wave, that is during the "vulnerable period" of the ventricular repolarization. Should this happen, it could result in ventricular fibrillation, which is a far more serious condition than that initially to be treated. Synchronization is achieved by obtaining the ECG signal and triggering the discharge during the appropriate phase of the cardiac cycle. This type of treatment is called **synchronized cardioversion** or **electroconversion**.

Defibrillator types

From a power supply standpoint, defibrillators can be categorized into three different groups. **Battery-operated defibrillators** are used as mobile units, for patient transport within the hospital or in ambulances. A great number of unsuccessful defibrillation attempts have been caused by failure to keep the batteries charged. Another common type of defibrillator is the **mains-operated** defibrillator with **integral batteries**, which are trickle charged as long as they are connected to the mains supply. When used as portable units, these defibrillators cannot be discharged as many times as ones with replaceable batteries. **Wholly mains-operated** defibrillators are intended for stationary usage only.

Techniques • Box 10:3

Defibrillator design

The basic principle of a defibrillator is illustrated in Figure 10:14. A capacitor is charged to the desired voltage level via a transformer and rectifier, supplied either by the mains system or by a battery. An inductance is connected in series with the capacitor, and its purpose is to ensure the appropriate pulse duration of 5 to 10 ms. Before the patient is treated, the capacitor is charged to a voltage level corresponding to the desired energy level. At the time of the defibrillation discharge, the high-voltage switch, which normally separates the capacitor charge from the patient, is closed.

The figure also illustrates how the defibrillation pulse when necessary may be synchronized with the cardiac cycle. With the switch set in the **without** synchronization position, the defibrillation will take place as soon as the manual trigger switch is pressed. In the **with** synchronization position, the synchronization circuit is connected serially with the trigger switch, and defibrillation can only take place during a certain phase of the cardiac cycle.

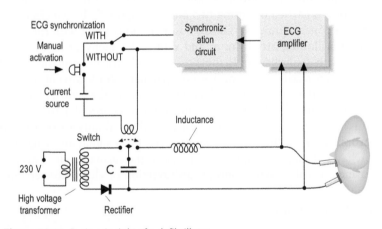

Figure 10:14 Basic principle of a defibrillator

From a functional viewpoint, defibrillators can be categorized according to their number of automatic features. With **manual defibrillators**, the user must assess the need for defibrillation and trigger the discharge by pressing the power switches on the electrode handles. **Semi-automatic defibrillators** are furnished with an advisory feature, consisting of software-integrated logic that analyses the ECG signal and indicates when defibrillation should be carried out. The semi-automatic defibrillators are available with or without automatic capacitor charging. If the defibrillator does not automatically charge the capacitor, then this step needs to be done manually before defibrillation can be carried out after the device has prompted the user to defibrillate. **Completely automatic** defibrillators will trigger the discharge without user intervention as soon as the logic has deemed that treatment is necessary.

Automatic and semi-automatic defibrillators are very valuable tools for paramedics and for others after training as they eliminate the need for interpretation of the ECG signal before defibrillation is carried out.

In the types of defibrillators described above, the current passes in one direction through the heart. Less energy is required if the direction of the current is changed once during the procedure, as it does in **biphasic defibrillators**. Because of the lower energy consumption such devices become smaller and more convenient to handle. The manufacturer's instructions for suitable defibrillation energies should be followed and not those that apply for monophasic defibrillators.

Since the patient's condition should always be assessed by interpretation of the **ECG waveform**, defibrillators are usually equipped with in-built **ECG displays**. By observing the waveform, the user can easily distinguish between ventricular fibrillation and asystole.

 Read the instructions for use for the defibrillator. If it operates on batteries, it is especially important to check how long the defibrillator may be used for ECG monitoring alone before the batteries need to be recharged.

CASE 10:4 Too much help

A middle-aged lady collapsed while away from home. An ambulance was called, but while waiting for it to arrive a local family doctor was summoned and started resuscitation. When the ambulance paramedic staff arrived, the lady was clearly cyanotic. Defibrillation pads were applied and the button on the defibrillator pressed to start the rhythm analysis sequence. The doctor was still giving chest compressions and was asked to stop. The analyser detected ventricular fibrillation, charged to 200 J and recommended a defibrillation shock. When the paramedic pressed the shock button on the defibrillator nothing happened, the defibrillator failed. He changed the device mode to manual, and delivered a successful 200 J shock. When the patient arrived at hospital she was sitting up and was talking.

Subsequent analysis of the stored defibrillation data indicated that the chest compressions had added noise to the ECG, resulting in the defibrillator being unsure of its previous decision. It then dumped the charge internally just before the paramedic attempted defibrillation, resulting in the failure experienced.

Defibrillation energies

- The American Heart Association has recommended the following energies for **external defibrillation:**

- Adults, first attempt 200 J; second attempt 200 to 300 J; third attempt 360 J.

- Children, first attempt 2 J/kg; thereafter 4 J/kg.

For **internal defibrillation:**

- 5 to 40 J regardless of body weight.

The European Resuscitation Council has recommended the following energies for external defibrillation in the following order for adults: 200 J, 200 J and 360 J. It should be noted that biphasic defibrillators can use lower energy outputs.

CASE 10:5   Confusion over defibrillator requirements

A patient was going to be defibrillated in a UK hospital. The personnel were accustomed to the ordinary monophasic defibrillators in general use at the hospital. When the patient suddenly went into ventricular fibrillation, confusion delayed treatment, since the available energy alternatives on the new biphasic defibrillator were lower than the generally recommended energies. The patient survived.

 Subsequent investigations of other similar incidents revealed that confusion occurred particularly when biphasic and standard defibrillators were available in the same clinical areas. Recommendations were made for better training, and for the use of a single type of device in any one clinical area.

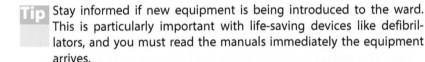 Stay informed if new equipment is being introduced to the ward. This is particularly important with life-saving devices like defibrillators, and you must read the manuals immediately the equipment arrives.

At energies of about 300 J, the current travelling through the patient is approximately 50 A. To achieve this high current, the contact between the patient's skin and the **defibrillation electrodes (defibrillation paddles)** must be extremely good. Then high-conductivity **gel pads (defibrillation pads)** or **self-adhesive electrodes** are chosen, which are easier to handle, especially during emergency transport. Previously, a special **defibrillation gel** was used to achieve good contact between the paddles and the skin. Older equipment may still exist in some places, and it is important to be aware of the pitfalls. If too much gel is applied, the gel might run and divert the electric current the wrong way – the current may even hit the operator via messy defibrillation electrodes. Furthermore, gel spills can result in reduced amounts of energy being conducted to the heart, as some energy gets wasted in warming the gel.

Gel pads must be stored flat and have a limited shelf life; dried-up pads cannot be used.

Patients with implanted pacemakers can be defibrillated, since the pacemakers are designed to withstand the strong electric shock. If possible, however, the defibrillation electrodes should be placed away from the pacemaker and perpendicular to an imaginary line between the pacemaker and the heart. The pacemaker needs to be checked after the defibrillation, as the programming may have been affected.

If done incorrectly, defibrillation may generate sparks, which can ignite resuscitation equipment used to administer oxygen. There have been cases where breathing bags have caught fire and patients have been burned. Touching the patient or the bed or patient trolley during defibrillation can be **fatal**. Defibrillators are potentially very dangerous devices, as the following example illustrates.

CASE 10:6 Ambulance driver killed

A patient was being transported in an ambulance, accompanied by an assistant nurse who had never previously carried out a defibrillation. The patient, who was suffering from a heart attack, went into ventricular fibrillation. The initial defibrillation attempt failed, but after the second attempt, normal rhythm was restored.

Soon thereafter, however, the patient again went into ventricular fibrillation, and the nurse administered CPR. The driver stopped the ambulance to assist with the resuscitation efforts. Afterwards, the nurse was not able to reconstruct exactly how the ambulance driver had been standing, but seemed to remember that he had told her to move one of the electrodes to a different location on the patient's chest.

During the defibrillation, the driver touched the nurse's right lower arm, and at this point the nurse felt a shock in her right hand, which became numb and temporarily paralysed. The ambulance driver fell backwards out of the ambulance and had generalized seizures with his mouth clamped shut as in an epileptic attack. The nurse was unable to resuscitate the ambulance driver in spite of administering CPR. The patient also died.

During the postmortem, it was found that the ambulance driver had a burn on one leg. The day following the accident, red lesions were noted on the nurse's right hand.

The ensuing technical investigation discovered two faults with the defibrillator, which was of an old type. One of the defibrillation electrode handles was cracked, which explains the injury to the nurse's hand. There was also a defective relay, which caused the metal casing of the defibrillator to become live during defibrillation, allowing the strong electric current to run from the defibrillator to the ambulance chassis.

The current had taken the following path: the electrode of the cracked handle – the nurse's hand – the driver's hand – arm – chest and heart – abdomen – leg – the ambulance metal chassis – the defibrillator.

This explains the burn on the driver's leg. Even if technical faults were partly responsible for the accident, the handling errors were also serious. The ambulance driver would not have died, had he not been in direct contact with the nurse.

 The person administering the defibrillation shock is responsible for making sure that no one else is injured in the process. An experienced specialist in intensive care medicine gives the following advice:
- If the patient is wet, dry the patient, so that the chest is dry at and around the defibrillation site.
- Use gel pads or self-adhesive electrodes. (If you have to use defibrillation gel, make sure you do not use too much gel between the electrodes and the patient's chest. An excessive amount of gel may run and thus create an undesired path for the electric current.)
- Remove all non-essential devices from the patient, but leave essential devices such as pulse monitors.
- Check the defibrillator settings. Be especially sure to check that it is not set for synchronized defibrillation.
- Do not charge the defibrillator until the patient is ready for the treatment.
- Make sure that all other personnel do not touch the patient or the patient bed eliminating any possible electric shock.
- Make sure that the patient really is unconscious before defibrillation.
- Make sure that both defibrillator electrodes are in good contact with the patient's chest via the gel pads, or that the self-adhesive electrodes, if used, are firmly attached to the chest cage along their entire surface. If self-adhesive electrodes are not being used, press down hard on the electrodes during the defibrillation – people inexperienced at carrying out defibrillations tend to feel intimated by the procedure and often hold the electrodes too lightly, which results in poor contact. Poor contact may lead to inadequate current being conducted through the patient's heart and to burns on the patient's skin at the contact site.
- Never discharge a defibrillator in order to test it, neither with the electrodes in the air at a distance from each other, nor with the electrodes in direct contact with each other. This can damage the defibrillator. (Defibrillator testing must be done with a suitable test unit consisting of a large resistor, capable of withstanding the high current. Defibrillators have an internal discharging facility.)

Many defibrillation attempts have failed due to poor technique and faulty devices. Defibrillators must therefore be checked frequently by qualified clinical engineers. The nursing staff are also responsible for making sure that defibrillators are kept in good working order. Cables must be intact, batteries kept charged and accessories easily accessible. The person carrying out the treatment must be proficient in the proper technique. There have been cases where improperly trained paramedics have actually defibrillated patients who were still conscious.

Implantable cardiac defibrillators (ICD)

An implantable defibrillator analyses the intracardiac signals and automatically detects when a treatable arrhythmia occurs, and then generates a defibrillation pulse. Defibrillation can be done with electrodes inserted intravenously into the cardiac chambers.

The defibrillator is often combined with an integrated antitachyarrhythmia/antibradyarrhythmia device. If the pacemaker is unable to prevent fibrillation from occurring, a defibrillation shock is triggered. Combining the defibrillator with an internal pacemaker is important, not only for improved treatment results, but also for minimizing the power consumption. The pacemaker can on some patients significantly reduce the number of defibrillations.

Implantable defibrillators are larger than ordinary pacemakers. This is because the defibrillator must accommodate capacitors, capable of storing the required pulse energy of up to 40 J (one million times greater than a normal pacemaker pulse), as well as the larger batteries. The batteries usually last for over 20 defibrillations.

Fitting patients with implantable defibrillators is an effective preventive treatment that can prolong the lives of patients who have previously been treated for sudden cardiac arrest or ventricular tachyarrhythmia. The treatment is, however, expensive.

MUSCLE STIMULATORS

When a motor nerve is damaged, the muscles supplied by the nerve are weakened. While the nerve fibres grow back, it is important that the muscle is stimulated so that it does not atrophy. Muscle atrophy can also develop during long-term immobilization, for example, in the treatment of fractures with casts. To prevent this, muscles may be treated with electric stimulators.

This is done by placing electrodes either directly over the muscle or over the nerve supplying the muscle. The positive electrode is placed proximally and the negative one distally. The electrodes, which can be made of conductive silicone rubber, are attached to the skin either with a conductive adhesive or an adhesive tape that ensures good skin contact.

The electrodes are connected to a small, battery-operated stimulation box, about the size of a cigarette pack. The muscle is stimulated using a series of repeated pulses, or **pulse trains**, lasting about 1 to 20 seconds each, during which time the muscle contracts. The treatment sessions usually last between 10 to 60 minutes, and are repeated up to several times a day, a couple of times per week.

NERVE STIMULATORS

Electric stimulation of nerves is used both to compensate for a physiological **loss of function**, for **pain relief** and to increase **peripheral blood flow**.

Functional nerve stimulators

It has already been described how electric stimulation can affect muscles, such as the heart muscle in pacemaker therapy. In other cases, the nerves supplying specific muscles that have been afflicted with functional losses may be stimulated. In certain types of respiratory disturbances, **phrenic nerve stimulation** can achieve a type of artificial respiration. In peroneal palsy, **peroneal nerve stimulation** can be used to assist the patient while walking.

Phrenic nerve stimulation

Patients with paralysed breathing muscles can be relieved from continuous ventilator treatment with a phrenic nerve stimulator, also called a **diaphragm pacemaker**. The most common cases arise from traffic accidents resulting in high spinal cord lesions, with injuries to the upper part of the cervical spinal cord. Cerebral haemorrhages and tumours can also cause treatable respiratory muscle paralysis.

Electrodes are implanted on the phrenic nerves on both sides of the neck and connected to a receiver, which is also implanted. A transmitter with an antenna, placed on the skin above the receiver, sends signals to the receiver through the intact skin, Figure 10:15.

One difficulty with this treatment is that the effect slowly wears off by a process called **adaptation**, which means that the nerves when receiving this type of monotonous stimulation get "worn out". For this reason, the stimulation is done on an alternating schedule, using the phrenic nerve on one side in the daytime, and on the other side at night.

The treatment results for phrenic nerve stimulation are good with increased mobility for the patient, who no longer is dependent on the ventilator. The patient's general health also improves as the blood gases normalize.

Peroneal stimulator

In **peroneal palsy**, or **drop foot**, the patient is unable to lift the sole of his foot off the ground while walking, and as a result the foot drags along

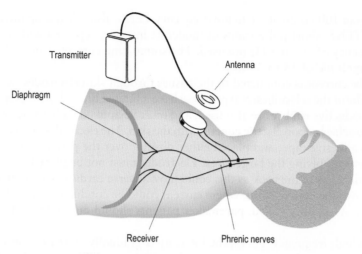

Figure 10:15 Phrenic nerve stimulation

the ground with each step. This can be caused by **cerebral haemorrhage, multiple sclerosis** and other diseases of the nervous system.

The peroneal stimulator consists of a battery-operated stimulator box, carried on the leg or hip, a heel switch beneath the foot, and two electrodes attached to the lower leg. As the leg swings forward while walking, the device sends stimulation pulses to the muscles in the lower leg, which then lift the foot upwards. As the foot is again placed on the ground, the heel switch breaks the circuit and the foot is lowered.

Pain relief and peripheral blood flow increase

Pain can sometimes be alleviated by local stimulation with electric impulses. The exact mechanism is not clear, but it is assumed that electric stimulation of large nerve fibres, which conduct afferent touch signals, to the spinal cord, block the incoming impulses in the fine afferent nerves that conduct the pain signals in the **gate control theory**. This results in decreased activation of the neurons in the ascending pathways going to the brain. The process resembles what some researchers believe happens when people scratch themselves because of an itch – the itch itself is not affected, but the incoming itch signals are blocked by the slight pain signals caused by the scratching.

In **transcutaneous nerve stimulation (TENS)** the stimulating electrodes are placed on the skin, whereas in **dorsal column stimulation (DCS)**, also called **spinal cord stimulation (SCS)**, the stimulating electrodes are implanted.

Transcutaneous nerve stimulation

Various types of electric current can be used for nerve stimulation. In **high-frequency TENS**, also called **conventional TENS**, alternating currents of about 100 Hz are used. In **low-frequency TENS**, also called **acupuncture-like TENS**, short pulse trains of moderate intensity repeated with a low frequency of about 2 Hz are used. The stimulating currents usually have a magnitude of 15 to 30 mA.

The current is conducted to the tissues through skin electrodes, which may be of the self-adhesive type (these have a limited life). Electrodes made of conductive rubber are also used, and must be applied with an electrode gel to achieve good electric contact with the skin. The electrodes are secured with adhesive tape, and placed either directly over the pain area or over a nerve supplying the target area. Electrodes must not be placed over the carotid sinus in the neck as this could have adverse cardiovascular effects, nor over the eyes or skull, where current could be conducted through the brain. As already stated, pacemaker patients should not be treated with TENS.

In high-frequency TENS, the intensity is gradually increased until the patient feels a tingling sensation. In low-frequency TENS, stimulation is increased until there is visible muscle twitching. Stimulation with low-frequency TENS can sometimes cause muscle soreness.

High-frequency TENS is usually attempted first. The pain relief may last about 2 to 4 hours after each treatment session, which lasts $\frac{1}{2}$ to 1 hour and is usually given 2 to 4 times per day. If a satisfactory response is not obtained, low-frequency TENS is attempted.

Dorsal column stimulation

An electrode is inserted into the dorsal region of the epidural space, and the spinal cord is stimulated. A flexible metal wire is inserted percutaneously by the same technique as that used when inserting an epidural catheter for anaesthesia or epidural administration of morphine. The electrode is connected to a receiver box, which may be placed subcutaneously below the costal arch on one side. The receiver is activated by an antenna coil placed on the skin next to the receiver. The coil is connected to a battery-operated pulse generator of the same type as that used for TENS. There are also completely implantable pulse generators that can be activated by the patient with the help of an external magnet.

During stimulation, the patient experiences paresthesias or tingling sensations in the body parts that are supplied by the same spinal segment as that which is being stimulated. To achieve effective pain relief, it is important that paresthesias are produced over the entire area of pain.

Medical use

Several types of pain can be treated with TENS, such as **nerve pain, back pain, pain due to fractures, menstrual pains, postoperative pain** and **labour pains**. During labour, some pain relief has been obtained during the first stage, but TENS has not been able to replace traditional pain relieving drugs. Psychogenic pain, pain where no objective findings explaining the origin of the pain can be found, responds poorly to nerve stimulation.

The disadvantage of this method is that not all patients obtain the same level of pain relief. Positive effects are achieved in about half of the cases, but better results have been demonstrated for menstrual pain.

Electric stimulation can also be used to **improve peripheral blood flow**. Therapy-resistant leg ulcers have thus been treated with electric stimulation.

Dorsal column stimulation works on the same principle as TENS, but is more effective. It is used for severe cases of **chronic back and sciatic pain** as well as for **peripheral neuralgias** and for patients with refractory angina pectoris that are not helped by any of the traditional treatments. The pain relief obtained may be a result of two processes, blocking of the pain signals and an increased oxygenation of the myocardium.

It may seem surprising that electric stimulation can be allowed in **angina pectoris**. The pain is the body's way of signalling that the heart muscle is suffering from a lack of oxygen – eliminating this warning signal of myocardial ischaemia ought to be dangerous. But experience has shown that increased blood flow results in a reduction in ST-depression on the ECG (Chapter 6). The treatment also improves the patient's quality of life.

Stimulation in the brain

In essential tremor, a disease of unknown cause, the patient suffers from shaking. In severe cases, this may be so pronounced that the patient has difficulty holding a glass of water or dressing himself. This condition is associated with changes in a pea-sized area in the brain. The condition can be alleviated by surgical ablation, or destruction of this area. This method can, however, produce severe side-effects. Another solution is to implant an electrode in the brain for electric stimulation. The patient is fitted with a subcutaneous pulse generator placed on the front of the chest. By placing a magnet on the chest, the patient can control the pulse generator until symptom relief is obtained.

DEATH CERTIFICATES

All types of implanted prostheses containing batteries must be removed before the body is cremated as the batteries **explode** when incinerated. This poses a hazard to the crematory staff. A large number of such explosions have happened during cremation of bodies with pacemakers. The physician signing the death certificate must make sure that no implanted devices containing batteries remain in the body.

11

Tissues and calculi

In various types of surgical procedures it is often necessary to destroy certain tissues in the body. Sometimes stones also need to be crushed, such as calculi that have formed in the kidneys or in the gall bladder.

Destruction of tissues and calculi can be achieved by applying various forms of energy. In **surgical diathermy** (also called **electrosurgery** or **high-frequency surgery**) the energy consists of a high-frequency electric current, whereas **laser surgery** is based on intense coherent light. Another special method, **ultrasound aspiration,** uses high-frequency sound. **Extracorporeal shockwave lithotripsy (ESWL)** relies on high-energy mechanical shock-waves to pulverize stones in the kidneys or gall bladder, so that the fragments can be eliminated through the body's natural orifices. A method that has been extensively applied in recent years is **balloon dilatation**, where mechanical force is applied to the tissue by means of a catheter.

Cryosurgery is another method less often used, where extreme cold is applied to freeze and thereby destroy the tissues. The opposite of cold, heat treatment in various forms, is used for a great variety of conditions. Severe depression can be treated with electric shocks, so-called **electro-convulsive therapy.** Many patients with malignant tumours receive **radiation therapy.**

Common to all these methods is the application of such amounts of energy that tissues are destroyed or affected. They must therefore be used with great prudence if unintended effects are to be avoided. Of these methods, diathermy requires the greatest vigilance, as the number of injuries in recent years has increased in spite of more advanced technology. With accumulated experience, many procedures have successively been modified to reduce the risks of unwanted effects.

SURGICAL DIATHERMY

Diathermy is technically complicated, and without special knowledge in electrical engineering it is not possible to understand the underlying mechanisms to the extent that all the hazards associated with this method become comprehensible (the techniques boxes contain brief descriptions of a few). This section outlines the general principles without the need to understand the details.

During diathermy, an electric current large enough to destroy the tissues by the heat generated is conducted through the tissues (Greek: *dia* = through, *terme* = heat). The tissue effects depend on the temperature produced. Below about 50°C there is no irreversible tissue damage. At about 50°C, the tissues coagulate, they are destroyed and the colour gradually changes from red to grey. At about 70°C, haemostasis is achieved. At approximately 100°C, the tissue water boils and vaporizes, known as **desiccation**, and the tissues shrink in size. At about 200°C, charring or **carbonization** occurs. The heat produced in the tissues depends on three factors:

The heat **increases** in proportion to
1. The square of current density
2. The duration of the current

The heat **decreases** in proportion to
3. The conductance of the tissue

Diathermy electrodes are designed to ensure a high current density where tissue is to be destroyed, and a low current density in other areas. A commonly used principle, the **monopolar technique**, is shown in Figure 11:1. The high current density is generated at the active electrode and the low current density at the patient return electrode, through which the current returns to the diathermy generator. The **bipolar technique** differs in that two electrodes of approximately equal size are used, and there is no large return electrode.

The electric power required depends on the field of application. In eye surgery a few watts will suffice, whereas wart removal requires a couple of tens of watts and general surgery typically about 50 to 100 watts. The highest power levels, 200 to 300 watts, are used in urology during bladder surgery.

To prevent the electric current from causing heart and other muscle contractions as well as stimulating the nerve tissues, a high frequency is used, 0.3 to 5 MHz. Currents of such high frequency, however, are not only conducted via metal conductors as is the case with the mains current which has a frequency of 50 or 60 Hz. They can take completely unexpected pathways, thereby causing injuries to the patient.

Radio waves are carried from transmitter to receiver without electric cables. Similarly, the diathermy current may travel to sites other than

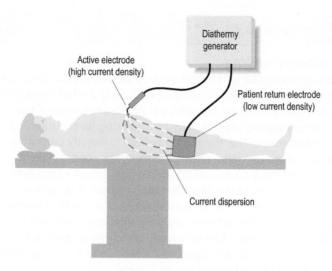

Figure 11:1 The most common set-up for surgical diathermy

those intended – sites that are not connected to the diathermy generator by means of a cable. Instead, the electric energy is transferred through **capacitive coupling,** Box 11:1. The diathermy current can also easily pass to the operating table or other connected devices such as an ECG monitor via the electrodes. If this happens, the patient could be burned in areas where the body is in contact with the operating table or beneath the ECG electrodes.

The practical solution to this problem is to ensure such good electric contact in the intended current circuit that the current through other possible pathways becomes low and harmless.

Types of tissue effects

Tissues can be destroyed in various ways. Diathermy is often used in place of a scalpel for **cutting** the tissues. In other situations, **coagulation** of the tissues may be the desired effect. A special form of coagulation is **fulguration,** where the superficial cell layer is destroyed by sparks that hit the tissue surface.

The various types of tissue destruction are determined by selecting the appropriate active electrode and diathermy current waveform (constant or intermittent). The waveform type is set on a dial marked for cutting (**Cut**) and coagulation (**Coag**). Experience has shown that the best cutting characteristics are obtained when the generator produces a current of constant amplitude. The best coagulating qualities, on the other hand, are achieved with an intermittent waveform with a high amplitude, and the current waveform is interrupted to generate short pulses.

Techniques • Box 11:1

Capacitive coupling

Direct current can be conducted only via electric conductors, such as a metal wire or water. Alternating current, on the other hand, can also be conducted via a capacitor, which in principle consists of two plates or conductors separated by an insulating layer (Chapter 3). The conductance of the alternating current is directly proportional to the size of the capacitor and to the frequency of the current.

Thus a diathermy current of 0.5 MHz is conducted 10,000 times more efficiently through a capacitor than the mains current with a frequency of 50 Hz. This is the reason why it is possible to perform diathermy procedures without applying a patient return electrode directly to the patient when only low output power levels are needed. The body has a certain low capacitance relative to its surrounding that is sufficient for adequate power transfer.

A capacitive patient return electrode can consist merely of a small plate located under the seat of the patient's chair. In these cases, the diathermy current is conducted through capacitive coupling between the patient and the return electrode. If no return electrode is used at all, it is the body's own capacitance to the diathermy generator that is utilized, Figure 11:2.

The body's capacitance to surrounding items is in principle not changed when a return electrode is connected directly to the patient,

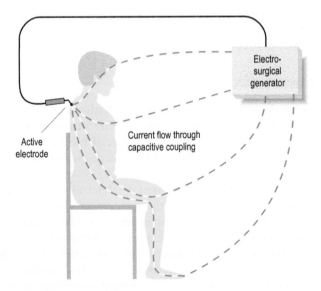

Figure 11:2 Capacitive coupling

Techniques • Box 11:1—Continued

as is often done during operations. Therefore, a certain amount of the diathermy current always travels back to the generator via such items (for example, the operation table or a connected ECG monitor). Hopefully, the conductance between the body and the patient return electrode will be much higher, resulting in the majority of the current taking this path.

However, in the case of poor contact between the patient return electrode and the skin, or a damaged patient return electrode cable, a greater part of the current will pass through other items. If any of these items are in contact with the body over a small area of about one square centimetre, a burn may occur at this site. It is therefore more dangerous to have a small contact area between the body and other items than a large area.

The tissue effects are not completely distinct in that even while cutting some superficial coagulation takes place, which is actually a desirable effect. Most generators also have an additional **blend** mode where the surgical effects of both dissection and haemostasis is obtained.

Cutting

During cutting, the tissues next to the active electrode are heated to such a high temperature that the tissue fluids vaporize and force the cells apart, Figure 11:3. As soon as gas is formed, the current is conducted to the tissue via sparks, and the tissue can be quickly transected.

There are two reasons why cutting is often done using diathermy instead of a scalpel. First, diathermy cutting causes less bleeding, as small blood vessels are coagulated during the heating process. Second, there is less risk of spread of bacteria and tumour cells from the surgical site to the surrounding tissue, which can happen when cutting with a scalpel. During diathermy cutting, the bacteria and tumour cells are destroyed by the heat.

For diathermy cutting, a small, thin active electrode is used. The electrode may be shaped as a thin blade or wire. The wire may be in the form of a loop, which can snare and cut pedunculated polyps, Figure 11:4, and plane off tissue sections, Figure 11:5. The output power is set at a level that produces the appropriate cutting effect, with a moderate amount of sparking generated and without the electrode adhering to the tissue.

The dial is not graduated in absolute numbers and each type of generator must be set individually for the appropriate output level. If the output power needs to be increased beyond the expected level, this may be a sign that the current is not being returned in the normal

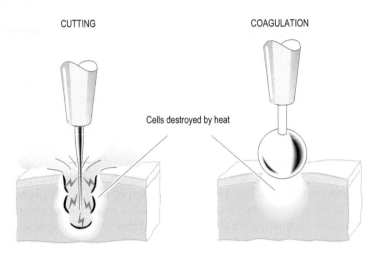

Figure 11:3 The two types of electrosurgery

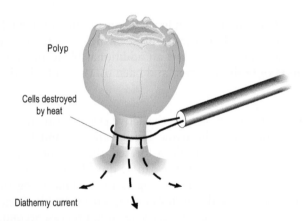

Figure 11:4 Removal of a polyp using a diathermy loop

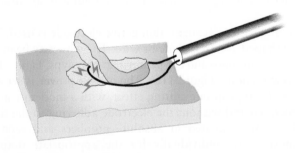

Figure 11:5 Use of an electrosurgical loop

fashion via the patient return electrode and that the situation needs to be investigated.

Coagulation

During coagulation, tissues are destroyed without being forced apart, as is the case during cutting, Figure 11:3. The tissues turn pale, almost white, and become desiccated. If the coagulation procedure continues at a high output power level, the tissues will be charred.

Coagulation can be achieved in two principally different ways, **monopolar** and **bipolar diathermy**. In the monopolar mode, Figure 11:6, the current is similar to that of cutting. Thus it passes from the comparatively small electrode to the large return electrode.

To coagulate the tissue, a somewhat larger contact area is created between the active electrode and the tissue than with cutting. For example, a ball-shaped electrode may be used, or a blade-shaped cutting electrode with a larger part of its surface area pressed against the tissues than that applied during cutting.

A disadvantage with monopolar diathermy is that the current must pass through the patient and back to the patient return electrode. As a result it may be difficult to assess exactly at what distance from the active electrode diathermy effects are obtained.

Many surgeons often use a haemostat or forceps as the active electrode when coagulating blood vessels to achieve haemostasis. The active electrode of the diathermy generator is simply pressed against the surgical instrument – sometimes called buzzing. Because of the relatively small tissue contact area, the current density becomes high enough to achieve

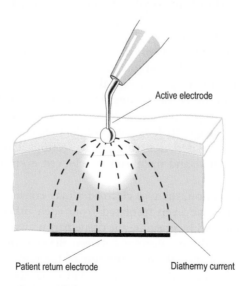

Active electrode

Patient return electrode   Diathermy current

Figure 11:6 Monopolar coagulation

coagulation. This is felt to be practical, especially if the haemostat is already clamped around a small, distinct tissue area. But the technique results in unnecessarily extensive thermal damage, as the diathermy current is concentrated mainly to the surrounding areas and not to the blood vessel itself. From a technical standpoint this technique is **incorrect**.

Surgical diathermy is a most valuable method in everyday use. But knowledge of how to handle the equipment is essential, among other things of how to put the pieces together. Numerous accidents have been reported of the following kind:

CASE 11:1 Patient's lip burned

A patient was going to have her tonsils removed. Surgical diathermy was used during the procedure. The patient obtained a burn on a lip.

The active electrode had not been fully inserted in the diathermy pencil. Hence an exposed part of the uninsulated post of the active electrode had come in contact with the patient's lip.

Some surgeons extend the length of the active electrode, particularly during throat surgery, by not fully inserting it in the handpiece. There is an obvious risk of causing a burn injury.

Tip Never ever extend the length of an active electrode by not inserting it fully. Longer electrodes are commercially available and should be used.

A specialized form of monopolar diathermy is **argon plasma coagulation,** where a stream of ionized argon is used as the active electrode. A fine stream of argon gas is directed towards the tissue surface, and a high voltage is generated between the metal tube from which the gas is flowing and the tissue. The argon gas hereby becomes ionized and conductive in the same way as the air during lightning. The advantage is that coagulation only becomes superficial, with a maximum depth of 3 mm. Further, the argon plasma is continuously moving towards new tissue areas not yet coagulated, as these conduct the current much better than the already coagulated, desiccated tissue sections. Large tissue areas can thus be coagulated and haemostasis achieved even in widespread, diffuse bleeding.

In **bipolar coagulation,** the two electrodes may consist of the tines of tissue forceps that have been insulated from each other, Figure 11:7. Coagulation is achieved by grasping the tissue part with the tissue forceps and applying the diathermy current between the two instrument jaws. The current does not pass through the rest of the body and no patient return electrode is needed. Bipolar coagulation is always used when highly localized tissue destruction is desired, such as in neurosurgery and

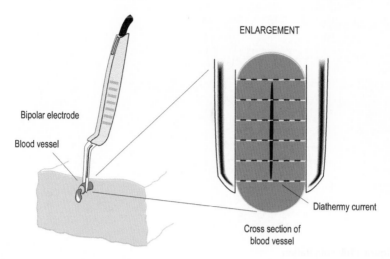

ENLARGEMENT

Bipolar electrode

Blood vessel

Diathermy current

Cross section of
blood vessel

Figure 11:7 Bipolar coagulation

microsurgery. The method ought to be used more extensively than is currently the case.

Use the **bipolar** method when **coagulating blood vessels**; monopolar diathermy results in unnecessarily extensive thermal damage, since the current passes through the tissues around the vessel.

The patient return electrode serves no function during bipolar coagulation, but it is still connected, as it is often difficult to know in advance whether or not the surgical procedure can be carried out using the bipolar mode only.

A difficulty when performing coagulation is knowing when adequate heating has taken place. If heated too long, the coagulated tissue will adhere to the electrode, and bleeding may then resume when the electrode is torn away from the tissue. An elegant solution to this problem is furnished by generators that record the current going through the tissue during the entire procedure and turn the current off when adequate coagulation has been achieved (tissue response technology). Thus such a feedback system reduces the need to adjust the power settings for different types of tissue.

Fulguration

For the removal of superficial skin lesions such as warts, the active electrode is passed back and forth above the wart surface – the surface is brushed as if using a paintbrush where the bristles have been replaced by sparks, Figure 11:8.

Great vigilance is required during diathermy procedures. It is necessary to keep track of the active electrode at all times so that inadvertent activation is avoided (compare Case 1:20).

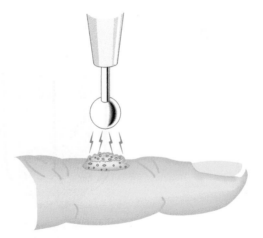

Figure 11:8 Fulguration

CASE 11:2 Something is burning

During a knee operation the surgeon suddenly smelled something burning. It was discovered that the active electrode had burned right through a sterile paper towel. The inside of the patient's thigh had also been burned.

The handle of the diathermy instrument, which had a trigger for activation of the diathermy current, had slipped down and become squeezed between the patient's thighs. The trigger was thus inadvertently pressed and the current activated.

Diathermy generators are equipped with an audible signal that alerts the user whenever diathermy current is being generated. In this incidence, nobody had heard the signal, as a ventilation system for bone cement preparation as well as a bone saw had both been running at the same time.

After the accident, no faults with the diathermy generator, the patient return electrode or the instrument handle could be noted. The reason for the incident was simply that the instruction had not been followed stating that the active electrode must be kept visible in a plastic holster when not in use.

Surgical diathermy must be distinguished from **electrocautery**, where a wire loop is heated by an electric current. The loop, which becomes burning hot, can be used to plane away tissue sections. During electrosurgery, it is primarily the tissues that are heated, not the electrode.

The patient return electrode

Depending on the area of use and whether it will be applied for high or low power output applications, the patient return electrode (also called dispersive electrode, neutral electrode or patient plate) can be designed in various ways.

Capacitive patient return electrodes

When only a low power output is required (>50 W), for example, when removing skin warts, a capacitive patient return electrode may be used. The diathermy current then returns to the generator **without a cable**, and is distributed over such a large area of the body surface that no thermal injury can occur. As pointed out above, when treating a sitting patient, the electrode may be placed under the seat of the chair.

If the patient touches a small area of the operating table, however, the patient may suffer small thermal injuries that feel like electric shocks. Similarly, the treating physician may experience unpleasant shocks if the patient is touched. A patient return electrode that is applied directly to the patient is preferable, since it conducts the current directly back to the diathermy unit.

Return electrodes applied directly to the patient

To determine the proper location for a patient return electrode, it is necessary to understand that different types of tissues have different specific conductance. Highly vascularized tissues have high conductance and allow the diathermy current to pass with a relatively low heat production. Fatty tissue has a low conductance, and bone even lower. Here high temperatures are quickly generated.

Patient return electrodes are often made of self-adhesive conductive foil with good adhesion and are easy to apply. The foil must adhere well to the skin, and excessive hair must therefore be shaved off prior to the application.

The patient return electrode must be placed relatively close to the surgical field, Figure 11:9. Thus, it should not be placed on the lower leg if used for abdominal surgery, for example. In this situation, the current density would become unnecessarily high in the knee, which consists primarily of bone with poor conductive properties. The current would become concentrated to the thin soft tissues of the knee, with overheating and possible burns as a result. Instead, the patient return electrode should be placed around the thigh. For the same reasons, the patient return electrode must not be placed around the lower arm during surgery in areas from which the current would travel through the elbow.

The patient return electrode should preferably be placed at a site that can be inspected during the operation, so that its position and application can be monitored, Box 11:2.

However, the patient return electrode must not be placed directly adjacent to the surgical field. This would lead to a concentration of the current at the edge of the patient return electrode, which would increase the risk of burns, Figure 11:9. The patient return electrode should if possible be placed opposite the surgical field, but not directly under the patient, where the pressure of the patient's weight could cause ischaemia

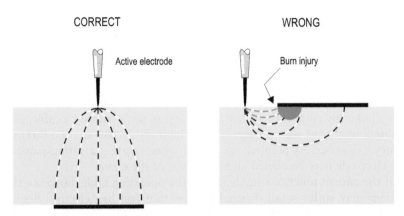

CORRECT   WRONG

Active electrode   Burn injury

Figure 11:9 The patient return electrode should whenever possible be positioned on the opposite side of the body relative to the active electrode

---

 Techniques • Box 11:2

Monitoring return electrode

As it is vital that the contact between the patient return electrode and the patient is good, several technical designs have been developed that trigger an alarm in the case of poor contact, and also deactivate the diathermy current.

An old, established design consists of a dual electric cable leading to the patient return electrode, Figure 11:10a. A low-frequency electric check current is conducted through the loop that is formed when the cables are electrically connected with the patient return electrode applied. If the patient return electrode is not connected or if there is a cable interruption, the circuit is broken and the generator will sound an alarm. The disadvantage with this method is that there is no guarantee that there is adequate electric connection between the electrode and the patient, as the patient return electrode does not have to be in any contact with the patient for the check current to still be able to pass.

In more recent designs, the patient return electrode is split into two parts and the two cables connected to one part each, to enable a high-frequency check current to pass via the patient, Figure 11:10b. This design is a considerable safety improvement, as the check current must always pass through the patient return electrode; if this does not happen, an alarm will sound and the diathermy current is shut off.

The latter design, however, does not prevent burns at other body locations. The safest generators are designed to check that an equal amount of current passes through the cable leading to the patient return electrode as through the cable leading to the active electrode, Figure 11:10c. If there is a difference in the amount of current passing

Techniques • Box 11:2—Continued

through the return and active electrode cables, this means that there is another, undesired current path. This will cause the current to be deactivated and an alarm will sound.

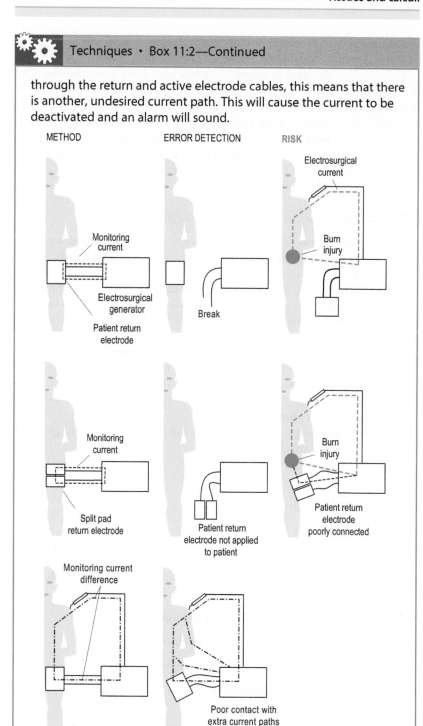

METHOD   ERROR DETECTION   RISK

Monitoring current

Electrosurgical generator

Patient return electrode

Break

Electrosurgical current

Burn injury

Monitoring current

Split pad return electrode

Patient return electrode not applied to patient

Burn injury

Patient return electrode poorly connected

Monitoring current difference

Poor contact with extra current paths

Figure 11:10 Patient return electrode contact-quality monitoring systems

in the tissues with resulting low tissue conductance, hence increasing the heat developed, as explained above.

Do not place the patient return electrode over bony prominences. The thin skin layer between the electrode and the underlying bone has high impedance, and at such sites, because of the irregular body contour, it is also difficult to achieve good contact with surrounding skin areas.

The patient must be insulated from the operating table and other metal objects; this could be achieved with at least three layers of cotton fabric, which must not be allowed to get wet during surgery.

CASE 11:3   Patient burned during abdominal surgery

In 1993, a patient was undergoing surgery for an abdominal aortic aneurysm. During the operation, the blood flow to the lower half of the body was temporarily shut off.

After the operation, it was discovered that the patient had a burn on his left buttock where the patient return electrode had been placed. No faults could be found with the diathermy generator or the patient return electrode.

The patient return electrode had been placed such that the patient had been lying on it, and the tissues had been squeezed between it and the table. This resulted in diminished blood flow to the tissues, and in addition, the entire blood flow to this area had been shut off during a large part of the operation. The resulting low conductance (high resistance to the current) had caused excessive heat production.

This incident prompted a revision of national regulations regarding placement of patient return electrodes.

Controls and colour coding

A diathermy generator is controlled via foot switches or switches located on the handpiece of the active electrode. A foot switch must be designed in such a way that the operator can always, regardless of the generator make or model, control the activation without having to actually look at the switches.

- **Left** foot switch activates the **cutting** mode
- **Right** foot switch activates the **coagulation** mode

Indicator lights are colour coded in the following fashion:

- **Green** – power supply switch on
- **Yellow** – cutting mode activated
- **Blue** – coagulation mode activated
- **Red** – fault condition

Diathermy during endoscopy

The risks of injuries are greatest when diathermy is being applied via endoscopes, and this is due to several factors. The small endoscope diameter makes it difficult to insulate the high-frequency current in a diathermy cable from the casing. Higher output powers are used, since some of the diathermy current is lost through capacitive coupling from the endoscope to the surrounding area.

Diathermy is often used during procedures carried out via flexible **gastroscopes** and **colonoscopes**. Both monopolar and bipolar electrodes are used. The bipolar technique is preferable whenever possible, as there is less risk of injury.

Endoscopes intended for diathermy resections, often called **resecto-scopes**, have been available in two principally different designs: either with an **insulated** or a **non-insulated** external surface. The noninsulated type has proven less reliable and should be avoided. Regardless of whether the insulated or non-insulated type is being employed, it is of vital importance that the correct type of lubricating gel is applied. Whereas non-insulated resectoscopes had to be used with conducting gel, insulated instruments must be used with a non-conductive gel to reduce the risk of localized burns. Should there be an insulation failure, the insulating gel reduces the amount of current leaking through the faulty endoscope insulation. Insulated resectoscopes must be inspected very carefully before use, to ensure that there are no insulation defects through which the electrical current could leak and cause a burn, for example, in the urethra, Figure 11:11. The insulation must also be tested at regular intervals. When using resectoscopes with external insulation, there is also a certain risk that some of the diathermy current might pass through the hands of the surgeon, as illustrated in the figure. This risk can, however, be avoided by using an S-cord (see below).

Resection of the prostate is often done via the urethra, so-called **TURP (transurethal resection of the prostate)**. This technique must be carried out with great care, as high output powers are required. The instrumentation must be in perfect condition. Components designed for single use must not be reused:

CASE 11:4 Patient suffers electric shock during TURP

During resection of the prostate the patient suddenly jerked, and it turned out that the non-insulated resectoscope was not working.

The ensuing investigation at the clinical engineering department showed that the diathermy generator was functioning properly. However, the resectoscope loop, which was part of a single-use set but nevertheless reused, had become short-circuited to the resectoscope casing. Hereby it had conducted the diathermy current. It was further discovered that fluids had penetrated between the loop insulation and the resectoscope cannula, causing further potentially harmful current paths.

This case demonstrates, besides the risks with noninsulated resectoscopes, the dangers of reusing components designed for single use only.

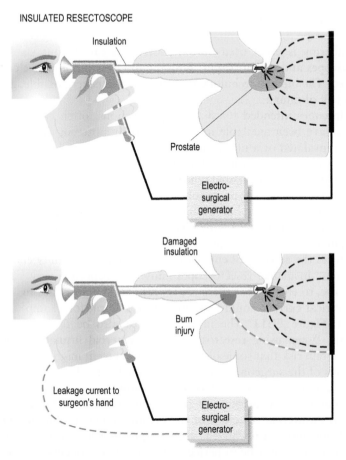

Figure 11:11 When using insulated resectoscopes, there must be no breach in the insulation

During surgery in body cavities such as the urinary bladder, the cavity must be filled with a low-conductance fluid so that the diathermy current is not short-circuited. For the same reason, the irrigation fluids used for removing tissue debris must also be of low conductance. Previously, a 2.2% isotonic glycine solution was used (an isotonic solution prevents the solution from being absorbed by the cells). But it has been shown that a glycine solution of this concentration can cause heart damage, and several deaths have been reported. Instead, for example, a mannitol solution could be chosen.

To prevent the diathermy electrode from sticking to the tissues, and to protect the tissues from injury due to ignition of the flammable gases that may be generated, a **protective gas** is sometimes used. This gas is made to stream around the active electrode. The protective gas often consists of carbon dioxide or argon. This application of argon must not be mixed up with the previously described technique of using ionized argon as the active electrode.

Diathermy injuries

Burn injuries are most frequently caused when the current through the patient return electrode is inadvertently concentrated to only a small area of this electrode.

Any electrically conductive object, such as temperature probes for monitoring and blood flow gauges, can cause burn injuries when the patient contact area is small enough to result in a high current density with high-frequency current leakage. Modern ECG machines designed for patient monitoring are equipped with special input circuit protective devices (choke coils), with a high impedance to the high-frequency diathermy current. This way, potential burns at the electrode placement sites are prevented.

Fluids that are allowed to spill and wet the fabrics intended for electric insulation of the patient from the operating table, anaesthesia screen holder, arm rests, stirrups, etc., present a risk of burn injuries, especially in cases of poor patient return electrode contact.

Several burns have been caused by inadvertent activation of the diathermy generator (see Case 1:20 and Case 11:2). To eliminate this risk, the electrode must always be kept visible in an insulated holster when not in use, so that current does not inadvertently flow to the patient. This might otherwise happen, if the electrode is placed by mistake on, for example, a wet surgical drape. To minimize the risk of inadvertent activation of the diathermy generator due to electric interference from external sources (Chapter 3), the generator must be turned on only when it is actually being used for the surgical procedure.

The diathermy cables must not be coiled up but should run straight, to avoid the risk of induction of diathermy currents in other cables, such as ECG cables. The diathermy cables must also be connected correctly:

CASE 11:5 Cables routinely misconnected

During endoscopic surgery of the colon, the patient suffered a modest burn at the site where a metal part of the colonoscope tubing connector had inadvertently been touching the patient's skin.

After the operation, it was discovered that the colonoscope grounding cable had been connected to the active receptacle on the diathermy generator instead of being connected to the patient return electrode. This erroneous way of connecting the grounding cable had been used routinely during many endoscopic surgical procedures without any previous injuries occurring. The generator had a floating output, which had previously avoided patients being injured by this major error.

Innumerable injuries, which have occurred in connection with diathermy procedures and have been interpreted as diathermy burns, were in reality caused by other factors, such as **pressure necrosis** and **chemical burns**. Other, "indirect" injuries have been caused by **explosions** due to ignition of gases and by the diathermy current having activated other **patient-connected devices**. A more trivial effect is the **muscle twitching** that can happen in both the patient and doctor during diathermy.

Pressure necroses

Pressure necroses can look deceptively like burns. They may arise at the patient return electrode site when this electrode has been inappropriately applied. Pressure necroses may also occur in many other locations and erroneously be interpreted as diathermy burns:

CASE 11:6 Assistant surgeon causes pressure necroses

A retired neurosurgeon was continuing his clinical practice at a private hospital. After a while it was discovered that all five patients operated on after a certain date had contracted ugly, nonhealing ulcers, which were interpreted as diathermy burns. Disfiguring necroses developed over the cheek bones on the patients that had been placed in the face-down position, and over the neck region on the patients that had been placed in the supine position. The surgeon had, during his very long career, never before encountered such injuries.

Several actions were taken. A new diathermy generator was purchased, but as this did nothing to alleviate the problem, a new earthed wall outlet was installed in the department at the recommendation of the generator supplier (this seems to have been an act of desperation, as it could hardly have affected the cause of these injuries). Rigorous routines were instigated, including meticulous checking of the placement of the patient return electrode and cables. Nothing helped.

A clinical engineer was consulted and found no faults with any of the devices. The head rest was made of thick rubber of poor conductance, intended for high-frequency applications, and it was not conceivable that any diathermy current of importance could possibly have passed through it. He then requested permission to personally observe the next operation, and discovered that the assistant surgeon was resting his hands very heavily on the patient's head during the operation.

The same surgeon, who was a new employee at the hospital, had assisted during all of the previous five operations. By advising the surgeon to release the pressure exerted on the patient's head at regular intervals, subsequent injuries were avoided.

Chemical burns

Intraoperative chemical burns due to chemical effects on the skin at the patient return electrode placement site are not uncommon. It is easy to understand why such injuries have been mistakenly interpreted as having been caused by incorrect diathermy procedures.

CASE 11:7 Patient injured by adhesives cleaned with petrol

During an operation a patient return electrode ("electrosurgery pad") was used. After the operation, adhesive residues from the patient return electrode were noted on the patient's buttock and thigh. The adhesive was removed with petrol (gasoline).

The next morning, a "burn" was discovered at the site where the patient return electrode had been placed. The lesion consisted of erythema and ruptured "burn blisters" in the middle of the lesion.

Since no burn had been noted immediately after the completion of the surgery, it was inconceivable that the diathermy could have caused the lesion. It was deemed that the cleaning and rubbing of the skin with petrol was the most likely cause of the injury.

Many liquids and solutions, which are normally harmless provided they are allowed to evaporate immediately, have, when improperly handled, been shown to cause chemical burns. This is the case if they are allowed to accumulate between the patient return electrode and the skin and remain there during the operation. It is therefore important to ensure that no disinfectants or skin preparation solutions are allowed to accumulate beneath the patient return electrode.

The lesions may resemble a first- or second-degree burn injury. A brownish discolouration of the skin often appears 2 days after the injury. Chemical burns usually heal without permanent scarring.

Explosions

Explosion of flammable intestinal gases is a serious but fortunately rare complication. The risk of oxygen fires in connection with diathermy has already been discussed (see Case 4:2). The following example emphasizes the problems encountered when performing surgery in an oxygen-rich environment:

CASE 11:8   Fatal burns to the larynx, trachea and epiglottis

A 72-year-old man was being treated for pneumonia in hospital. In spite of extra oxygen administration, his oxygen saturation was unsatisfactory. In order to start respiratory support with a ventilator, a tracheostoma (an opening to the windpipe on the front of the throat) needed to be created. During this procedure, a "fault with the diathermy generator" occurred, whereupon a fire erupted around the tracheostoma opening. The patient's trachea, larynx, epiglottis, oral cavity and lips were burned and he died a few minutes later.

Using diathermy while the patient was breathing oxygen was a fundamental error.

The same risk exists for flammable liquids, such as alcohol, which can ignite during diathermy (see Chapter 4 and Case 4:9).

Gas emboli

To improve visualization during various endoscopic surgical procedures, gas is often insufflated into the body cavities. This carries a risk of gas emboli, as the gas is under pressure and an endoscopic procedure always leads to some degree of vascular damage.

Carbon dioxide is the gas normally used as it quickly dissolves in the blood should it penetrate to the vascular system. Therefore, carbon dioxide emboli are fortunately rare. Because of the fire hazard, oxygen must of course never be used. Argon gas is highly unsuitable as it has low blood solubility; however, this gas is used in argon plasma coagulation.

Injuries caused by other connected devices

The high-frequency currents during diathermy may interfere with other devices through capacitive coupling. This may have particularly serious implications when the patient's life depends on other devices, such as a ventilator or heart–lung machine. The following example illustrates the importance of inactivating or disconnecting other devices during diathermy whenever possible:

CASE 11:9   Runaway heart–lung machine kills patient

When heart operations are completed, the blood in the heart–lung machine is returned to the patient and the pumps are shut down. The tubing to the patient is clamped off with a haemostat to prevent the air in the now air-filled machine from entering the patient.

In one case, when diathermy was used right after the heart–lung machine had been stopped, the blood pump suddenly started again, pushing air past the haemostat and into the tubing connected to the patient's arterial system. The patient died.

Through capacitive coupling the diathermy generator had affected the control circuit for regulating the pump motor speed of the heart–lung machine, causing the pump to start up again. This happened in spite of the pump control knob having been turned to the stop position. This accident would have been avoided if the power to the heart–lung machine had been disconnected before starting the diathermy, thereby preventing the inadvertent restarting of the pump.

Diathermy currents cannot drive an electric motor directly; they can, however, affect sensitive electronic circuits, such as the motor control circuit.

To make matters even worse, the distribution of information about this accident was highly unsatisfactory, resulting in yet another two such accidents in the same country – one of which occurred at the very same hospital.

Pacemakers can be damaged by diathermy current. Certain precautions are therefore necessary before pacemaker patients may undergo surgery. An external pacemaker must be at hand ready for use, should the patient's own pacemaker stop working. To minimize the risks, diathermy should never be carried out at a distance shorter than 15 cm from the pacemaker. The patient return electrode must be placed on the same side of the heart as the surgical site, to prevent the entire diathermy current from passing in close proximity to the pacemaker electrodes. The direction of the diathermy current should be perpendicular to the line between the pacemaker box and electrode, so that the power transmitted to these is minimized. If possible, the bipolar technique should always be applied as well as the lowest possible output power.

Interference to diathermy generators from other devices can also occur, resulting in the generator being activated without any action by the surgeon. For example, an operating table remote control has been shown to interfere with a diathermy generator of a certain make, due to inadequate electromagnetic compatibility (EMC, Chapter 3).

Muscle twitching

Even though high-frequency currents do not affect muscles or nerves, muscle contractions sometimes still occur. This happens when the high-frequency current is rectified to some extent during contact at the surgical area.

The surgeon may also experience electric shocks during the operation. This usually occurs during buzzing, touching tissue forceps or haemostat with the active electrode for haemostasis. Surgical gloves are too thin to offer protection against the high-frequency voltage that can develop because of inappropriate connection of the diathermy generator. Glove insulation will break down from disruptive discharges. A clinical engineer should always be consulted in such cases. The electric shock can sometimes be felt even outside the surgical area:

CASE 11:10   Surgeon suffers electric shock to the foot

A surgeon was accustomed to using monopolar diathermy to coagulate the tissue by buzzing common tissue forceps. A surgical assistant on one occasion activated the diathermy generator before the surgeon had had time to touch the forceps with the active electrode. At this time, the surgeon inadvertently put her foot against the operating table, whereupon she received an electric shock that passed through her body. Fortunately, neither the surgeon nor the patient was hurt.

The combined leakage currents emerging from the diathermy generator exceeded the limit value. If the surgeon had been touching the forceps with the active electrode prior to activation of the diathermy generator, she would not have received a shock. It would have been even better if she had used bipolar diathermy.

When applying insulated endoscopic instruments, muscle twitching can be eliminated by conducting the high-frequency current through a cable, an **S-cord**. This cable is connected between the patient return electrode and a metal part of the endoscope.

The risk of muscle twitching increases with any insulation failures in the diathermy generator resulting in arcing between the metal parts. Generators that cause an unusual amount of muscle twitching should therefore be sent to a clinical engineering department for inspection.

The large number of diathermy accidents during the last couple of decades has prompted several revisions of regulations. This illustrates the difficulty in preventing diathermy accidents, which still form a major part of the accidents within health care.

 Before every surgical procedure, remember to do the following:
1. Verify that the cable insulation and cable connectors are intact. Before connecting the diathermy generator, check to make sure that an audible signal sounds when the generator is activated.
2. If the diathermy generator is equipped with an alarm circuit, verify that the alarm is working by turning the generator on and then testing it according to the accompanying operation manual.
3. Connect the cable between the diathermy generator and the patient return electrode before it is applied to the patient.

When the patient is placed on the operating table, remember to do the following:
1. The patient should have all skin areas completely insulated from any metal objects. You can use three layers of cotton drapes, which must be covered by a waterproof sheath – they must not be allowed to get wet during the operation.

2. Avoid having two skin areas touching each other, such as the patient's hand touching his thigh or keeping the heels together.
3. Select a location for the patient return electrode with an under-lying muscle layer (avoid bony prominences). The patient return electrode must be placed relatively close to the surgical site, and the diathermy current must not pass through the elbow or the knee. The site selected must be located at a distance of least 15 cm from any ECG electrodes. The patient return electrode must be accessible for inspection during the entire operation.
4. If there is excess hair at the location for the return electrode, shave the skin. Apply the patient return electrode in such a way that its entire contact area adheres to the skin.
5. Place the diathermy cables away from the patient and operating table and let them hang in an arch in the air. Do not roll up the cables and do not attach them with drape clamps that may damage the insulation.
6. If the patient has a pacemaker, select a placement site where the patient return electrode will be at a greater distance from the heart than from the surgical site. Consult a cardiologist and get instructions as to what you should do if any pacemaker compli-cations arise.

During the operation, remember the following:
1. The diathermy generator must only be turned on when in use; turn the generator off when it is not being used. Ensure that the foot switch cannot be stepped on by mistake.
2. Allow all flammable disinfectants to evaporate completely before diathermy is used.
3. Always use bipolar diathermy whenever possible. (This considerably reduces the risk of burn injuries and minimizes unnecessary thermal tissue damage in the surgical area.)
4. Always store the active electrode visible in an insulated holster when not in use.
5. If the patient is repositioned during the procedure, check the position of the patient return electrode.
6. If the output power needs to be increased more than usual, check the patient return electrode position and its cable connections. The operating surgeon must be actively involved in the checking procedure.
7. When diathermy is used, disconnect all other devices that are not indispensable for patient life-support or monitoring.

Finally, remember that if an accident has happened, all medical technical devices must be left intact (settings must not be changed), electrodes and cables kept, and the clinical engineer in charge be contacted.

Unfortunately, this last rule is often overlooked, which makes it difficult or impossible for the clinical engineers to determine the cause of the accident. This in turn may lead to further patients getting injured.

LASER SURGERY

A laser emits a very special kind of light, which is concentrated to a thin parallel beam with very high output power. Because of these characteristics, lasers are applied extensively within medicine for the destruction of superficial tissues.

The output power varies greatly with the area of use, and it amounts to about ten or a few tens of watts. Since the heat can be dissipated during the time that the laser beam hits the target tissues, there is less thermal effect on the tissues when the output power is distributed over a large area than when it is concentrated on a small area. For this reason, the total output power is of less importance than the actual power density. The unit for power density is watts per square centimetre.

Effects

Laser light has different characteristics depending on the specific type of laser being used, Box 11:3. We differentiate between **thermal effects, photochemical effects** and **photodissociation.**

Thermal effects

The thermal effects result in direct heat generation in the tissues. Proteins coagulate and nucleic acids are broken down in a process called **photocoagulation.** If the output power density is increased to the point where the temperature approaches 100°C, **evaporation** occurs. At even higher power densities the tissues are **charred.** The latter phenomenon poses a problem during surgical applications, as the soot absorbs the laser light and thus impedes the continued treatment.

When short laser pulses with high power density are applied, the thermal effects progress to becoming explosive. **Mechanical acoustic destruction** of the tissues occurs due to the immediate, explosion-like expansion during the instantaneous evaporation – a plasma formation. Surgical incisions with laser light is based on such mechanical acoustic destruction. But this effect can also be of disadvantage, as it can make it difficult to preassess the extent of the actual tissue destruction.

Photochemical effects

For selective effects in certain tissues, special agents can be administered, which have a tendency to accumulate in the target tissue and which also have a high absorption of specific laser light. With this type of **photodynamic therapy (PDT)** it is possible to treat certain tissues without damaging the surrounding areas.

Techniques • Box 11:3

Types of medical lasers

The carbon dioxide laser emits light within the infrared spectrum with a wavelength of 10,600 nm, far away from the visible spectrum. Water has a high absorption of this type of laser light, and for this reason only very superficial coagulation is possible. The light cannot be conducted through fibre optics. Carbon dioxide lasers are used to cut the skin and to coagulate superficial blood vessels. The penetration depth is only about 0.2 mm maximum.

The erbium laser also emits light within the infrared spectrum, and has replaced the carbon dioxide laser for certain types of applications.

If deeper penetration of about 5 to 7 mm is desired, light from the Nd-YAG laser is used (this laser consists of an yttrium–aluminium–garnet crystal, where some yttrium ions have been replaced by neodymium). This laser emits light with a wavelength of 1064 nm, within the infrared spectrum, which is close to the visible spectrum. This light can be conducted through light conductors and can be used for various endoscopic treatments. The penetration depth can be brought down to 0.5 to 1 mm by placing a sapphire lens at the tip of the light conductor, which concentrates the light to a focal point, while being dispersed over a larger area beyond the focal point.

The argon laser emits light within the wavelength interval of 488 to 514 nm, which is within the blue-green area of the visible spectrum. This light is absorbed to a high extent in the blood and by other pigments (whose red colour is the complementary colour of blue-green).

There are several types of excimer lasers, which emit light in the ultraviolet spectrum, for example, at 351, 308, 248 and 193 nm. This light has a very shallow penetration depth, and by dividing it into short pulses, it produces high energy in thin superficial tissue layers by photodissociation. Light from excimer lasers can cut through hard tissues, such as calcified areas, and it is especially useful in surgery as it can cut without heating the tissues.

Dye lasers have the advantage of being able to emit light within a very broad spectral range, depending on the concentration of the dye in the liquid where the light is generated.

There are also helium–neon lasers with very low output power that emit red light at 632 nm. These are used to align various other instruments, such as therapeutic laser devices before the therapeutic laser is activated.

One example of photodynamic agents is the **haematoporphyrin derivative (HPD)**, which accumulates in tumours. Upon irradiation with 635 nm laser light, this agent produces toxic substances that kill cells. These substances exert their action on the tumour cells within the following 24 hours after the treatment – the irradiation used is not powerful enough to immediately kill the cell.

Photodissociation

Photodissociation is the breaking of chemical bonds upon irradiation with ultraviolet light. When used in medicine, this effect is called **photoablation,** and enables the removal of very thin tissue layers without bleeding or scarring.

Risks

To avoid accidents during laser procedures with hazardous power outputs, rigorous safety regulations have been imposed. It is especially important to prevent the laser beam from shining directly into anyone's eyes, as the eyesight could be damaged instantly. The injuries are of three different kinds. A moderate output power laser will destroy the illuminated area of the retina. If the fovea (the central area of the retina, responsible for colour and critical vision) is hit, the result is an incapacitating loss of vision.

The second injury type is even worse: this occurs when high output powers within the visible or shortwave infrared range are generated, causing such rapid evaporation that the eye explodes from the resulting shockwave. Thankfully such injuries are rare.

The third injury type is only caused by lasers that generate ultraviolet light. This can cause acute damage to the cornea, and a long-term effect resulting in lens opacifications and cataracts.

For these reasons, everyone present in the treatment room must use laser protective eyewear whenever lasers of a certain minimum output power are generated. These glasses possess a high light absorption at the particular laser wavelength, but do not absorb other wavelengths within the visible spectrum. It goes without saying that the correct type of protective eyewear must be selected for each specific laser type.

Tip Whenever new laser equipment is used for the first time or new protective glasses are put on, check that they absorb at the correct wavelength.

During destruction of tissues by laser light, irritating and bad smelling gases (surgical smoke) is produced, which must be eliminated with special types of evacuation systems.

Other devices and objects that might be exposed to laser light must be especially customized. For example, surgical instruments must have a nonreflecting satin finish that will not reflect the laser light, and all materials that might be hit by the laser beam must not be flammable. However, such exceptional precautions are not required for all applications. Often only low power output lasers are needed, where simple safety precautions suffice.

Gases, disinfectants and plastics must be selected for their nonflammable characteristics. The maximum permissible airway oxygen level is 30%, but if possible, the level should be lowered to 21%, the concentration in air.

CASE 11:11 Burns to the throat

A patient was undergoing laser surgery for a vocal cord lesion. The patient was intubated in the normal fashion with a metal reinforced tube and the tracheal cuff positioned just below the vocal cords. To minimize the fire hazard, a water-saturated strip was initially placed below the vocal cords, but it had to be removed as it obstructed the view. The administrated anaesthetic gas mixture consisted of 6 litres of oxygen and 5 litres of nitrous oxide per minute. The laser was a carbon dioxide laser set at 3 watts.

As the breathing bag was being filled to increase the gas inflow, pure oxygen accidentally filled the endotracheal tube and the larynx. At the same time, the laser was activated and the endotracheal tube ignited. It was immediately removed and replaced by a new tube. The patient had contracted burns to the oropharynx and upper larynx, but later recovered.

Using a mixture of oxygen and nitrous oxide for this anaesthesia was clearly inappropriate, as nitrous oxide supports combustion in the same way as oxygen.

Thanks to the rigorous laser regulations, accidents are uncommon. There are different regulations depending on laser type – the lasers can be divided into four major hazard categories called the Laser Hazard Classifications (I, II, IIA, IIIA, IIIB and IV). Laser surgery is a safe method.

Areas of use

The tissue penetration depth is determined by the wavelength of the laser light. Thus the choice of laser type is determined to obtain an appropriate penetration depth. Another factor to be considered is the type of physical effects desired.

Ophthalmology

One of the complications of **diabetes** is a deterioration of the blood circulation to the retina in the eye – the body tries to compensate for this by forming new blood vessels, **diabetic proliferative retinopathy**. But the new blood vessels are abnormal and rupture easily, causing bleeding into the vitreous body of the eye and loss of vision. By laser photocoagulation the newly formed vessels can be destroyed, leading to a slow down, and sometimes even to a halt of the progression of eye complications.

If **retinal detachment** is caught early, before the retina has started bulging into the vitreous body, the retina can be fixed by photo-coagulation. The laser light produces a scar tissue that fixes the retina to the underlying tissue layers.

Elevated intraocular pressure has been considered to be one factor for developing glaucoma, although **glaucoma** in some patients develops in spite of a normal pressure. The pressure is increased due to impaired fluid drainage, which normally takes place via the trabecular meshwork between the cornea and the iris. In open-angle glaucoma, a large number of small openings in the trabecular mesh are therefore created by laser photocoagulation, **trabeculoplasty**. This improves the fluid drainage. The immediate result is usually good, with adequate lowering of the intraocular pressure; the effects may, however, subside over time.

Clouding of the vitreous body and of the lens capsule following cataract surgery may also be treated with laser. Even one single treatment can produce dramatic improvement.

Refraction errors in the eye can be corrected with laser **refractive surgery**. The central part of the cornea is exposed to light pulses from an **excimer laser** – about 0.2 μm of tissue is removed for each exposure. The illumination of the cornea is controlled by a computer with a series of such pulses, resulting in planing of the cornea and improvement of the patient's myopia. Refraction errors between approximately –1.5 and –15 diopters can be treated this way. Astigmatism, a condition where the cornea has an irregular curvature and as a result focuses the light differently along different planes, can be treated. There are concerns about the safety of the procedure in the long run.

Tumour treatments

A number of different types of superficial, small tumours, or precursors to these, can be removed. Malignant or benign lesions in, for example, the **urinary bladder, genital organs, airways** and **skin** can be treated with laser surgery with very good results. In the **oesophagus** and **stomach** this can be performed without the need for open surgery.

Genital condyloma, which is otherwise difficult to get rid of, can be removed. The laser method carries the advantage of eradicating viral accumulations beneath the skin. Cell changes on the cervix of the uterus can also be removed. Cancer of the larynx is another condition where laser surgery is beneficial.

Haemangiomas or fire marks were previously incurable without large surgical reconstructions that would leave ugly scars. But today, haeman-giomas can often be removed with laser. Not every case may respond, however, and the treatment is usually first tested in a small area to assess the chances for success.

If the tumour has spread deeply into the tissues where the laser light cannot reach, actual healing cannot be achieved. In such cases, the method can still be used for palliative treatment. In cases of oesophageal tumours, for example, laser surgery can aid in keeping the oesophagus patent. Similarly, large tumour masses in the airways can be reduced, saving the patient from suffocation.

Wound healing

Light from lasers has been found to have documented effects on the cellular level. Light of certain wavelengths can speed up wound healing.

The circulatory organs

In cases where standard balloon dilatation (see below) of the coronary arteries has failed to produce satisfactory results, **percutaneous transluminal laser angioplasty (PTLA)** has combined the standard procedure with laser therapy. A light cable is introduced into the vessel and the stenosis is either illuminated directly with laser light via a focusing sapphire lens, so that blood clots and fibrous tissue are vaporized, or the laser light is focused onto a metal tip, which then heats to about 400°C with the same tissue effects. Thus the lesions are burned away, resulting in a widened or re-established vessel lumen. The usefulness of this method is, however, still under discussion.

Stenoses in other blood vessels are common, and similar techniques can be used.

Dermatology

In addition to the treatment of haemangiomas discussed above, pigmentations and tattoos can also be removed with laser. The pigment particles are **fragmented**, and the body's immune system then clears away the fragments.

Laser lithotripsy

When other methods fail, calculi can be crushed with laser light. Gallstones can be reached either via an orally introduced choledochoscope, or via a catheter introduced percutaneously through the abdominal wall. A laser light cable is inserted by either route until it is in contact with the stone. For treating calculi in the ureter, the laser light cables are inserted via the urethra and urinary bladder.

Laser pulses are generated by a dye laser at a rate of approximately five pulses per second until 1000 to 8000 pulses have been produced. The bile ducts are then flushed with normal saline for 24 hours following the treatment to remove the remnants of the crushed stones.

ULTRASONIC SURGICAL ASPIRATION

During surgery in highly vascularized tissues such as the liver, kidneys and brain, bleeding often occurs and can be difficult to control. In such cases, ultrasonic surgical aspiration can be useful. The tissue parenchyma with its high water content is fragmented, while blood vessels, skin and bile ducts remain intact.

The instrument consists of a 20 to 50 kHz ultrasound transducer connected to a conical resonator (handpiece) made of titanium, for transmission of the ultrasound to the tissues. Normal saline is continuously administered. The solution is needed partly to achieve the acoustic coupling to the tissues, and partly to emulsify the tissue fragments for elimination via an internal channel in the resonator.

Two mechanisms are responsible for the fragmentation. First, **high accelerations** (>300,000 g) are generated just next to the titanium tip, resulting in only small fragments being able to oscillate along with these movements, while areas at a greater distance remain immobile. This leads to the fragmentation of fragile tissues. Second, in a process called **cavitation**, dissolved gases form microscopic bubbles synchronous with the sound pressure changes, which fragment the fragile tissues. The effect is proportionate to the water content, which explains the selective fragmentation with disintegration of parenchyma, while fibrous tissue and larger blood vessels are spared.

By choosing the appropriate ultrasound output level, parenchyma in the brain, liver and kidneys can be dissected (skeletonized) from an intact network of blood vessels. The blood vessels can then be ligated or coagulated with diathermy.

LITHOTRIPSY

Calculi in the kidneys and gall bladder are common diseases. The stones can be removed with conventional surgery, but this carries the risk of complications and necessitates long hospital stays. Today it has become standard practice to crush the stones with shockwaves, which allows the resulting fragments to be eliminated from the body via the natural orifices. This method is mostly used for kidney stones, but can also be applied for removing gallstones.

In **extracorporeal shockwave lithotripsy (ESWL)**, mechanical shockwaves are focused on the stone. The shockwaves are produced by various methods, for example, by discharging a voltage of about 20,000 volts in an electrode that resembles a spark plug of a car. The discharge takes place in water, causing a sudden vaporization, with electrohydraulic shockwave generation. With an ellipsoid reflector the wave is focused to a volume of about one cubic centimetre at the location of the stone, Figure 11:12. The patient is acoustically connected to the device by means of a water-filled balloon, which is pressed against the patient's body, allowing the transfer of the shockwave to the patient. Some 300 to 2000 such shockwaves are needed before the fragments have become small enough to pass through the ureter.

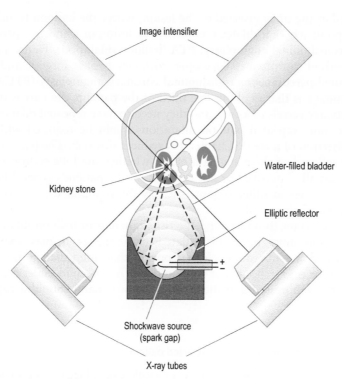

Figure 11.12 Shockwave lithotripsy

The device is focused on the stone with the help of biplanar fluoroscopy. During the treatment, repeated checks are made to ensure that correct positioning is maintained. Usually only sedation, and sometimes painkillers, are required during the treatment.

An alternative method consists of **percutaneous electrohydraulic lithotripsy (PEHL)**, where the skin is penetrated and a probe advanced to the stone under fluoroscopy guidance. The probe is equipped with two insulated electrodes, and a series of electrical discharges takes place between these. The integrated optic system enables the physician to check that the electrodes remain in contact with the stone. The result can be verified immediately and the stone fragments eliminated by irrigation and suction.

A third possibility is **percutaneous ultrasound lithotripsy (PUL)**, where ultrasound is applied to the stone via a probe under endoscopic visualization.

BALLOON DILATATION

Arteriosclerotic lesions in blood vessels cause impaired blood circulation. It can often be restored with angioplasty. A catheter with a balloon attached at the tip is inserted to the lesion, where the balloon is inflated to the point where it dilates the narrowing lesion or stenosis – **percutaneous transluminal angioplasty, PTA (balloon dilatation)**, Figure 11:13. This method can often replace open coronary bypass surgery, and it is then called **percutaneous transluminal coronary angioplasty (PTCA)**. A disadvantage is that in about one third of the patients the narrowing of the coronary vessels reoccurs, and they need to have repeated dilatations. One or more repeated balloon dilatations might be required within a year. Insertion of a stent (Chapter 10) reduces this risk. The patients are largely relieved of their angina attacks; whether the long-term survival rate is actually improved or not depends on the patient's general health status. Stenoses in other organs, such as the oesophagus, can also be treated with balloon dilatation.

It is important to understand the risks inherent in balloon dilatation. The balloon must never be inflated with air, as it may explode. Compressed air has an explosive power that immediately is transferred to the organ should the balloon burst. But a liquid under pressure cannot be compressed and therefore will not expand should a rupture occur.

CASE 11:12   Air in the pleural cavity killed patient

A patient suffering from many years of swallowing difficulties was undergoing balloon dilatation of a stricture in the oesophagus. As the balloon was being inflated, a sharp bang was heard. When the balloon was withdrawn, it was discovered that it had ruptured.

The operating physician could not detect any definite signs of the oesophagus having ruptured, but later the same day, the patient developed chest pains

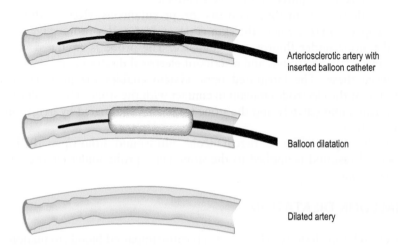

Arteriosclerotic artery with
inserted balloon catheter

Balloon dilatation

Dilated artery

Figure 11:13 Percutaneous angioplasty

and an X-ray examination revealed that air had penetrated to the pleural cavity. The patient died.

In the instructions for use for the device it was clearly stated that the balloon must be emptied of all air and inflated with either sterile water or a contrast medium. The physician had not read the instructions for use.

CRYOSURGERY

Tissues can be destroyed if frozen to adequately low temperatures. The treatment is carried out either by applying a freezing agent directly to the tissue, or more commonly, by pressing a **cryoprobe** against the tissue. The cryoprobe consists of a tube-shaped device through which the freezing medium can circulate. After freezing, the tissues are again allowed to thaw, and the necrotic parts gradually fall off.

This method has several advantages. It is not very painful and can be performed under local anaesthesia. Connective tissue, bone and blood vessels can withstand cryotherapy without going into necrosis. Thus these tissue parts are revitalized following cryotherapy for removal of a tumour, and the tissues heal with surprisingly little scarring.

Mechanisms

The effects of low temperatures on the tissues differ somewhat depending on the speed at which the tissues freeze. When frozen slowly, ice crystals form predominantly extracellularly and fluids are osmotically driven out of the cells, and this causes a rise in the intracellular electrolyte concentrations to toxic levels. This leads to cell death.

In rapid freezing, ice crystals are formed both intra- and extracellularly, resulting in destruction of cell structures. Histologically a cryolesion resembles an infarction with a central necrosis and infiltration of leucocytes at the margins.

During the freezing process the tissues become white due to the formation of ice. It is therefore easy to determine how much superficial tissue has been treated just by looking at it; but determining the extent of deeper effects is much more difficult. If the tissue is homogeneous and does not contain any large blood vessels through which heat can be added, it can be assumed that the ice formation will extend hemispherically; the depth of the affected tissue is approximately half of the diameter of the superficial frozen tissue layer.

Destroying normal cells requires a temperature of at least –20°C and destroying tumour cells at least –30°C. Repeated freeze–thaw cycles increase the likelihood of all the cells being killed.

The tissues are demolished to such an extent that a histopathological examination is pointless. This is one of the definite drawbacks of this method, as is it not possible to histopathologically determine whether the surgery has been radical enough to eliminate all infiltrating tumour cells.

Types of cryodevices

The most commonly used freezing medium is liquid nitrogen, which boils at −196°C. The nitrogen is kept enclosed in a thermos flask. During application, an immersion heater is used to increase the pressure in the flask, forcing the nitrogen to rise up through an insulated tube to the tip of the cryoprobe. Such devices are expensive to buy but cheap to operate.

A more inexpensive alternative is to utilize the fact that when a gas expands, it also cools (air blown through tightly squeezed lips onto the hand feels cold). Nitrous oxide, which has a boiling point of −89°C, or carbon dioxide, with a boiling point of −78°C, is made to expand rapidly at the tip of the cryoprobe or in direct contact with the tissue. But this technique merely offers limited cooling capacity, enabling only a smaller tissue volume to be treated.

To determine the extent of the cryoeffects in deeper tissue layers, the temperature can be measured using straight or curved needle-shaped thermocouples. Another possibility is to measure the electric impedance, which increases sharply when the tissue water freezes to ice. Furthermore, the cryotherapy effect can also be monitored by ultrasound imaging.

Risks

The release of cryogas presents an occupational safety hazard. Oxygen is avoided, due to the fire hazard. When large amounts of nitrogen are released, the operating theatre ventilation system must be effective enough to ensure that the oxygen level in the room air does not become unacceptably low. The same goes for carbon dioxide, and room air gas levels that could affect respiration must be avoided. Nitrous oxide must also be evacuated by means of specialized equipment.

Area of use

Cryosurgery is mostly applied for the treatment of tumours. The method is particularly suitable for palliative treatment, for example, removal of tumours causing localized symptoms, such as metastases that are growing in locations where they cause discomfort for the patient. The technique is especially valuable for treatment of skin tumours, and treatments in body cavities that can be visualized, enabling direct inspection of the freezing process. Internal organs such as the prostate can also be treated – the extent of the freezing is then monitored with ultrasound imaging.

Cryosurgery has also been successfully applied for curative treatment of localized prostate cancer. The method is gentle to the patient, and therefore suitable for patients unable to withstand alternative methods.

HEAT TREATMENT

Heat can be transferred to the tissues by various methods, such as **electromagnetic high-frequency energy** and **ultrasound energy**. It is a common misconception that there should be no therapeutic difference between these two methods as long as the tissues are equally heated. Such a conclusion is unwarranted since high-frequency energy is absorbed by atomic and molecular processes, whereas ultrasound is absorbed by the tissues that are mechanically vibrated. The mechanical movement may, for example, be more effective in removing local pain substances.

Electromagnetic high-frequency energy

Alternating currents of high frequency are absorbed by the tissues while simultaneously generating heat. This phenomenon has been utilized in various situations, for example, to increase the radiation sensitivity of tumours by heating the affected tissues in combination with radiation therapy, **hyperthermia treatment**. Microwaves are conducted to the tumour, resulting in a temperature increase to 43°C. The temperature is continuously monitored and the output power automatically controlled, so that the desired heating is achieved.

When this method is applied for treatment of prostate enlargement (prostatic hyperplasia), it is called **transurethral microwave thermotherapy (TUMT)**. The microwaves are conducted to the prostatic region via an instrument inserted through the urethra. This treatment often results in a shrinking of the prostate, thereby alleviating the patient's urination problems. The method is simpler than a standard prostate operation, and it requires shorter hospital stays. But there are differing views as to the long-term usefulness of this therapy.

Some cardiac arrhythmias where the heart is beating too fast are caused by a malfunction in an anatomically well-defined cardiac structure. These structures can be found with the help of a catheter equipped with an ECG electrode at the tip. By applying radio-frequency energy at the catheter tip and thereby destroying the abnormal tissue, **radio-frequency ablation**, the cardiac arrhythmia can be efficiently treated.

Heat therapy by means of electromagnetic waves (such as shortwave or microwave radiation) has sometimes been used in attempts to treat various pain conditions in the joints and muscles and to improve the joint range of motion. In some countries this method has not been applied for about two decades as they considered it to have no therapeutic effect, and also because it caused several types of unwanted side-effects. Therapeutic diathermy is contradicted for patients with active implants:

CASE 11:13   Two combined treatments kill

A patient with a deep-brain neurostimulator was being treated with radio-frequency therapeutic diathermy for chronic scoliosis. The therapeutic energy resulted in tissue heating beside the stimulator lead, causing severe and irreversible brain damage. The patient died.

Both the stimulator and therapeutic diathermy device were found to be working correctly. The interaction between the devices caused the problem. It was noted that a similar result could have occurred even if the stimulator had been switched off, or had previously been surgically removed and the stimulator lead left in place.

Ultrasound energy

Ultrasound has been shown to have a definite effect on pain conditions in joints and muscles, in connection with physical exercise. Heat therapy alone does not produce any lasting pain relief or increased range of motion.

The heat generated by the ultrasound in the tissues probably increases the blood flow, and this facilitates the elimination of pain-releasing substances from the tissues. The ultrasound also has purely mechanical effects, for example, resulting in bruises clearing up faster following treatment. Thanks to the temporarily reduced sensitivity to pain, the patient is able to participate more efficiently during the ensuing physical exercise.

The heat produced during ultrasound therapy becomes concentrated at the bone/soft-tissue interface. The treatment should therefore be applied with caution, as there is a risk of high local temperature increases that could cause cell damage.

Even the therapist may be exposed to high doses of ultrasound, especially when the treatment is done underwater, and is at risk of unintentionally immersing a hand in the water.

ELECTROCONVULSIVE THERAPY

Severe melancholic conditions accompanied by suicidal tendencies, anorexia and delusions can be treated with electricity. During electroconvulsive therapy (**ECT**), an electric current is conducted through the head by means of two electrodes placed at the temples at opposite sides of the head. The current is divided into alternating positive and negative pulses of about 1 ms with a frequency of 50 pulse pairs per second. The current is limited to less than 1 ampere, and the electric energy applied is about 15 to 25 J. The therapy triggers an "epileptic" attack of the grand mal type.

Prior to therapy, a light general anaesthesia is administered and a muscle relaxant is also given to prevent the body's muscles from contracting during the grand mal attack; the patient could otherwise develop vertebral fractures from contractions of the back muscles. The procedure is usually repeated two to three times per week for a total of six to eight therapy sessions.

There has been no neurophysiological explanation as to why ECT alleviates depression. The method carries the disadvantage of causing memory loss for the time period surrounding the treatments – in some cases a complete memory loss covering several weeks prior to the electro-convulsive treatment. ETC does not prevent relapse of the depression.

In general, electroconvulsive therapy tends to be looked upon more favourably by psychiatrists than by the patients themselves or their families.

RADIOTHERAPY

In **radiotherapy**, also called radiation therapy, the genetic material in the cells is damaged by exposing it to ionizing radiation. If the radiation dose is high enough, all cells within the irradiated area will be killed; a so-called **lethal** dose. After a lower, or **sublethal** dose, the cells are able to repair the damage and recover after the irradiation.

With surgery alone, it is often difficult or even impossible to remove the entire tumour without simultaneously having to remove important organs that have been infiltrated by the tumour. Radiotherapy, however, uses the fact that healthy tissues often have a greater capacity than tumour cells for self-repair following a sublethal radiation dose. The total dose is therefore administered as a low-intensity dose over many hours or days, so-called **protracted radiotherapy**, for example, by placing radioactive radiation sources inside the tumour, or dividing externally applied radiation over a longer period of time, for example, 30 treatments over the course of 6 weeks – **fractioned radiotherapy**. This way, it is possible to destroy cancer cells with infiltrating growth patterns while preserving the normal tissues.

Different types of both normal tissues and tumour tissues have highly differing radiation sensitivity. Organs rich in epithelial and nervous tissue, such as the eyes, spinal cord, kidneys and skin are highly sensitive to radiation, whereas organs consisting of muscle and connective tissue are less sensitive. The most malignant and rapidly growing tumour types are generally also the most sensitive. But this does not mean that they are the easiest to cure, as their high propensity to metastasize results in rapid spread to many locations throughout the body.

Radiation doses

The unit **gray**, abbreviated **Gy**, is used to measure the radiation dose, and is defined as the amount of energy, expressed in joules absorbed per kilogram of tissue (J/kg).

Since different types of ionizing radiation exert different effects on biological tissues, another unit is used for radiation protection purposes, the **dose equivalent**. This is measured in **sieverts** (Sv), and is calculated by multiplying the dose expressed in Gy by a factor specific to the type of radiation in question. One sievert is a large dose: at about 3 to 4 Sv, 50% of irradiated individuals would die. Therapeutic radiation doses are therefore mostly expressed in terms of mSv (millisievert).

Radiation therapy devices

The ionizing radiation used almost exclusively consists of photon radiation (electromagnetic quanta) or electron radiation. Photon radiation can be generated by **X-ray tubes, telegamma devices** (also called **isotope machines**) and **high-voltage accelerators**. Electron radiation can be generated only by the latter types. Photon radiation is gradually attenuated as it penetrates the tissue layers, in the same way as the light becomes dimmer under the sea with increasing depth. Electron radiation on the other hand has a definite range limit – just like the shot of a shot-putter it cannot go beyond a certain maximum distance.

The radiation from **X-ray tubes** using acceleration voltages of up to about 300 kV is of low energy and thus has poor tissue penetration. Its use is therefore limited to treatment of superficial tumours. The disadvantage with the energy being so low is that the greatest radiation dose is absorbed by the skin, and the skeletal dose also becomes relatively higher than the dose absorbed by the surrounding soft tissues. This leads to latent damage to the skeletal structures, with the accompanying risk of among other things subsequent fractures.

Tumours located at a greater depth can be treated with **teletherapy units**. One such device contains cobalt 60, which is produced in nuclear reactors. This isotope, which emits photons with energy levels of about 1 MeV (mega electron volt), is sealed inside the unit treatment head, which is furnished with a massive radiation shield. The photons can only pass through a collimator system, which focuses the radiation field so that it hits only the part of the body to be treated.

Brachytherapy is another special method to obtain a high radiation dose in the tumour while limiting the exposure to the surrounding tissues. Then the radiation source consisting of a radioactive isotope is placed inside or very close to the tumour. The isotope can be contained in tubes or needles, which can be introduced in the organ either manually or by special automatic remote loading devices to minimize the exposure to the medical staff. Tumours in hollow organs such as the uterus are highly suited for brachytherapy. But the method is not limited to such applications since the isotope in the form of seeds, needles or wires can be inserted directly into tumour tissues, **interstitial implantation**.

There are several types of high-voltage accelerators, such as **linear accelerators, betatrons** and **microtrons**. All these accelerate electrons to high velocities. By varying the energy level to which the electrons are accelerated, the tissue penetration depth, the tissue depth at which the greatest radiation dose is absorbed, can be selected. The greatest radiation effects are thus not obtained at skin level, but deeper inside the body. This is of value because of the relatively high radiation sensitivity of the skin.

Dose planning

The treatment goal is to obtain as large a dose as possible in the tumour, and as small as possible in surrounding normal organs. The varying radiation sensitivity of the different tissue types and the importance of the organs must be taken into consideration. Thus, the gonads in individuals of fertile age must be protected from exposure to unnecessary radiation that could damage the genetic material. To achieve the optimal effect, an appropriate combination of the **radiation type, radiation energy, fractioning** and **radiation field distribution** must be made. Radiation beams are often focused on the tumour from various angles, so that the dose is distributed over a large area of the skin surface while being concentrated inside the tumour. Dose planning is based on highly complicated computer calculations. The calculations take into account the external body contours as well as the various tissue densities, determined via computerized tomography or magnetic resonance (Chapter 7).

During the treatment, control readings are also made, for example, by measuring the dose exiting the patient and comparing it with the entry dose. These checks are performed a number of times during the treatment period of several weeks.

To minimize the risk of incorrect device settings during the repeated treatment sessions, modern devices are equipped with a computerized control system, so-called **check and confirm**. The computer checks that all settings, usually as many as 10 to 12 for each treatment, are within certain predetermined limits before the radiotherapy can begin.

12

Computers in health care

Information technology (IT) or medical informatics has been used with mixed success in health care. Patient administration and the processing of laboratory test results are some of the simpler routines that have been computerized. The technology has also been very successfully applied in various forms for anaesthesia and intensive care. Computers have also long been used to determine the optimal radiation therapy for the treatment of tumours.

The possibility of making diagnoses with artificial intelligence (AI) have often been discussed – but this term gives an exaggerated impression of the capabilities of the computer. The term medical expert system is more appropriate. Assembling all the necessary patient information to create a computerized patient record has proven to be a tough problem. The internet, one of the greatest achievements of information technology, is gaining an ever-increasing significance in medicine, and provides the possibility of communicating via email. Before we go on to describe these applications, some basic facts about computers are given.

The computer

A computer has two main components: the hardware, which comprises all the physical parts with its numerous electrical and mechanical components, and the software, which is the programs that control the actions of the computer. The everyday user needs to know neither how the computer is constructed nor programmed.

In a ward or in a laboratory, staff can access the central computer via a terminal and a server, Figure 12:1. It is equipped with a memory where

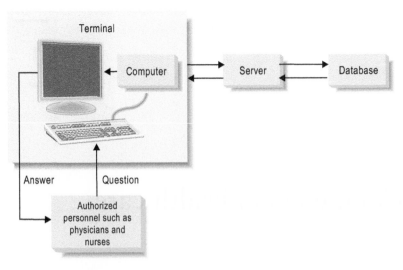

Figure 12:1 Through the terminal authorized personnel have access to databases

large amounts of data are stored in **databases**. The data can quickly be accessed from the terminals. A database is like a box of cards with notes about the patients. Other databases may contain other information, such as waiting lists for hospital admission and systems for financial audits. Several databases can be interconnected, enabling communication between them. The databases can also be accessed simultaneously by several users. Almost all data about out-patients is stored in such databases, and for in-patient care database utilization is steadily growing.

A database is thus a huge archive from which data can be easily retrieved. The data may consist of text (e.g. a patient's medical history), numerical data (e.g. laboratory values) and images (e.g. X-ray images). By analysing these **data, information** is gathered about the patient. The information is thus personal interpretation of these data.

Communication with the central computer is made possible by a **network,** which physically connects all the terminals and other components of the computer system. Thanks to this network, doctors and nurses can instantaneously access a patient record at their own terminals. Similarly, special investigations may be ordered at the user's own or another hospital, and confirmations received immediately as to when they can be scheduled. Test results from the clinical chemistry, bacteriology and pathology laboratories can be reviewed on screen as soon as the results are ready. Prescriptions can be transmitted to the pharmacy terminal, so that medicines may be prepared in a timely manner and kept ready for the patient to pick up.

A handheld computer is a lightweight version that communicates with the network through wireless transmission. Special care needs to be taken with access and confidentiality, but such computers will offer convenient opportunities for doctors and others to have easy access to patient data. At the same time they can enter new data.

A **personal computer** is a complete unit that operates independently, without the help of a central computer. On a personal computer, texts are easily composed and edited with the help of word-processing software, and numerical calculations can also be carried out. On a personal computer, smaller databases for the user's own use can be kept, eliminating the need for connection to the central database. Most personal computers are, however, electrically connected in a network, which among other things enables access to larger databases as well as to other personal computers. In the absence of a network, a **modem** is required, so that the personal computer may be connected by dialling up via the telephone system.

Data acquisition

Much of the work done at a terminal or personal computer consists of data entry. The data for the most part need to be typed in manually ("keyed in"). There are, however, some tools that both facilitate and make the data transfer more secure. Blood bags and samples can be more securely identified with the help of a **barcode reader**, thereby eliminating the risk of a mix-up between patients – this is done in the same fashion as when groceries are checked out at the cash register. The barcode system thus helps to reduce the risk of a mix-up, which is one of the major hazards in health care.

Laboratory analysers can be directly connected to a computer, so that all calculations and sorting of lab results are done automatically. Images from an X-ray investigation can similarly be stored in the database just as a digital camera can store images. Larger amounts of data and programs can easily be transferred to a personal computer from **CDs** or other storage media.

Another method for entering, storing and retrieving data is **smart cards**. These could possibly gain considerable practical significance. A smart card is the same size as a standard credit card. It is equipped with a memory that can store as much data as would be contained in a few thousand typewritten pages. The obvious advantage with such cards is that patients can carry with them important information about previous and current illnesses, allergies and drugs previously and currently used. In principle, the patient could carry all the records from his entire life in his wallet. Another great advantage with smart cards is that they could potentially ensure much greater confidentiality – since it is the patient who carries the information, sensitive data theoretically need never be stored in a central database from where they might be sent to the wrong places via the network. The greatest hurdle would be to convince all patients always to carry their cards.

The introduction of IT within health care has at times met with opposition. Whenever computerization is introduced, organizational changes have to be made, and the nature of the work carried out by the health care staff also has to change, at least in part. Processing of all the data necessitates the introduction of new routines. System development is tedious work, which is often met with scepticism due to the fact that many workers will be required to undergo further training.

Confidentiality

Medical data must never be allowed to leak out to unauthorized persons. Patient records may contain sensitive information such as venereal and psychiatric disease. The records must only be available to a few authorized individuals. Inadequate confidentiality could potentially prevent patients from seeking care. Therefore procedures have been developed that check the authorization of anyone who tries to access any data.

There are different authorization levels, so that, for example, social welfare personnel may only access a very limited amount of information such as address, telephone number and sick leave period. Ward nurses may access a wider range of information about the patients in their wards, to which nurses at other wards do not have access. The patient's physician, on the other hand, is authorized to access all the information. Confidentiality is thus implemented with the help of authorization codes, which may also be used in combination with ID cards. Authorization can also be made with a personal swipe card. Every new entry in the patient record should be signed, preferably by means of a secret personal code, so that it is evident who made the entry.

A patient record stored in a computer can be made very secure against unauthorized access; the problem with this is that the system becomes quite cumbersome. All these requirements need to be balanced against each other. In order to increase the sense of accountability, all who access the information in a patient record are automatically registered.

PATIENT DATA

Administrative data

Most administrative routines can be made simpler with the help of computers. Information from a patient record can be easily accessed using a patient identity number, address or telephone number. Scheduling of doctor appointments at health care centres and hospitals are nowadays routinely made with computers.

Recording referrals and follow-up of referred patients also becomes easier. Thanks to computerization, diagnoses may be compiled and statistically processed, such as the number of treated cases of a certain disease, or the cost of health care for each disease category.

Laboratory results

Thanks to the application of computer technology, significant advances have been made in the clinical laboratories, especially in clinical chemistry. When samples are collected, the test tubes are labelled with barcode labels which have been printed out automatically and ensure that correct sample identity is maintained during the entire assay procedure. Print-outs are obtained in the form of **cumulative results** lists, where results from earlier testing of the same patient with the same assays are already recorded. This way, monitoring of changes in the patient's condition is facilitated.

Computer technology also provides means for ongoing quality control of laboratory assay procedures. By generating daily reports of mean values obtained from standardized controls, early detection of any systematic errors in the assay methods is facilitated.

For bloodbanks, computerization has become an important tool for all work stages, from calling blood donors to documentation of trans-fusions, so that each unit of blood can be tracked from donor to specific recipient. The latter possibility is especially important for tracing any infection that may have been transmitted.

Anaesthesia and intensive care

When a patient is anaesthetized during surgery, and during postoperative intensive care, large quantities of data are collected. Even in other forms of intensive care, such as coronary care units, the large amount of information that needs to be stored would be difficult to handle without the help of computers. This care includes **monitoring** data.

Computer support is required for several reasons. It is important to create a **log**, much in the same way as the flight recorder in an airplane records data about the pilots' actions and the plane's behaviour during the flight. When complications arise during an operation, there is no time to write down all the values for blood pressure, pulse rate, respiratory rate, medications administered and other actions taken. It is very important to document everything that happens in such situations, and this can be achieved with the help of automated data acquisition, Figure 12:2.

A computerized patient record makes it easier to assess whether there are systematic changes to certain parameters – the computer can analyse **trends**. The respiratory rate is normally irregular and depends on many external factors, not least psychological ones. When treating asthma patients, it is of interest to monitor any slowly occurring changes of the respiratory rate. Such a change can be detected by computers, and would be much harder to discern just by repeatedly assessing the respiratory rate. A trend analysis can be performed for several monitored parameters simultaneously, depending on the patient's condition (such as pulse rate, blood oxygenation, respiratory rate, temperature and blood pressure),

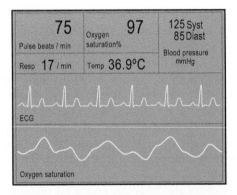

75 Pulse beats / min	Oxygen saturation% 97	125 Syst 85 Diast Blood pressure mmHg
Resp **17** / min	Temp **36.9°C**	

ECG

Oxygen saturation

75 Pulse beats / min	Oxygen saturation% 97	125 Syst 85 Diast Blood pressure mmHg
Resp **17** / min	Temp **36.9°C**	

Alarm limits:	Upper	Lower	Alarm	Store
Pulse	130	50	🔔	ON
Oxygen saturat.	100	85	🔔	ON
Respiration	30	7	🔔	OFF
Systolic press.	140	90	🔕	ON
Diastolic press.	100	50	🔕	ON

75 Pulse beats / min	Oxygen saturation% 97	125 Syst 85 Diast Blood pressure
Resp **17** / min	Temp **36.9°C**	Trends

	13:00	13:05	13:10	13:15	13:20
Pulse	81	82	79	74	75
Oxygen saturat.	92	93	95	98	97
Respiration	21	22	20	18	17
Temp	37.5	37.3	37.1	37.1	36.9
Systolic press.	140	135	125	130	125
Average press.	116	113	107	107	105
Diastolic press.	93	91	89	85	85

Figure 12:2a An example of the presentation of data used in monitoring in intensive care

Figure 12:2b Through a simple selection on the displayed screen, an alarm can be activated and alarm thresholds set. The crossed out bell indicates that the alarm function for blood pressure has been inactivated. The "Alarm" column shows which alarms are active. The upper part of the screen displays the current values, i.e. the same parameter values as in Figure 11:2a

Figure 12:2c By selecting another option on the displayed screen, the trends for a specific period can be displayed and reviewed. The same data can also be displayed in curve format

Figure 12:2c. Trend analyses provide much more information than single measurements. A decreasing pulse rate in itself may not be alarming, but in combination with decreasing blood oxygenation it can be a sign of heart failure.

Another use is for monitoring fluid balance and calculating the required infusion volumes and concentrations that need to be administered. This relieves personnel from tedious work.

ECG readings are often obtained in intensive care. A great deal of effort has been put into developing various methods for automatic ECG interpretation (Chapter 6). It is especially important to monitor for any arrhythmias. Thanks to computerization, this can now be done with a high degree of accuracy.

Radiation therapy

Before a tumour can be treated with radiation, **dose planning** must be completed. The location of the tumour is determined and the most optimal collimation and alignment of the radiation beam is calculated, ensuring maximum radiation to the tumour while sparing surrounding tissues. A three-dimensional calculation (cranio-caudal, medio-lateral and ventro-dorsal) is very complicated and could not be done without the help of computers.

Dose planning is based on the tumour location and the thickness of surrounding tissues along various directions of the radiation beam, as well as the tissue composition, such as the amount of bone and air present in the tissue. For this purpose, images obtained by standard X-ray, computer tomography and magnetic resonance tomography (Chapter 7) are used. From these data, the optimal distribution of the radiation field, including appropriate radiation type, radiation energy, field shape and incident angle is calculated. Such optimization problems are solved by making thousands of repeated attempts at finding the best alternative in a very short amount of time. Safety features preventing dose miscalculations are always included in the program.

Even though computerized dose planning is superior, there is always a risk of an accident:

CASE 12:1 Computers programmed to kill

A patient had had a tumour removed from his back and was given a series of radiation treatments to destroy any remaining cancer cells. At normal doses, such treatment is not noticeable by the patient. One day, however, the patient felt a burning sensation.

The radiation machine displayed a code that meant that the dosage was either too low or too high. This and other error codes usually appeared about 40 times a day, and this particular code appeared frequently due to the fact that the radiation energy was often somewhat lower than it should be. The operator, who had got used to just pressing a key and continuing the treatment whenever this code appeared, did so also at this time, since the dosage always used to be too low. The result was that the patient was burned several times, but eventually succeeded in moving away from the beam.

No defect could be found in the radiation machine and the patient was sent home. The next day the patient began to cough up blood and it was suspected wrongly that this may have been be due to an electric shock. The patient's condition gradually worsened and he died of radiation damage 4 months after the treatment.

A couple of weeks after the first case, a similar episode occurred with another patient who died 1 month later.

Once this became known, reports of similar cases with severe radiation damage which had occurred in other places both before and after the two fatal ones, began to emerge. All cases had happened with a certain type of radiation machine and with the same computer program. The error occurred only occasionally, which is evidenced by the fact that more than 500 cases had been treated by the machine that killed the two patients.

It was a highly insidious error. It would only occur if the operator pressed certain keys in a certain sequence, whereupon the radiation dosage became many times higher. The direct cause was a programming error.

The example also illustrates another, indirect fault with the program – it was written in such a way that it was difficult to use. No one can manage 40 error codes a day, especially if the error codes can have two entirely opposite meanings, such as the dose being either too low or too high – technology at its worst.

EXPERT SYSTEMS

Computers can be used as diagnostic aids and can provide suggestions for treatments. Such programs are called **medical expert systems**. These systems are based on the knowledge of how an expert would assess a certain situation, and the system attempts to mimic how a very experienced physician would solve the problem, including using some simple rules of thumb. The technology is based on user-friendly communication with the computer. The computer asks questions, perhaps suggests that several tests be done and then suggests a number of possible diagnoses with the statistical probability of each diagnosis. In this way **decision support** is obtained.

Such systems are based on statistical material collected from a large number of cases of each disease. The percentage occurrence of all symptoms is calculated and weighted, and a numerical value is obtained that indicates how much consideration should be given to each particular symptom. For an individual patient, the weightings are combined, yielding a certain probability that the patient suffers from the disease in question. Thus, in an expert system for children's diseases, the weighting for the symptom of headache in connection with measles is very low, while the weighting for Koplik's spots in the mucus membranes of the mouth is maximized, as this symptom only occurs in this disease.

There are expert systems for several disease groups that fall under categories such as general practice, haematology, rheumatology, allergy and pulmonary medicine. There are also programs that assess fluid and electrolyte imbalances and drug interactions. An example is a system that can handle more than 700 disease profiles in internal medicine, and 7000 related symptoms, signs and laboratory findings. The diagnostic capability of the system is as good as that of a well-trained doctor.

Expert systems can also alert the user when certain ominous combinations of values occur. Systems have also been designed for surgical and medical patient monitoring. If a patient is being treated for heart failure and the blood tests show a low serum potassium level, the program immediately triggers an alarm, as this combination constitutes a risk of cardiac arrest. Potassium can then immediately be given to the patient, which otherwise may not happen until the doctor reviews the test results the following day.

Expert systems have an obvious value when it comes to rare diseases, such as those of tropical origin when occurring in countries outside the tropics. Expert systems are also of particular value in the ongoing training of doctors, as they didactically explain how the system has arrived at the diagnosis by weighting the various symptoms. Unfortunately, as yet, these systems are not heavily used.

TELEMEDICINE

Telemedicine means that telemedia – telephone and radio transmissions – are used for medical consultations. This way, experienced and specialized doctors can collaborate remotely in the care of patients at health care facilities that lack such competence on-site.

The advantages are a higher quality of care, shortened hospital stays and avoidance of unnecessary hospital visits to specialists. Such a system, when fully developed, may reduce the cost of health care. Telemedicine can be used to communicate across the entire nation, and should competence be required that is only available in other countries, this can also be easily accessed.

Such consultations imply remote diagnostics and decision support, so that a less experienced person can receive help in uncertain situations. The information is transmitted with video cameras and computers to the recipient's monitor, by telephone or internet connection and the two users can simultaneously confer with each other with the help of speaker phones. This way, the distances in the chain of care are diminished.

Initially, telemedicine was mostly applied within radiology to transmit X-ray images. Such image transmission within hospitals has long been possible with the **Picture Archiving and Communication System (PACS)**. In this type of system, several computerized workplaces, or **work stations**, are connected to each other and to a centralized image archive via a technically advanced network. The images can be transmitted with high resolution. In radiology, telemedicine has meant that the usable network has been expanded to encompass an entire country.

In pathology, telemedicine usage started early. The microscope is fitted with a video camera, enabling transfer of tissue section images.

Telemedicine is routinely as well as experimentally used in most major medical disciplines. Some examples are teledermatology, telecardiology and telephysiology.

One of the most useful applications of telemedicine, seen from the perspective of lives saved, is during ambulance transport. At the first contact with a patient with a suspected myocardial infarction, paramedics can obtain an ECG. The ECG is then transmitted to the doctor at the hospital for detailed analysis. The ECG can be transmitted as a 12-lead ECG or as selected electrocardiogram leads. If there are signs of an infarction, the paramedics can administer thrombolytic treatment as prescribed. Mortality can thus be reduced by about 50% compared with the situation where no such treatment is given; administering this treatment at the hospital after 2 to 3 hours reduces the mortality only by about 25%.

COMPUTERIZED PATIENT RECORDS

Conventional patient records consisting of stacks of papers have important disadvantages. Data are difficult to find. Important information, for example, regarding allergies and current medications, can be missed by a new doctor. Patient records vanish – in large hospitals with central archives it has been reported that up to 15–20% of the records cannot be found when needed and up to 5% are never retrieved. Such archives furthermore require large amounts of space – it has been estimated that paper patient record archives grow in the order of 2000 metres of shelving per million inhabitants per year. The cost of managing the records, that is, writing, storing, sorting, searching and archiving the records reached the equivalent of some 10 million euros per million inhabitants before computerization.

A **computerized patient record** consists of:

- a patient administration section (consultation scheduling, payment, etc.)

- a medical record (the text in which the doctor describes the clinical findings, test results, diagnoses, treatment, etc.)

- care record (the text where the actual care is described)

- referral reports (results from clinical chemistry and bacteriology laboratory tests, biopsies, radiological investigations, etc.)

- pharmacy referrals (automatic transmission of prescriptions)

- a reference section (normal values for laboratory results, lists of drugs, drug interactions, medical reference literature, etc.)

The **demands** on a computerized patient record are the following:

- user friendly, easily read

- good security, with information held confidentially and ethically

- follow-up and quality assurance

- easy retrieval

A computerized patient record is the hub in the care of the patient. It has many advantages as the record can be accessed on a monitor in a few seconds. Previous illnesses, laboratory results, consulting specialist reports and administered drugs can be accessed quickly. Trends can be reviewed easily in diagram formats, such as recent blood pressure readings in a trend curve format. Such information can be retrieved when patients call and reviewed while they are still on the line. Another advantage is that patients appreciate not having to repeat their entire medical history from the very beginning every time. A picture of the patient or other medical images, such as photos of skin lesions, or X-ray images, are easily accessible.

Once these systems are sufficiently developed, the resulting administrative rationalization will free up time that can be used for actual patient care. The number of nurses with administrative duties can be reduced, as less time will be required for sorting papers. There are thus many advantages and such systems are nowadays routinely used in primary health care clinics and by some doctors in private practices.

However, there are also several disadvantages with computerized patient records. During a power failure, no information can be accessed. System development is very complicated and has been met with scepticism by many doctors and nurses.

For in-patient care, there have been great problems because of the large amounts of information that the system must be able to manage. The actual rationalization gains during the 1990s did not meet the expectations. Many attempts at introducing computerized patient records in hospitals were therefore initially unsuccessful, as they instead brought about a great deal of extra work for the hospital staff. The development work began in the 1960s, but it was not until the latter half of the 1990s that the process of abandoning paper-based records could be initiated at a few sites. Development is, however, inevitable, and fully computerized patient records will eventually be introduced at all hospitals.

STANDARDIZATION WITHIN HEALTH CARE

Extensive international efforts are going on to standardize medical informatics. The worldwide International Organization for Standardization (ISO) and the International Electrotechnical Commission (IEC), along with bodies such as the European Comité Européen de Normalisation (CEN) have the responsibility to coordinate efforts. The standardization is important for several reasons, among other things to enable different systems to communicate, and enable security and quality assurance procedures.

THE INTERNET

From the perspective of health care, the **internet** constitutes an expansion of the hospital network to encompass the whole world. Via the internet, literally hundreds of millions of other computers can be reached. This global network is called the **World Wide Web,** or **www** for short. Every computer has a unique address. Text, pictures, sound and video films can be transferred between these computers.

To use the internet, in addition to a computer with the appropriate connection, a **browser** is needed, which is a program that enables the user to receive and send information to and from the computer. With the browser, web pages containing text and pictures can be displayed on the computer screen. The web pages often contain **hyperlinks** presented in underlined blue font when they appear in the body text. These links act like the special buttons on telephones, which are pre-programmed to call a specific number when pressed. By clicking the mouse (pressing a mouse button) in this position, a connection is made to another web page that has been created by someone else at another computer somewhere in the world.

To target and optimize the search for information, special **catalogues** or **search engines** can be used to access the desired information. Catalogues are lists organized by subject areas; the disadvantage with these, however, is that they are not always kept up to date.

When using a search engine – the most popular is Google – the user enters one or more search words. This results in a listing of web pages that contain the word or words. It is important to select the words carefully and combine them in such a way that the intended search is actually executed, otherwise too many web site addresses could be returned, or none at all. Search techniques are, however, very easy to learn, thanks to the help functions that are included at the search engine sites.

The user can also subscribe to mailing lists, to continuously receive information within a specific subject area so that it is always up to date. A problem with the internet is that there is little verification of the data available.

Home pages and sites

A combination of web pages from a single source is called a **site**. Every site has a specific address which may start with http://www (but it is sufficient to start the search with only the "www" prefix). The page that provides entry to a site is called the **home page**. Most organizations and government authorities have home pages. These are usually free but not all are. Some sites of medical interest contain:

- medical products
- drug and device alerts
- scientific journals
- publications
- medical advice
- nursing information

Specific web sites can be found when entering such terms in a search engine.

Email

The ability to send mail to other computer users is one of the great advantages introduced by the internet. **Email** addresses have an @ symbol in them. The symbol is pronounced "at". The first author's email address was once bertil.jacobson@labtek.ki.se. From the address itself, it is often easy to see in which country the person lives and sometimes even where the person works. The address ending .se denotes the country domain of Sweden, and the .ki denotes the organization domain, in this case the Karolinska Institute. Such addresses are underlined and often appear in blue on the computer screen.

When everything works as it should, an email can be sent to another computer anywhere in the world within a minute. Large text documents, pictures and sound clips can be attached. Replies can be received at the same speed.

Email is progressively replacing ordinary "snail mail". The advantages for health care, and not just for in-patient care, are significant. With the help of a laptop computer and a modem, primary care doctors and nurses can contact their primary health care centre and thus retrieve necessary information via the mobile telephone net when away from their home base.

User groups

There are a vast number of **Usenet Newsgroups** on the internet, where any topic can be discussed. These function as open bulletin boards, where other users can answer a question or contribute to the discussion. Participation in such user groups is normally free of charge, and can, for example, be of value for the continuing education of doctors. There is a generous sense of camaraderie in such newsgroups, and most people seem keen to contribute and share their own experiences.

LIMITATION OF INFORMATION TECHNOLOGY

Modern computer technology was one of the most important technical achievements in the 20th century. For medicine it meant among many other beneficial things that it revolutionized the possibility to disseminate knowledge.

The free access unfortunately also had disadvantages. An information hungry public was not always qualified to sort out the good from the bad. "Cyber doctors" made information available on their sites; many were both competent and responsible and have given sick people excellent help. But some have failed miserably and in their own interest have given quack advice to critically ill people.

CASE 12:2 Internet can kill

On the internet a 55-year-old patient asked for advice about a skin problem. The day before many fluid-filled painful blisters had appeared on a broad streak of reddened skin on his chest. He also stated that he had received a kidney transplant recently and had to take a particular named drug every day.

Initially he had intended to just wait and see if the blisters disappeared, but his son urged him to seek advice on the internet. Help was requested from 17 different US-based medical websites. Answers were obtained from 10 doctors, of whom three abstained from giving an answer because dermatology was not their area of expertise. Some answers were medically correct, telling the patient to seek medical treatment immediately. But one doctor recommended homeopathic medicine and vitamin C. From two other cyber doctors he received totally incorrect advice that could have killed the patient.

The patient did not die, nor had he ever existed in the real world. He was made up by two German doctors who wanted to check the quality of advice offered on the internet. Their conclusion was that consumers should be protected from quacks and healers without medical training who made themselves available for consultations on the internet.

In every situation within health care and at every level within any organization the key issue is always to act with responsibility.

13

Responsibility*

In the early days of aviation, two pilots were placed in each aircraft to increase safety. But a couple of times the result was quite the opposite. Planes crashed because the pilots were not sure who was actually flying the plane – both thought that the other one was doing it. Such incidents led to the introduction of new routines, so that accidents could not happen because of unclear distribution of responsibility. The pilots knew who was flying the plane.

The distribution of responsibility within the health care system has still not reached aviation standards. Numerous accidents and near accidents have been the result of poor distribution of responsibility, both with regard to medical devices and the health care system as a whole.

As technology becomes increasingly more sophisticated, the risks of accidents increase. The more complicated the device, the greater the number of individuals will be involved in the procurement, training, use and maintenance of the device. The number of patients using complex equipment in the home is increasing. This places high demands on administrative management competence.

CASE 13:1 Radiation equipment crushes patient

A patient was to receive radiation therapy for a tumour in the neck region. Due to a break in the stand, the 1.5 tonne encased cobalt radiation source

---

This chapter was originally based on lectures by Göran Liedström, Medlaw Consulting HB, Sweden, who kindly edited two Swedish editions, contributed to the editing of the present chapter and devised Figure 13:1.

fell down on the patient's right upper arm and head. The patient, trapped underneath until a rescue squad could arrive with lifting equipment, died from the injuries.

The clinical engineers had never carried out any preventive maintenance or inspection of the device, since they felt that this was the responsibility of the manufacturer.

The manufacturer had never been contracted for this task, and no maintenance agreement had ever been signed.

During the investigation of the case described above, it was found that the lack of maintenance had not necessarily been the cause of the accident. The investigation revealed that the lack of a clear distribution of responsibility nevertheless was a significant problem.

In the next case there is, however, no doubt that the lack of a clear distribution of responsibility caused the death of the patient.

CASE 13:2 Kidney patient dies during dialysis

A patient was to undergo his regular haemodialysis treatment. After just half a minute of treatment he lost consciousness and subsequently died.

During the investigation, it was revealed that the dialysis machine had been disinfected as usual, using a 2% formaldehyde solution, but that the solution had not been rinsed out of the machine prior to the initiation of treatment.

The direct cause of the death was that formaldehyde residues had remained in the dialysis machine. The indirect cause was that nobody had been given the responsibility for ensuring that the prescribed rinsing was always performed.

CASE 13:3 Computer not reprogrammed for 33 patients

The drawback with radioactive radiation sources used for the treatment of tumours is that they gradually weaken. Eventually, the radiation sources have to be replaced by new ones.

At a hospital, such a depleted radiation source was replaced, but the computer used for dose planning was not reprogrammed, which resulted in wrong calculation of durations of treatments. Before the error was discovered, 33 patients had received radiation overdoses.

Although the health care system still has a lot to learn from aviation, many steps have been taken in the right direction thanks to directives within the European Union. Unfortunately the requirements for personnel competency with medical devices have not increased as this issue lies outside the scope of the Union to regulate. Medical devices must now be assessed according to extensive requirements, and a system for reporting of accidents and near accidents has been created. More human resources have been allocated for quality improvement and experiences from other member states have been pooled.

A number of statutes have been revised to achieve a **harmonization** of these activities within Europe. Harmonization means that all EU Member States employ similar requirements for certain activities. Thanks to these harmonized **standards**, according to the Medical Devices Directive, design and manufacture of medical devices have improved.

Systems for quality assurance have been introduced in the EU and the distribution of **responsibility** within the health care system has largely been clarified. Managers at all levels possess the right, under certain conditions, in certain countries to **delegate** tasks. Organizational prerequisites have also been established that designate which managers are authorized to order the acquisition of specified equipment and what routines they must follow. This chapter describes these issues. Summaries in the form of **checklists** for various personnel categories are provided in the next chapter.

STANDARDS

A standard is a written agreement on how an item should be designed and manufactured or a task performed. Standards are of great benefit to consumers. When people go on holiday in their home country, they know that the plug of their razor or hairdryer will fit into the wall outlet. Both the plug and the wall outlet are manufactured according to a standard. Unfortunately, the standards are not always the same from country to country, which they discover when they travel abroad and the plugs do not match. This can easily happen, as there are about 20 different standards for plugs in Europe. If the standards for electrical wall outlets and plugs were harmonized, the same plugs could be used in all EU countries.

Harmonized standards have been developed by **CEN** (Comité Européen de Normalisation, or European Committee for Standardization) and **CENELEC** (Comité Européen de Normalisation Electrotechnique, or European Committee for Electrotechnical Standardization) to aid manufacturers of CE-marked medical devices. Provided the manufacturer follows the standards, the products will conform to the **essential requirements**. The manufacturer's ability to demonstrate product usability and safety is thus facilitated.

Harmonized standards for medical devices are also of great value for the purchaser and user. The products are thus becoming safer. By looking at the labelling, the user can more easily discern whether a product is manufactured legally. As mentioned earlier, the CE mark (Chapter 1) indicates that the manufacturer has constructed and built the device according to the essential requirements applicable for the **specified use**. Although devised for EU use, the CE marking has become a useful symbol internationally. It is, however, important to understand that the CE mark is not a sign of quality – it is an indication that the device fulfils the requirements. Great responsibility has been assigned to the manufacturer. However, the user must bear equally great responsibility – the device must be used as intended and the specified use must not be deviated from.

There are standards not only for the manufacturing of devices, but there are also a great number of standards for how certain procedures are to be carried out. ISO 14155, for example, specifies how new medical devices are to be tested clinically. Also ISO 13485 is important for medical devices as it confirms an independent assessment with a quality management system.

When staff carry out their tasks according to current standards, they demonstrate responsibility for their actions; there should be very good reasons for any nonadherence to a particular standard.

MEDICAL DEVICES

People occupied with everyday, practical work within the health care system do not need to possess very detailed knowledge of the complicated set of rules surrounding medical devices. But it may be necessary to at least be familiar with the fundamental rules that apply when, for example, connecting several devices to each other; or connecting several devices to the same patient. Medical devices are grouped into three different categories, depending on their use:

- **Active implantable medical devices (90/385/EEC)**, such as pacemakers.

- **Medical devices (93/42/EEC)**, devices in general, such as X-ray equipment, dental equipment, aids for the handicapped and disposables.

- **In vitro diagnostic medical devices (98/79/EC)**, such as reagents and certain analytical products.

Medical devices are in turn divided further into four **classes**, depending on the risks associated with the use of these devices. The more serious the potential injury during use of a particular product, the more important it is that there are detailed regulations for the construction and **intended** use of the device.

- **Class I** includes the least hazardous products such as reusable surgical instruments and handicap aids. Most products belong to this class.

- **Class IIa** includes many diagnostic devices, e.g., devices for ECG and diagnostic ultrasound, monitors and pulse oximeters.

- **Class IIb** includes many **life-saving** devices, e.g., incubators, ventilators, infusion sets and transfusion sets.

- **Class III** includes products in contact with the central circulatory system, e.g., artificial heart valves, products in contact with the central nervous system, and products which exhibit a biological effect, such as copper intra-uterine devices (IUDs).

The manufacturer is responsible for classifying and CE-marking the product. The manufacturer must verify or have verified the significant requirements applicable to the product class in question. The manufacturer must also specify any "adverse effects" and the risks associated with the use of the device. Products of Class IIa and higher are verified by one of the "notified bodies", independent testing organizations appointed to carry out these tasks. Only then can the product be CE-marked. Many notified bodies are international organizations, and within each EU country they are formally monitored by a single government-appointed competent authority. Within the UK this is the Medicines and Healthcare products Regulatory Agency, within France the Federal Ministry of Health and Social Security, within the Netherlands the Healthcare Inspectorate, and within Italy the Ministry of Health.

The manufacturer thus bears a great responsibility. If its product fails to meet the requirements, its use can be restricted or even prohibited by the competent authority, even if the product is CE-marked, and the fact be notified to the EU Commission.

Anyone packaging, processing, labelling or putting on the market CE-marked medical devices has the same responsibilities as the original manufacturer.

Even if a company is responsible for the product during the entire life of the product, the user must apply and maintain the product correctly, according to the manufacturer's instructions. Regular maintenance carried out by qualified personnel as per these instructions, may thus be necessary.

The liability might be transferred to the user if the product is used:

- for nonintended purposes (including reuse, such as resterilization of disposable single-use products)

- together with a product that has not been approved by the manufacturer (e.g., wrong tubing set used with an infusion pump)

- with a product that has not been approved, even if that product has itself been CE-marked

Medical devices that have reached the end of their useful lives must always be **disposed of** in an environmentally friendly manner. Risks of infection must be recognized. Sometimes infectious blood and other fluids run down along the inner sides of the devices, which health care personnel are unable to clean. Such devices must be sent to the hospital clinical engineering department for further processing. Devices which possibly contain environmentally hazardous components, such as rechargeable batteries, must be disposed of correctly.

QUALITY MANAGEMENT

Quality management stands for the systematic efforts at improving health and medical services and the utilization of resources. Quality management should lead to **quality assurance**. However, this term is not very appropriate, as medical procedures can never be rendered absolutely safe. A more realistic term for the same concept would be **quality improvement**. Health care can only improve through continuous effort.

The internationally recognized standards procedure ISO 9000 can be used to establish a quality management system. Upon compliance with the requirements, a clinical chemistry laboratory, for example, can become **certified** after **an audit** by an **accredited body**.

Among medical specialities, the clinical laboratory departments are the ones in which international standards have been most extensively applied. Thus to become an accredited laboratory in general it has to conform to ISO/IEC 17025 and for a medical laboratory to ISO 15189. The difference between the two standards is that 15189 is written with terminology that is specially applicable for medical laboratories, whereas 17025 is not.

The goal of the quality assurance system is to achieve established procedures and targets and thereby prevent mistakes from happening. Much of what is said in this book is really geared to achieving such quality assurance, for the provision of health and medical services, in a responsible manner and using common sense.

The responsibility for quality assurance at the clinical department level falls primarily on the hospital management and the head of department or ward. Procedures must be documented. After an accident or near accident this helps in the investigation of the cause.

The most important goal from a practical point of view is, however, not to fill a number of binders with minutes from meetings. Rather it is for all health care personnel to develop a positive and responsible attitude to their work.

The quality management process may be carried out in various ways, and often starts in smaller **quality groups**. Personnel of different categories meet and discuss the various problems that may exist within health care, including, among other things, problems related to the use of various types of device. Suggestions for improved work procedures are put forward. The aim is not to simply discuss an incident that has already happened, but to try to anticipate things that could happen. The causes are, however, often difficult to anticipate, and a great deal of imagination is necessary.

The quality assurance process encompasses so much more than just outlining and eliminating risks involving medical technical devices. However, technical problems are among the most important ones to discuss, as most accidents happen when devices are involved.

The purpose of the quality assurance process is not to find scapegoats, but to develop work procedures where "medical errors become medical assets". An understanding of the cause of an error is an asset if it helps to prevent another similar error. The goal is to do things right the first time. This can sometimes be difficult even in familiar situations:

CASE 13:4 Operated on instead of examined

An elderly woman with impaired hearing was to undergo gastroscopy for gastrointestinal problems. When the next patient was called in from the waiting room, she thought the nursing assistant was looking at her. She accompanied the assistant to the examination room, where she told the staff that she had very poor hearing. A dentist and an oral surgeon, who according to the patient, did not introduce themselves, placed her in a dental chair, whereupon a green surgical drape was placed over her face. She protested, but was told that access was only needed to the mouth. She was not surprised when given local anaesthesia, as she had received it before during a previous gastroscopy.

The oral surgeon then started carrying out a surgical procedure on the patient's jawbone. The patient tried to protest, but couldn't, because the surgeon had his fingers in her mouth the whole time. When the presumed jaw bone lesion was not found, the surgeon enlarged the incision. Since no pathological changes could be found, the surgeon asked the patient her name. It was then discovered that they had the wrong patient and the incision was closed.

All personnel in the operating theatre had believed that they were treating a patient for a lesion of the jaw.

The patient was transferred to the gastroscopy room, where the originally planned examination was performed.

Patients are often eager to cooperate and are anxious to come in and see the doctor. Mix-ups of patients are an ever-present and well known risk. When mix-ups still happen, it demonstrates a flagrant lack of a quality assurance system. In this case, simply asking the patient to state her name and personal identification number before initiating the surgery would have sufficed.

Each report regarding an incident or a potential accident hazard must be followed up and discussed; if this is not done the reporting person will lose interest in participating in the ongoing quality assurance process.

RISK MANAGEMENT

The magnitude of a particular risk depends partly on what can go wrong, and partly on the probability of the fault occurring and the severity of the consequence:

$$\text{risk} = \text{probability} \times \text{consequence}$$

Even if all mankind would be wiped out if a large comet hit the earth, the risk for each individual to be killed by a comet is still very small, as it is extremely unlikely that such a comet will enter the earth's orbit during their lifetime. Even if almost everyone catches colds, the risk of death upon catching one is still small, as it is rare for anyone to suffer serious consequences from the disease. However, the risk from smoking is high, as too many people smoke and it is a known fact that many serious diseases can develop or be aggravated by smoking. When conducting a risk analysis, it must be considered that there may be many different reasons for the risk to increase:

- Faulty devices (construction or manufacturing error).

- Unclear, or difficult to understand, or even incorrect instructions for use (IFU), or no instructions at all.

- Inadequate training in device use.

- Inadequate maintenance.

- Inadequate management.

A risk must be weighed against the benefit resulting from the use of the device. A few hazardous situations:

- Non-functioning (defibrillator, infusion set, ventilator, incubator).

- Mechanics (falling device parts, patient lift, crushing between parts of a power-operated device).

- Gas (leakage of gaseous anaesthetics, wrong gas, explosion).

- Fire (oxygen, heating element, short-circuiting, inflammable solutions with surgical diathermy).

- Heating (heating pads, blood warmers, incubators).

- Electricity (macroshock, leakage currents in connection with devices in close proximity to the heart, diathermy).

- Chemicals (harsh or allergenic substances).

- Ionizing radiation (X-ray and isotope examinations).

- Non-ionizing radiation (laser, ultrasound).

A common cause of accidents is that the devices are difficult to use. Unsatisfactory ergonomics is unfortunately common. Training is therefore of vital importance. In some hospitals, the equivalent of an "**operator's licence**" has been introduced for certain special devices. This means that everyone using certain complicated equipment must pass the equivalent of a test before being allowed to operate it without supervision. These should include infusion pumps and diathermy generators. This training is often conducted with the assistance of the hospital clinical engineering department or the manufacturer or agent. Older colleagues also often participate. It has been suggested, however, that there may be a danger in issuing such "operator's licences", in that it may offer a false sense of security by making the users overestimate their proficiency – most car accidents happen with young, inexperienced drivers who have just obtained their licence. The same may be true within health care.

 Do not think that you can handle all situations because you have received an "operator's licence" for a certain device. Do not hesitate to ask those who know and have more experience using the device.

TYPES OF RESPONSIBILITY

Responsibilities come in various types. Five different responsibilities are discussed below, and although there is much interaction between different types of responsibility, these five types do give a framework for understanding the important issues involved.

Legal responsibilities

Everyone is responsible for upholding the laws in the countries where they live. These laws may differ from country to country, but countries tend to have the same underlying concerns. All countries have general laws relating to health and safety. In addition, many have specific laws dealing with medical devices, and in Europe this comes under the Medical Devices Directives. Then to ensure that these directives are upheld, the governments in European countries nominate a competent authority to regulate medical device issues.

Political responsibilities

The population elects politicians, who in turn are responsible for allocating money for health care, and for ensuring that the population has access to good health care. It is a responsibility of the political system to provide these resources and hence guarantee that health care is available. This is not an easy matter as it is subject to restraints imposed by economic and other conditions that affect the availability of resources.

Administrative management responsibilities

Once resources are allocated to health care, it is vital that these resources are managed efficiently and effectively. This is undertaken at the local health care or hospital level by administrative management, which encompasses planning, leadership and organization of work, as well as monitoring work performance. Within the administrative hierarchy, supervisors must provide their staff with advice, guidance and training. If this training is not provided by the manager personally, it must be provided using the assistance of other trained personnel. Such specialized training is organized very often before medical devices are put into clinical use.

Overall administrative management responsibilities lie with the health care director or hospital director. No director could possibly supervise all work personally, and responsibility has to be borne by others in the organization. When responsibility is transferred to others it is very important for everyone to be clear about who has accepted and holds which responsibilities. Within the nursing hierarchy in the UK, responsibility is transferred from the chief hospital nurse, to ward nurses and others. Other countries may have other organizations.

Medical and other professional management responsibilities

Responsibilities for the care of patients lie with the medical profession, that is, physician, dentist and nurse. There are concurrent administrative responsibilities for planning, training and organizing. Senior management positions exist in units providing medical diagnosis, treatment and care. If the head of department or ward is medically qualified, the person in this position carries both the medical and administrative management responsibility. A head of department or ward is among other things required to oversee the personnel allocated to them, and make sure that medical tasks are performed correctly. This includes ensuring that medical devices are used correctly, and hence provide maximum patient benefit.

CASE 13:5 Infant burned by electricity

A baby girl in a neonatal department had been connected to an infusion pump in battery operation mode, as well as to an ECG monitor using chest electrodes. At one point, when the mother was holding the baby, these devices were disconnected. On putting the baby back in her cot, the mother asked the paediatric assistant nurse to reconnect the monitor.

When the nurse connected the cables, she did not receive a signal from the ECG monitor, and therefore tried connecting the pins at the end of the cable into various holes. After a moment smoke began to emanate from the baby girl, and she noticed a burning smell. The electrodes had partly melted, and the girl had received severe burns.

The investigation demonstrated that the nurse had connected the ECG electrodes to the infusion pump power cable. It was connected to a live wall outlet at one end with the other end unconnected, since the infusion pump had been operated by the integral battery. According to the infusion pump instructions, when not in use the power cable must be kept coiled up on the pump cable holder. It must not be connected to the main power supply. This instruction had been added following a similar accident in the United States in which a 23-day-old infant was electrocuted when two apnoea monitor electrodes were connected directly to a power source.

The investigation found that formal decisions by the hospital management had made no less than five different doctors responsible for the medical management and three for administrative management. In addition, the head of department had the overall administrative management responsibility. The responsibility of the chief administrative nurse was limited to administrative duties. The head nurse for the ward was responsible for personnel guidance and training, as well as for ensuring that safety regulations were being followed. The multitude of persons supposedly responsible resulted in no one really bothering to assume responsibility.

When patients are discharged from hospital there can be a gap in assuming responsibility for those patients. Health departments in many countries have now issued directives regarding physician responsibilities when patients are referred to other health care professionals. It is the responsibility of the discharging physician to ensure that the patient is actually transferred to a doctor who will take over the care of the patient. If the patient, on discharge, requires any type of technical aid, such as an oxygen concentrator or ventilator for home use, it is necessary to ensure that a designated and identifiable doctor assumes the continued responsibility for this treatment.

Personal responsibilities

Every manager must be able to accept responsibility for the work carried out in their area. The physician responsible for the patient is also responsible for patient safety. According to codes of practice for physicians, every doctor must provide clinical advice or treatment in accordance with scientific knowledge and proven effectiveness of the treatment. This obligation is part of a moral responsibility, and there exists a grey zone between formal and moral responsibilities, Figure 13:1.

One example of these moral responsibilities is the task of caring for the relatives of a deceased patient. The relatives must be treated with respect and concern, but the extent of the task is not clear. The patient is

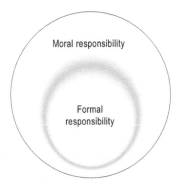

Figure 13:1 There is a grey zone between formal and moral responsibility (after Göran Liedström)

dead, the physician is no longer required to care for the patient, and the relatives are not consulting the doctor because of any illness of their own. But the doctor and any other health care personnel are still caring for the relatives.

Every person working within the health care system must be competent to perform the tasks allocated to them. In relation to medical devices, workers must be able to perform functional tests on medical technical equipment before connecting equipment to a patient, and they must possess the necessary competence to use the equipment in question independently. Anyone who feels they lack the necessary competence should notify their supervisor, who then must assume the responsibility until training is complete.

With technology becoming increasingly more complicated, not everyone can be expected to handle every device. In hospitals, nurses and other staff are trained in the use of specific devices. Sometimes nominated individuals can take a lead role with specific medical devices.

Liability

Offences of varying degrees can lead to certain sanctions, either under criminal law, where fines or even prison sentences may be imposed, or the offender may be held liable for damages in a civil court. Personnel considered to have violated their medical responsibilities may also be subjected to a reprimand or warning, or have their licence to practice revoked following a decision by a disciplinary board of a professional body or health care authority.

Any investigation of an accident or near accident can be among the most disturbing and unpleasant things in a person's life. Unfortunately, it often results in many people trying to blame each other. Everyone must do all they can to avoid the accidents happening in the first place.

DELEGATING

In some countries it is legally important to distinguish between giving someone an **order** to carry out a certain task and **delegating** a task. This is dependent on the qualifications of the persons involved.

Health care personnel can be qualified to different levels. Qualifications can relate to education or training, and most health care workers will have both types of qualification. Education can result in a certificate or a university degree. Also, the levels of training can be very different. Some are trained to undertake a specific function, while others have undertaken substantial training, usually over several years, resulting in a professional qualification that indicates their competency in specific clinical areas. This is essentially the worker's "licence to practice".

Health care requires many tasks to be performed correctly and safely. Training in these tasks is often undertaken locally in the hospital or health care institution, and will not result in any formal qualification, but is often based on many years of professional experience. There will be no certificate, but the person has obtained real practical competence. These staff are said to have nonformal qualifications.

These qualifications are important for the smooth functioning of any complex organization such as a hospital. After in-job training to the required level of competency, the health care personnel are then allowed to carry out these special tasks under certain conditions.

 The following restrictions apply for delegating jobs:

- Tasks can be delegated only by a person with formal qualifications. A person with nonformal qualifications thus may not further delegate the task in question.
- Delegation of tasks may only be done within the same organization; tasks may not be delegated to someone at another unit for which the delegating person is not formally responsible.
- A delegated task is personal, and a substitute or successor in the position may not automatically assume the delegated tasks in question.
- The delegating person must ensure that the person to whom the task is delegated is practically competent.
- The person to whom the task is delegated must consider themselves to be practically competent and also be willing to assume the task.
- The duration and extent of the delegated task must be clearly stated. The task may be delegated for a single occurrence, a limited time period or indefinitely. Such delegation may be revoked at any time.
- Delegation should be in writing, which is beneficial to both parties, should an accident occur. Such delegation can be done using a simple form.

- Existing statutes may prohibit the delegation of certain tasks, such as the prescription and handling of drugs; however, no such limitation exists when it comes to the handling of medical devices.

A person who has accepted overall management responsibilities may not informally delegate their supervisory responsibilities:

CASE 13:6   Air injected into infusion tubing

A 9-month-old girl with pyelonephritis was receiving antibiotics via an infusion pump. At one point, the pump alarm went off as the container was empty.

A substitute paediatric assistant nurse disconnected the pump. So as not to waste the remaining infusion solution in the tubing, she connected a 50 ml syringe filled with air, and injected the air into the tubing. As no end cap was available for sealing off the tubing end, she simply left the tubing open.

After telling the nurse on duty about what she had done, the nurse ran in to the patient and closed the open infusion tubing, but air had already been sucked into the vein. The patient developed dyspnoea, which lasted for half an hour, but survived.

The paediatric assistant nurse had not been delegated the task of operating the infusion pump, and had therefore exceeded her authority.

 Delegation must be distinguished from work supervision, where the responsibility remains with the supervisor.

PROCUREMENT

With the increasing complexity of medical technology, it is no longer possible for the responsible medical management to judge the medical and economic consequences when **purchasing** new equipment. Such technical evaluations must include clinical engineers, who often have access to reports from many other hospitals, **test houses** and **product assessments** both within and outside the country. The users, such as doctors, nurses and laboratory personnel, should participate in the purchasing.

When purchasing equipment, all these functions must be involved when proposals are acquired and when the contracts are written. The purchasing procedure must be preceded by a **requirements specification**: a list specifying the necessary performance of the equipment, its application, functions required, frequency and periods of use. In many cases, the standards to be met need also to be specified. During the evaluation of standards, it is important to read the section "Scope", which describes what the standard covers. The technical requirements that must apply over and above the given standards must be specified in detail. It is helpful to divide the requirements into **must have** that must be fulfilled, and **ought to have** that ought to be fulfilled. Throughout the purchasing process due attention must be given to existing rules and regulations for public procurement.

As discussed in Chapter 1, new equipment must go through the hospital clinical engineering department for **initial inspection** and registration. After installation, it is often necessary to **instruct** the personnel in the use of the devices.

In this instruction session, the clinical engineer can also make sure that the **instructions for use (IFU)**, which accompany the device really are clearly understandable and suitable. **Preventive maintenance** and **repairs** must also be planned.

Tasks that are beyond the competence of the administratively responsible doctor must be scheduled with a clinical engineer.

All users must know with certainty that each device is of an approved type (usually in Europe it bears a CE mark), that it has passed the initial inspection, and that it is regularly serviced. A simple way to administer this is to provide all devices that fulfil these requirements with an **asset tag**, with a device number. If the device has such a tag, the device can be used with confidence.

A **log** should be created for each of the more complex types of devices procured. The log should, among other things, be used to register details about operational maintenance, calibration data, deviations and correctional steps taken.

Special risks arise when a **new type of equipment** is being tried out at the hospital or when some device is set up **on loan**. Such devices must also pass through the hospital clinical engineering department, and their use be approved.

STATUTES AND OTHER PUBLICATIONS

There are different types of rules: **laws, ordinances** and **regulations**, which must be followed, and **general guidelines**, that should be followed. There must be very good reasons not to do so. From a practical point of view, it is of lesser importance in the daily operations which type of rule regulates the action. But should an accident occur it will have implications for the consequences.

There are in all countries laws concerning the use of medical devices. The importance of following the law is obvious, as otherwise, legal punishments may be imposed. Such risk can be avoided by knowing the fundamental principles and learning from the mistakes of others. Reading the examples in this book should help.

During recent years there has been a decreasing interest in finding scapegoats. A Chief of Air Staff in the USA once altered the attitude to accidents – he asserted successfully that there are no pilot errors, only system faults. Mistakes made must lead to better work routines, so that similar accidents can be prevented.

The responsibility for medical **devices** within health care is specified in countries by listing the people responsible and their positions. Where the position of head of department exists, this person carries the overall responsibility; in other cases the personnel carrying out the patient care, such as the qualified nurse, physiotherapist or occupational therapist become responsible. Those responsible for medical devices must ensure that:

- only suitable products are used
- products are checked before use
- personnel are competent to use the product
- the product is serviced regularly
- user manuals and technical documentation are available
- products are disposed of when they are no longer within the "use by" date, have been damaged, or are no longer sterile

OVERALL RESPONSIBILITY

The greater the number of officials who are to be responsible for medical technical installations, the greater the risk that no one assumes the overall responsibility, and that accidents and near accidents occur. Contrary to all earlier examples in this book, the one described below is created by bringing together various incidents and near incidents which have occurred in hospitals in several countries.

Figure 13:2, which demonstrates the assumed hospital organization for this case history, may appear confusing. Although this is typical for the organization in any well-organized large hospital, a similar type of organizational chart is likely to be available in most hospitals. If this is not the case, the responsibility pathways are not defined, and this makes it possible for administrators to put blame on subordinates. The constructed example differs from virtually all other real case histories in the previous chapters; here we take account of management duties. In practice a nurse or a doctor is often blamed, and they have to take all the legal and moral responsibility, although management is more often at fault.

CASE 13:7 Complicated distribution of responsibility

In a modern hospital, medical gases are distributed through gas pipes to the various places requiring gas, such as surgical and obstetric departments and

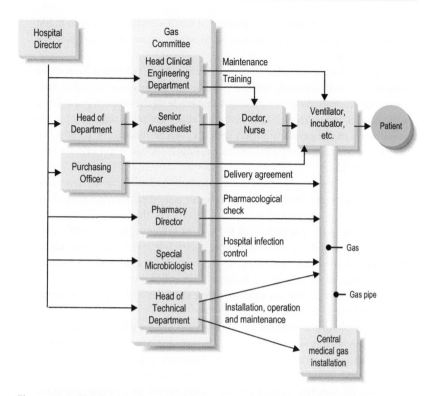

Figure 13:2 Distribution of responsibilities for a central gas installation system

other departments for patient care. The installation of such gas pipes cannot be done in the same manner as in industrial installations, and detailed instructions for central gas installations are given in documents available to all hospitals.

A patient under general anaesthesia was, as usual, being administered oxygen from a gas mixer connected to a ventilator. Initially, the oxygen level was set at 40%. Suddenly the patient became cyanotic and despite further opening of the oxygen valve, the patient's condition quickly worsened. Another ventilator was connected, but the patient had already suffered permanent brain damage.

The investigation revealed that the gas mixer had stopped working because of oxide flakes in a needle valve. The filter that normally should have prevented the accident was damaged because of a manufacturing defect, resulting in the oxide flakes being able to clog the gas mixer.

During a routine check of an anaesthetic machine before the accident, the clinical engineering department had discovered large quantities of debris in a filter. This was reported to the senior anaesthetist who, however, paid it no attention. (Relations between the head of the clinical engineering department and the senior doctor were not the best, as they on several earlier occasions had held opposing views with regard to various procurement issues.)

During the weeks before the accident, a small alteration had been made to the hospital gas distribution system to renew a part of the hospital gas conduit system.

Proposals for the installation of gas pipes had been obtained from three suppliers. A small company was less expensive than the other two. Decisions on minor renovations were routinely being made by the hospital purchasing officer, who, for reasons of cost economy, chose the small company for the installation of the gas distribution network. No verification as to whether the company was aware of the existing norms for medical gas installations had been made.

The head of the hospital technical department had sent a written message regarding the planned renovation to the senior anaesthetist (no gas committee according to the regulations had been instituted at the hospital). Since the reconnection of the gas pipes was to be done at night, the gas supply only needed to be shut down for a short time during one night. The notice about the planned work had ended up at the bottom of a pile; and a written approval was never sent to the hospital technical department.

The investigation did not explain why a gas filter with a manufacturing defect had been installed in the gas mixer.

An example of the distribution of responsibility for a hospital gas distribution system is shown in Figure 13:2. By not clarifying the responsibilities to the involved parties, neglecting to establish a gas committee at the hospital and by failing to ensure that existing regulations were being followed, the **hospital director** carried a large part of the responsibilities for the accident.

The **purchasing officer** also carried a large responsibility, as he had failed to obtain information from the hospital technical department regarding existing regulations. The head of the hospital technical department had yielded to the purchasing officer's wish to accept the cheapest proposal; he had, however, verbally expressed reservations regarding the consequences if the installation was to be performed without the use of protective gas during soldering. The purchasing officer failed to realize the importance of this. The purchasing officer had even neglected to ensure that the supplier being used had sufficient qualifications to carry out the renovation.

The **head of department** had not fulfilled his obligation to ensure regulations were being followed, especially with regard to the establishment of a gas committee.

The **senior anaesthetist** had failed his responsibilities by not paying attention to the alarming report from the clinical engineers about the debris in the gas distribution system. He had also failed in his review of the competence of the substitute nurse-anaesthetist, who was given the responsibility of handling the anaesthesia, despite her lack of experience. She was obviously not experienced enough to react swiftly and adequately in the situation that arose.

The **head of the clinical engineering department** had failed by not reporting his observations to higher authorities when the clinic director did not pay attention to the information about debris in the gas system. The head of the technical department should have supervised the installation and insisted on a written approval of the renovation from the senior anaesthetist.

The only people free of responsibility in this case, were the pharmacy director and hospital special microbiologist, since, in this particular case, they had not received any information about the renovation. There was therefore no reasonable way that they could have realized the risks and were therefore not held responsible for the accident.

The example above could as well have been constructed around the mix-up of gas pipes. As reported in Cases 4:6 and 8:4, a mix-up of gases can lead to tragic events. A further two accidents involving four patients in a single European country can also be noted. The first involved two patients who died in quick succession under anaesthesia because the oxygen and nitrous oxide gas pipes had been mixed up during repair. Thus the death of the first patient did not prevent the second patient being put under a fatal anaesthesia. Despite these two deaths, which became well-known in the country, an identical incident occurred soon after at another hospital, also involving two deaths.

The example also illustrates something that does not often come to light in official investigations of accidents and near accidents – behind such events there are often personal conflicts – in this case between the senior anaesthetist and the head of the clinical engineering department. It seems that such conflicts often result in safety aspects being more readily ignored.

No one deliberately wants to make a mistake; but everyone does. Realizing this was how aviation achieved its excellent safety standard. For medicine there is no other way than to realize that there is a wealth of information in the many unnecessary accidents that have occurred, and that this information must be retrieved from those who caused them. Punishment will never achieve this; forgiveness may well do.

14

Checklists

In the history of aviation, no single measure for improving safety has had any greater impact than pilots using checklists before take-off and landing. When accidents have occurred, they have sometimes been caused by pilots failing to follow this simple requirement. But accidents within commercial aviation are exceedingly rare in view of the many millions of passengers transported worldwide each year – in 2004 no passenger was killed. Checklists are of great value. Within health care much could be gained if personnel at all levels used checklists.

Countless checklists have been written within health care, but they have generally been intended for special applications, particularly within device-intensive specialities such as anaesthesia. It is well accepted that one of the unfortunate consequences of using anaesthetic techniques can be hypoxic brain damage or death. Even though these events are rare, when they happen they do cause much distress. Throughout the world, anaesthetists have discussed how best to tackle this problem, and many groups have come to the conclusion that checklists are the way forward. To take one example, the Association of Anaesthetists of Great Britain and Ireland produced a document "Checklist for anaesthetic equipment" detailing how to deal with 11 separate device areas. But even if checklists are available they are not always followed:

CASE 14:1 Explosions during cremation

Even after death, loved ones want their deceased relatives to be handled with respect. One of the last things they want to hear is that the body has exploded. Unfortunately, this has happened many times. If a pacemaker or automatic implantable defibrillator is not removed before cremation, explosions can result. Naturally information on specific people is not publicized, but a high proportion of crematoria report such explosions, often with some damage created.

If the death certificate with its associated checklist had been correctly filled in by the doctor responsible, these events would not have happened.

The type of checklist suggested below is of a more general nature than those referred to above, and they are intended to facilitate effective management rather than specific medical procedures. The lists summarize the earlier sections in this book, and are suggestions that might be helpful in developing local checklists for various categories of personnel. The checklists refer only to procedures dealing with medical devices.

Asset tags for medical devices are mentioned in the checklists. As described earlier, the fact that a device has been supplied with such a tag implies that it has been:

> inspected and checked upon delivery
> registered in the hospital medical device database
> installed in the department
> accepted with a suitable user manual

HOSPITAL DIRECTOR (OR HEALTH CARE DIRECTOR)

In every organization the person holding the highest position has the main responsibility for the organization and can never delegate this overall responsibility to a lower level. The chief executive or hospital director must consider the following questions:

1. Are all **heads of department** and others with leadership responsibilities aware of their own senior responsibilities and how responsibilities are distributed across the organization?

2. Is there written **documentation** for medical devices, for procurement, installation, operation, maintenance, and training?

3. Have **collaborative groups** been established for patient activities that extend across several departments? These may include medical gas distribution, control of infection, fire prevention, isotope use and radiation protection.

4. Are issues of **ownership and maintenance** of medical devices clear, so that equipment does not end up in "no man's land" between two units? An example is mobile X-ray units used in the X-ray department or clinic.

5. Have the **boundaries between the responsibilities** of clinical engineering and hospital estates or technical engineering been determined? In general, hospital engineering is responsible for permanent installations, while clinical engineering is responsible for medical devices. For example, the boundary between the gas installation and the ventilator is at the gas outlet in the wall. Special care must be taken when any function is provided by an external company.

6. Are heads of clinics and laboratories aware of the regulations applying to **internally manufactured** products?

7. Is there a process for a **review** of operations, so that personal conflicts, among other things, can be identified at an early stage?

8. Are there routines for how **deviations** from standard practice should be handled?

9. Is there a **quality management** system for medical devices?

10. Has education about relevant current **statutes** been arranged for those in supervisory positions?

PURCHASING OFFICER

1. When purchasing a medical device, is there a **requirement specification** with clear descriptions of functional, medical and technical requirements, and standards to be fulfilled? The list should separate "need to have" from "ought to have".

2. Before an order has been placed, has the requirement specification been **evaluated** by those who will be involved in its use? They should include head of department, representatives of all categories of user, and clinical or hospital engineering department.

3. Has the cost included consumables and maintenance, and so included **life cycle cost (LCC)** analysis?

4. Has the supplier performed a satisfactory **risk analysis**?

5. Have **training and maintenance**, both during and after the warranty period, been decided?

6. Is the law on **public procurement** being applied?

HEAD OF DEPARTMENT OR WARD

1. Has the responsibility for training, maintenance and operation of medical devices been **delegated** to **competent** personnel, and in writing?

2. Have all **newly delivered devices** been passed through clinical engineering? Asset tags will confirm this.

3. Are all devices in the clinic **suitable for use?**

4. Are all personnel **qualified?** Is there a routine review to check that all personnel are **trained** in the handling of medical devices?

5. Are all devices checked before use for **damage** or **contamination,** and are supervisors aware of their responsibility to ensure that all devices receive regular **maintenance?**

6. Are **functional checks** of medical devices always carried out when needed?

7. Are all personnel aware that all **internally modified or manufactured devices** must be examined by independent medical technical personnel for an evaluation of safety and for written approval for use?

8. Have practical routines been developed for **risk analysis?**

9. Are all doctors, nurses and other supervisors aware of the procedure that must be followed when an **accident** or near accident occurs, so that if possible device settings are left intact, accessories safeguarded, the device quarantined, and the accident or incident **reported.**

10. Are **areas of responsibility** clearly defined with written delegation, so that no doubt exists over who has the right to do what?

11. Are products that are **no longer suitable** discarded?

12. Are staff aware that **stress** and **personal conflicts** can lead to accidents?

HEAD NURSE

1. Have all devices passed through the **clinical engineering** department before being put into use? Usually an asset tag guarantees that this has been done. Devices that have not been used for some time may pose special safety hazards and may need to be sent to the clinical engineering department before reuse.

2. Have all subordinate personnel been **trained** in the use of the devices in their area?

3. Are **user manuals** easily accessible to all personnel?

4. Is the distribution of **responsibility** unequivocally clarified when devices can be operated by several people? Examples of devices with shared responsibilities are those that before use go through a process of disinfection, such as anaesthetic machines, ventilators and dialysis equipment.

5. Is **communication** between personnel good, ensuring that procedures are not ignored and stressful situations reported?

6. Do all subordinate personnel know that when an **accident** or a near accident occurs, all device settings are to be left intact if possible, all settings noted, all accessories safeguarded, the device quarantined, and the accident or incident **reported**?

USERS

1. Are you **qualified** to use the device? User manuals may have to be read several times, and **practical training** must be given by teachers and by experienced colleagues to whom the responsibility for providing training has been delegated.

2. Are you aware that when there is even the slightest **doubt** about the use of the device, you must inform your immediate superior? Refuse to use the device if you do not have necessary qualifications or training.

3. Have you checked that new devices are **approved for use**? Generally an asset tag on the device will confirm that this is the case, but locally other systems may be used.

4. Do you know that you are required to make sure that **damage** and other **defects** on the device must be repaired before use and regular **maintenance** is being carried out? For example, damaged electrical cables must be reported.

5. Do you know that you are required to carry out **functional tests** before each use of **certain complicated medical devices**?

6. Do you realize that **stress** and **personal conflicts** can lead to accidents, and that you must take steps to rectify such problems?

7. Are you aware that when an **accident** or near accident has occurred, all device settings are to be left intact, if possible, and that you should note these settings and safeguard all accessories? The device must be quarantined, and in some countries marked with a "Do not use" tag? Finally, the event and associated circumstances must be reported, so that similar incidents can be collated and appropriate action taken to avoid further accidents or incidents.

CASE 14:2 Incident reporting saves lives

A patient with heart rhythm problems had an implantable cardiac defibrillator (ICD) inserted surgically in his chest to prevent sudden cardiac death from ventricular fibrillation. His clinical history indicated that this was likely without intervention.

Some time later he attended a hospital cardiology outpatient clinic for a routine follow-up. To the astonishment of the cardiology staff, tests indicated that there was no energy left in the internal battery of the ICD, in spite of the history of use indicating that energy should still exist. The unit was explanted and replaced.

This incident was reported to the national Department of Health and to the manufacturer. Collation of reports from elsewhere, including other countries, indicated that this was not an isolated failure. These reports culminated in the modification of the manufacturing and production processes, the provision of enhanced software to check battery current consumption and provide battery voltage history at follow-up outpatient visits, and clinical recommendations to explant and replace ICDs in certain conditions.

Reporting single device failures helps other patients.

People needing medical treatment have often no choice. If they fail to accept treatment the result could be disability, and for some fatal. The numbers of patients requiring and accepting treatment is huge. For example, in the UK, annual patient visits to National Health Service general medical practitioners is about 300 million, and hospitals have 9 million admissions and 12 million new outpatients. These figures can be compared with the population of the UK, which is about 60 million.

To determine how to improve safety, the UK Department of Health published a report "An organisation with a memory" to encourage health care staff to learn from past events. It reported that about 400 people die or are seriously injured in adverse events involving medical devices each year, that is about 7 per million inhabitants. Many could not have been prevented, but other estimates suggest that half could have been.

These deaths are well below those for smoking or road accidents, and even much lower than the best estimate of deaths from passive smoking. But any death or injury is one too many. Incidents involving medical devices must by all means be prevented.

Index

Please note that page numbers in *italics* refer to boxes, figures or tables

Printed and bound by CPI Group (UK) Ltd, Croydon, CR0 4YY

03/10/2024

01040847-0016